MW01120974

REDUCING THE BURDEN OF HEADACHE

FRONTIERS IN HEADACHE RESEARCH
VOLUME 11

FRONTIERS IN HEADACHE RESEARCH SERIES

Published by Lippincott-Raven:

Published by Oxford University Press:

Reducing the Burden of Headache

EDITED BY

J. Olesen
*Department of Neurology, Glostrup Hospital,
University of Copenhagen, Denmark*

T. J. Steiner
Division of Neuroscience, Imperial College, London

and

R. B. Lipton
*Departments of Neurology, Epidemiology and Social Medicine,
Albert Einstein College of Medicine, New York, USA*

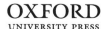

OXFORD
UNIVERSITY PRESS

OXFORD

UNIVERSITY PRESS

Great Clarendon Street, Oxford OX2 6DP

Oxford University Press is a department of the University of Oxford.
It furthers the University's objective of excellence in research, scholarship,
and education by publishing worldwide in

Oxford New York

Auckland Bangkok Buenos Aires Cape Town Chennai
Dar es Salaam Delhi Hong Kong Istanbul Karachi Kolkata
Kuala Lumpur Madrid Melbourne Mexico City Mumbai Nairobi
São Paulo Shanghai Taipei Tokyo Toronto

Oxford is a registered trade mark of Oxford University Press
in the UK and in certain other countries

Published in the United States
by Oxford University Press Inc., New York

A catalogue record for this title is available from the British Library

Library of Congress Cataloging in Publication Data
(Data available)

ISBN 0 19 8515898 (Hbk)

10 9 8 7 6 5 4 3 2 1

Typeset by Integra Software Services Pvt. Ltd, Pondicherry, India
www.integra-india.com

Printed in Great Britain
on acid-free paper by
Biddles Ltd, Guildford and King's Lynn

Preface

Headache disorders have been slow to gain recognition. They were not clearly classified or operationally defined until 1988 and, therefore, valid epidemiological data have been accumulating only over the last decade. Yet such data are an obligatory requirement for reliable determination of the burden attributable to headache. It follows that studies of the burden of headache have taken place only within the last 5–10 years and no book has been devoted to this topic, and how to reduce this burden, until the present volume.

This publication analyses the costs, financial and otherwise, of headache disorders, the disability and suffering they cause and the impact they have on the quality of life and well-being of those directly affected, their families, friends, and colleagues. The figures are astounding. Migraine, in the calculations of the WHO, is number 20 of all diseases with regard to years lived with disability. In terms of lost work-days due to health problems, headache accounts for approximately 20% in a Danish study. Migraine, to the great surprise of many, has more impact on quality of life than a range of other chronic diseases generally considered to be more serious.

What can we do about this enormous personal and public burden of headache? Because of the apparent information gap, intensified teaching of primary-care physicians is absolutely necessary. The know-how is there, but the traditionally poor recognition of headache disorders seems negatively to affect the teaching of them and, therefore, also the treatment given to patients with migraine and those with other common and burdensome headache conditions. Studies from the EU have shown that patients with migraine are generally poorly treated because modern drugs are only slowly taken into use. A three-tier system for the care of those with headache is envisioned, which must reach out to the many who for whatever reason do not seek medical help. Given appropriate education of general practitioners, the great majority of headache patients can be managed well in family practice. The next tier is the specialized unit which, according to resources available and the local health system, may be staffed by neurologists or by specialist primary-care physicians or others so long as they have a well-developed interest. The ideal third tier is a highly specialized academic headache centre with teaching and research obligations. Such centres are now emerging in North America and the EU.

The bad news brought by this book is that physicians are slow to accept headache disorders as biological and to see a need for and apply modern treatment. The good news is that, with judicious use of existing resources and treatment possibilities, there is room for huge improvement of the lives of those affected by headache disorders world-wide.

Jes Olesen
Timothy Steiner
Richard Lipton

Contents

Contributors

R. Alberca	Hospital Virgen del Rocío, Seville, Spain
F. Andrasik	Institute for Human and Machine Cognition, University of West Florida, Pensacola, Florida, USA
J.P. Auray	University of Lyon, 1–27 Bld du 11 Novembre 1918, 69622 Villeurbanne Cedex, France
F. Baldinetti	Pfizer, Italy
Alice S. Batenhorst	GlaxoSmithKline, PO Box 13398, Five Moore Drive, Research Triangle Park, North Carolina 27709, USA
Birgit Bauer	Department of Anaesthesiology, University of Münster, 48129 Münster, Germany
M.S. Bayliss	Measurement Sciences Group, QualityMetric, Inc., 640 George Washington Highway, Lincoln, Rhode Island, USA
W.J. Becker	Department of Clinical Neurosciences, University of Calgary and Calgary Regional Health Authority, Foothills Hospital, 1403 29th Street NW, Calgary AB T2N 2T9, Canada
E. Berndt	Massachusetts Institute of Technology, Sloan School of Management, Cambridge, Massachusetts, USA
V. Besançon	Emergency Headache Centre, Lariboisière Hospital, Paris, France
J.B. Bjorner	National Institute of Occupational Health, Copenhagen, Denmark
Joseph Bleiberg	Headache Care Center/Clinvest, Inc., Springfield, Missouri, USA
M.C. Borrell-Wilson	Department of Neurology, University of South Florida, HeadachePain Treatment Center, Tampa General Hospital, Tampa, Florida, USA
M.G. Bousser	Department of Neurology, Lariboisière Hospital, Paris, France
Gunnar Bovim	Department of Clinical Neuroscience, Section of Neurology, Norwegian University of Science and Technology, Trondheim, Norway
Naomi Breslau	Department of Psychiatry, Henry Ford Health System, 1 Ford Place, 3A, Detroit, Michigan 48202–3450, USA
Anne Bülow-Olsen	Danish Migraine Association, Postboks 115, 2610 Rødovre, Denmark
T.A. Burke	Formerly Glaxo Wellcome Inc, Research Triangle Park, North Carolina, USA
Peter Buschmann	Allgemeine Ortskrankenkasse AOK, Schleswig-Holstein, Edisonstrasse 70, 24145 Kiel, Germany

G. Bussone	C. Besta National Neurological Institute, Via Celoria 11, 20133 Milano, Italy
Roger K. Cady	Headache Care Center/Clinvest Inc., Springfield, Missouri, USA
C. Cahill-Wright	Department of Neurology, University of South Florida, HeadachePain Treatment Center, Tampa General Hospital, Tampa, Florida, USA
A.E. Cassedy	Headache Research Unit, Department of Family Medicine, University of Cincinnati, College of Medicine, 141 Health Professions Building, Alberg Sabin Way, Eden Avenue, Cincinnati, Ohio 45267, USA
T. Catarci	Pfizer, Italy
C. Chaffaut	AstraZeneca, Rueil-Malmaison, France
B. Charlesworth	AstraZeneca, Macclesfield, UK
S. Chauvet	The City of London Migraine Clinic, London, UK
G. Chazot	Hôpital Neurologique, Neurology Department, Bld Pinel, 69394 Lyon Cedex 03, France
Joseph J. Chmiel	Abbott Laboratories, USA
Virginie Chrysostome	Federation of Clinical Neurological Sciences, Hôpital Pellegrin, Place Amélie Raba Léon, 33076 Bordeaux Cedex, France
Carl G.H. Dahlöf	Gothenburg Migraine Clinic, Sociala Huset, Uppg. D, S-41117 Gothenburg, Sweden
D. D'Amico	C. Besta National Neurological Institute, Via Celoria 11, 20133 Milano, Italy
Jean François Dartigues	Unité INSERM, U. 330, Epidemiologie, Santé Publique et développement, Université Victor Segalen, Bordeaux 2, 146 rue Léo Saignat, 33076 Bordeaux Cédex, France
Sergio De Filippis	Internal Medicine, Headache Centre, II School of Medicine, University 'La Sapienza', Sant'Andrea Hospital, 00189 Rome, Italy
M. Diamond	Diamond Headache Clinic, Chicago, Illinois, USA
Hans-Christoph Diener	Department of Neurology, University of Essen, Germany
A. Dimitriadis	Outpatient Headache Clinic, 1st Department Internal Medicine, General Hospital 'Ag. Dimitrios', Thessaloniki, Greece
Todd A. Dimsdale	GlaxoSmithKline, PO Box 13398, Five Moore Drive, Research Triangle Park, North Carolina 27709, USA
R. Djomby	Emergency Headache Centre, Lariboisière Hospital, Paris, France
V. Domigo	Emergency Headache Centre, Lariboisière Hospital, Paris, France
A. Dowson	Kings College Hospital, London, UK

A. Ducros	Emergency Headache Center, Lariboisière Hospital, Paris, France
G. Duru	University of Lyon, 1–27 Bld du 11 Novembre 1918, 69622 Villeurbanne Cedex, France
Mohamed El Amrani	Hôpital Lariboisiére Neurologie, 2 rue Ambroise Paré, 75010 Paris, France
Abdelkader El Hasnaoui	Laboratoire GlaxoSmithKline, Economic Affairs and Pricing Department, 100 Route de Versailles, 78163 Marly-Le-Roi Cedex, France
Stefan Evers	Department of Neurology, University of Münster, Albert-Schweitzer-Str. 33, 48129 Münster, Germany
Kathleen Farmer	Primary Care Network, 1230 E Kingsley, Springfield, Missouri 65840, USA
M.D. Ferrari	Department of Neurology, Leiden University Medical Centre, PO Box 9600, 2300 RC Leiden, The Netherlands
S. Finkelstein	Massachusetts Institute of Technology, Sloan School of Management, Cambridge, Massachusetts, USA
Pietro Folino-Gallo	Institute for Population Research, Italian National Research Council, Rome, Italy
Paula A. Funk-Orsini	Pfizer Pharmaceuticals Group, New York, USA
W.H. Garber	QualityMetric, Inc., 640 George Washington Highway, Lincoln, Rhode Island, USA
A.F. Gaudin	Laboratoire GlaxoSmithKline Economic Affairs and Pricing Department, 100 Route de Versailles, 78163 Marly-Le-Roi Cedex, France
Hartmut Göbel	Kiel Pain Clinic, Heikendorfer Weg 9–27, 24149 Kiel, Germany
Ingrid Gralow	Department of Anaesthesiology, University of Münster, 48129 Münster, Germany
F. Granella	Institute of Neurology, University of Parma, Parma, Italy
L. Grazzi	C. Besta National Neurological Institute, Via Celoria 11, 20133 Milano, Italy
Knut Hagen	Department of Clinical Neuroscience, Section of Neurology, Norwegian University of Science and Technology, Trondheim, Norway
Michael T. Halpern	Exponent Inc, Alexandria, Virginia, USA
S. Harmoussi-Peioglou	Out patient Headache Clinic, 1st Department Internal Medicine, General Hospital 'Ag. Dimitrios', Thessaloniki, Greece
Lora A. Hasse	Headache Research Unit, Department of Family Medicine, University of Cincinnati, College of Medicine, 141 Health Professions Building, Alberg Sabin Way, Eden Avenue, Cincinnati, Ohio 45267, USA
Axel Heinze	Kiel Pain Clinic, Heikendorfer Weg 9–27, 24149 Kiel, Germany

Patrick Henry	Federation of Clinical Neurological Sciences, Hôpital Pellegrin, Place Amélie Raba Léon, 33076 Bordeaux Cedex, France
Jayasena Hettiarachchi	Pfizer Pharmaceuticals Group, New York, New York, USA
Ingo W. Husstedt	Department of Neurology, University of Münster, Albert-Schweitzer-Str. 33, 48129 Münster, Germany
H. Igarashi	Department of Neurology, Kitasato University, 1–15–1, Kitasato, Sagamihara, Kanagawa 228–8555, Japan
M. Iigaya	Department of Neurology, Kitasato University, 1–15–1, Kitasato, Sagamihara, Kanagawa 228–8555, Japan
Bengt Jönsson	Stockholm School of Economics, Stockholm, Sweden
Robert Kaniecki	University of Pittsburgh Headache Center, University of Pittsburgh, 120 Lytton Avenue Suite 300, Pittsburgh, Pennsylvania 15213, USA
M. Kosinski	QualityMetric, Inc., 640 George Washington Highway, Lincoln, Rhode Island, USA
Steinar Krokstad	HUNT Research Unit Verdal, Faculty of Medicine, Norwegian University of Science and Technology, Trondheim, Norway
Joachim Krüger	Howaldtswerke Deutsche Werft AG, Werftstrasse 112–114, 24143 Kiel, Germany
W. Jackie Kwong	GlaxoSmithKline, PO Box 13398, Five Moore Drive, Research Triangle Park, North Carolina 27709, USA
M.J.A. Láinez	Hospital Clínic Universitari, University of Valencia, Valencia, Spain
Michel Lantéri-Minet	CHU de Nice, Hôpital Pasteur, Neurology Department Pain Service, 30 Av de la Voie Romaine, 06002 Nice Cedex, France
L.J. Launer	Neuroepidemiology Section, Laboratory of Epidemiology, Demography, and Biometry, National Institute on Aging, Bethesda, Maryland, USA
R. Leira	Hospital Xeral de Galicia, Santiago, Spain
M. Leone	C. Besta National Neurological Institute, Via Celoria 11, 20133 Milano, Italy
Volker Limmroth	Neurologische Universitätsklinik Essen, Essen, Germany
Richard B. Lipton	Departments of Neurology, Epidemiology, and Social Medicine, Albert Einstein College of Medicine and Headache Unit, Montefiore Medical Center, Bronx, New York and Innovative Medical Research, Stamford, Connecticut, USA
C. Lucas	Hôpital Roger Salengro, Neurology Department B, 59037 Lille Cedex, France
E.A. MacGregor	The City of London Migraine Clinic, London, UK
Joan Mackell	Pfizer Pharmaceuticals Group, New York, New York, USA

J.E. Magnusson — Department of Clinical Neurosciences, University of Calgary and Calgary Regional Health Authority, Foothills Hospital, 1403 29th Street NW, Calgary AB T2N 2T9, Canada

Morris Maizels — Department of Family Practice, Kaiser Permanente, 5601 DeSoto Avenue, Woodland Hills, California 91367, USA

Lisa K. Mannix — Cincinnati, Ohio, USA

Gian Camillo Manzoni — Headache Centre, Institute of Neurology, University of Parma, Parma, Italy

Paolo Martelletti — Internal Medicine, Headache Centre, II School of Medicine, University 'La Sapienza', Sant'Andrea Hospital, 00189 Rome, Italy

Bradley C. Martin — University of Georgia, Athens, Georgia, USA

Frank Meyer — Howaldtswerke Deutsche Werft AG, Werftstrasse 112–114, 24143 Kiel, Germany

Robert Miceli — Pfizer Pharmaceuticals Group, New York, New York, USA

Philippe Michel — C.C.E.C.Q.A., Hôpital Xavier Arnozan, 33604 Pessac Cedex, France

Bruno Mihout — CHU Département Neurologie, 76031 Rouen, France

M.J. Monzón — Hospital General Universitari, Valencia, Spain

F. Morales — Hospital Clínico, Saragoza, Spain

L. Morin — Emergency Headache Centre, Lariboisière Hospital, Paris, France

Fatima Nachit-Ouinekh — Laboratoire GlaxoSmithKline, 100 route de Versailles, 78163 Marly-Le Roi, France

Bertold Nicola — Abteilung Gesundheitsökonomie, GlaxoWellcome, Alsterufer 1, 20354 Hamburg, Germany

Jes Olesen — Department of Neurology, Glostrup Hospital, University of Copenhagen, Ndr. Ringvej, 2600 Glostrup, Denmark

Fabio Palazzo — Institute for Population Research, Italian National Research Council, Rome Italy

J. Pascual — Hospital Marqués de Valdecilla, Santander, Spain

Dev S. Pathak — The Ohio State University, Columbus, Ohio, USA

Marianne Petersen-Braun — Bayer Vital Consumer Care, Scientific Department, 51149 Cologne, Germany

Frederico Polano — Abteilung Gesundheitsökonomie, GlaxoWellcome, Alsterufer 1, 20354 Hamburg, Germany

A. Pradalier — Hôpital Louis Mourier, Internal Medicine Department, 178 rue des Renouilleres, 92701 Colombes Cedex, France

G. Pransky — Liberty Center for Disability Research, Hopkinton, Massachusetts, USA

Elke Püffel — Allgemeine Ortskrankenkasse, Schleswig-Holstein, Edisonstrasse 70, 24145 Kiel, Germany

Birthe Krogh Rasmussen   Department of Neurology, Hilleroed Hospital, 3400 Hilleroed, Denmark

Dennis Reeves   Headache Care Center/Clinvest Inc., Springfield, Missouri, USA

P.N. Richey   Department of Sociology, University of Cincinnati, Cincinnati, Ohio 45267, USA

A. Rigamonti   C. Besta National Neurological Institute, Via Celoria 11, 20133 Milano, Italy

C. Roos   Emergency Headache Center, Lariboisière Hospital, Paris, France

D.J. Rudawsky   Headache Research Unit, Department of Family Medicine, University of Cincinnati, College of Medicine, 141 Health Professions Building, Alberg Sabin Way, Eden Avenue, Cincinnati, Ohio 45267, USA

F. Sakai   Department of Neurology, Kitasato University, 1–15–1, Kitasato, Sagamihara, Kanagawa 228–8555, Japan

Ann I. Scher   Department of Epidemiology, Bloomberg School of Public Health, The Johns Hopkins University, Baltimore, Maryland and Neuroepidemiology Branch, National Institute for Neurological Disorders and Stroke, and National Institute on Aging, National Institutes of Health, Bethesda, Maryland, USA

Curtis P. Schreiber   Headache Care Center/Clinvest, Inc., Springfield, Missouri, USA

Marc Sharfman   Headache and Neurological Institute, Winter Park, Florida, USA

Stephen D. Silberstein   Department of Neurology, Director, Jefferson Headache Center, Thomas Jefferson University, Philadelphia, Pennsylvania 19107, USA

Elizabeth P. Skinner   GlaxoSmithKline, PO Box 13398, Five Moore Drive, Research Triangle Park, North Carolina 27709, USA

Alain Slama   Laboratoire GlaxoSmithKline, 100 route de Versailles, 78163 Marly-Le Roi, France

L. Ben Slamia   Emergency Headache Centre, Lariboisière Hospital, Paris, France

Robert Smith   Headache Research Unit, Department of Family Medicine, University of Cincinnati, College of Medicine, 141 Health Professions Building, Alberg Sabin Way, Eden Avenue, Cincinnati, Ohio 45267, USA

A. Solari   C. Besta National Neurological Institute, Via Celoria 11, 20133 Milano, Italy

T.J. Steiner   Division of Neuroscience, Imperial College, London, UK

Walter F. Stewart   Department of Epidemiology, Bloomberg School of Public Health, The Johns Hopkins University, Baltimore,

	Maryland 21205, and Innovative Medical Research Inc, Towson, Maryland, USA
Giuseppe Stirparo	Institute of Biomedical Technologies, Italian National Research Council, Rome, Italy
Lars Jacob Stovner	Department of Clinical Neuroscience, Section of Neurology, Norwegian University of Science and Technology, Trondheim, Norway
E. Díez Tejedor	Hospital la Paz, Madrid, Spain
S. Tepper	The New England Center for Headache, Stamford, Connecticut, USA
G.M. Terwindt	Department of Neurology, Leiden University Medical Centre, PO Box 9600, 2300 RC Leiden, The Netherlands
F. Titus	Hospital Valle Hebrón, Barcelona, Spain
Paola Torelli	Headache Centre, Institute of Neurology, University of Parma, Parma, Italy
S. Usai	C. Besta National Neurological Institute, Via Celoria 11, 20133 Milano, Italy
D. Valade	Emergency Headache Center, Lariboisière Hospital, Paris, France
Lars Vatten	Department of Community Medicine and General Practice, Norwegian University of Science and Technology, Trondheim, Norway
G. Vlachogianni	Out patient Headache Clinic, 1st Department Internal Medicine, General Hospital 'Ag. Dimitrios', Thessaloniki, Greece
J.E. Ware Jr	QualityMetric, Inc., 640 George Washington Highway, Lincoln, Rhode Island, USA
Nicholas E.J. Wells	Outcomes Research, Pfizer Global Research and Development, Sandwich, Kent CT13 9NJ, UK
Paul K. Winner	Palm Beach Headache Center, Palm Beach, Florida, USA
John-Anker Zwart	Department of Clinical Neuroscience, Section of Neurology, Norwegian University of Science and Technology, Trondheim, Norway

Section

I

Headache-related disability

1
Overview of headache prevalence, burden, and management

Richard B. Lipton, Ann I. Scher, and Walter F. Stewart

Introduction

Headache is a symptom of a range of systemic and neurological disorders. Headache disorders encompass a group of conditions, usually characterized by recurrent episodes of head pain and associated symptoms. Although headache is a nearly universal human experience, headache disorders vary in incidence, prevalence, and duration. As we attempt to understand the prevalence and societal impact of headache, we begin with the epidemiological studies.[1,2]

Epidemiological data describe the scope, distribution, and burden of the public health problem caused by headache.[1-3] Understanding sociodemographic, genetic, and environmental risk factors helps identify those groups at highest risk for various headache disorders and may ultimately provide clues to preventive strategies or disease mechanisms. Epidemiological studies have identified a number of conditions that are comorbid with migraine (that is, occurring with migraine at a higher frequency than would be expected by chance). Comorbidities for other headache disorders are less well established. Comorbidity must be considered in formulating treatment plans and may provide insights into the mechanisms of disease.[4]

Epidemiological studies assess individuals, whether or not they seek care for their headache disorders. This approach is important since fewer than half of individuals with active migraine actually see a doctor each year for headache and consultation rates are even lower for tension-type headache.[5,6] As a consequence, substantial selection bias occurs in clinic-based studies, where factors that predispose individuals to consult may be mistaken for attributes of the disease.

It is useful to distinguish between clinical and public health perspectives on headache. Clinicians are concerned with the diagnosis of individual patients as a prelude to effective treatment. From a public health perspective, the distribution of diagnoses in a defined population is of importance. While clinicians are interested in the burden of headache disorders imposed on each individual patient, from a societal perspective the direct and indirect costs of illness are priorities.

In this chapter, we will review the epidemiology of migraine and tension-type headache, emphasizing the population-based studies using standardized diagnostic criteria. We will highlight descriptive epidemiology, burden of disease, patterns of diagnosis and treatment, as well as approaches to improving health-care delivery for headache. We focus on migraine and tension-type headache because they are the most important primary headache disorders from the perspective of societal burden. We also focus on studies based on the criteria of the International Headache Society (IHS) because they are more explicit and rigorous than earlier criteria.[1,2,7–13]

Principles of epidemiology

Precise case definitions are essential to facilitate reliable and valid diagnosis and to measure the distribution of disease.[1,2] While there is no true diagnostic gold standard for the primary headache disorders, the IHS criteria provide operational definitions that have been widely used in epidemiological research.[7] For primary headache, the most difficult boundary to identify is the one between migraine and tension-type headache.[14–19]

Epidemiological studies often focus on the incidence and prevalence of disease. Incidence refers to the rate of onset of new cases of a disease in a given population over a defined period. Prevalence is defined as the proportion of a given population that has a disease over a defined period. Prevalence is determined by the product of average incidence and average duration of disease. For example, migraine prevalence may increase because either incidence or duration of disease is increasing. Prevalence may also be affected by demographic shifts in the population if the proportion of the population at high risk for a disease increases. For example, the ageing of the population may increase the prevalence of the headache disorders most common in the elderly (for example, headache secondary to intracranial disease, giant cell arteritis).

Epidemiology of primary and secondary headache

Rasmussen, Olesen, and co-workers were the first to apply the IHS criteria in population studies. They examined the population distribution of all headache disorders using in-person clinical assessment in a large, representative community sample in the greater Copenhagen area.[2,8] The lifetime prevalences of various headache disorders from this population are summarized in Table 1.1.

Tension-type headache is a far more common primary headache than migraine.[8] Cluster headache is relatively uncommon, with a prevalence of 0.1% of this population.[8] Of the secondary headaches, fasting headache (a headache precipitated by missing meals) is the most common type, followed by the headache due to nose/sinus disease and headache secondary to head trauma. Non-vascular intracranial diseases, which include infections and brain tumours, are rare. The rest of the chapter will focus on the two most common primary headache disorders, migraine and tension-type headache.

Table 1.1   Lifetime prevalence of primary and secondary headaches*

Type	Prevalence (%)
Primary	
Tension-type headache	78
Migraine	16
Secondary	
Fasting	19
Nose/sinus disease	15
Head trauma	4
Nonvascular intracranial disease	0.5
(brain tumour and other disorders)	

*After ref. 8.

Migraine

The incidence of migraine is best evaluated in longitudinal studies of persons at risk for migraine; cross-sectional data can also be used to derive incidence estimates. Stewart *et al.* estimated migraine incidence using prevalence data.[20] In males, the incidence of migraine with aura peaked at around 5 years of age at 6.6/1000 person-years; the peak for migraine without aura was 10/1000 person-years between 10 and 11 years. New cases of migraine were uncommon in men in their twenties. In females, the incidence of migraine with aura peaked between ages 12 and 13 years (14.1/1000 person-years); migraine without aura peaked between ages 14 and 17 years (18.9/1000 person-years). Thus, migraine begins earlier in males than in females and migraine with aura begins earlier than does migraine without aura.

Stang *et al.*[21] used the linked medical records system in Olmstead County, Minnesota to identify migraine sufferers who sought medical care for headaches. Their incidence is lower (probably because many people with migraine do not consult doctors or receive a medical diagnosis)[5,6,22] and their peaks are later than those identified by Stewart *et al.*[20] (because medical diagnosis may occur long after the age of onset).

Migraine prevalence studies

The published estimates of migraine prevalence have varied widely (for reviews see refs 1, 2, and 23). In 1995, a meta-analysis of 24 studies that met inclusion criteria included only five that used IHS criteria.[24] This meta-analysis revealed that case definition, along with the age and gender distribution of the study samples, explained 70% of the variation in migraine prevalence among studies. In a second meta-analysis confined to studies using the IHS criteria, in gender-specific models (females and males were modelled separately) age and geography accounted for much of the variation in prevalence as described below.[1] Because case definition so powerfully influences prevalence estimates, we will focus on studies that used the IHS criteria for migraine.

In the previously mentioned study based on the greater Copenhagen area, for men the lifetime prevalences were 93% for any kind of headache, 8% for migraine, and 69% for tension-type headache.[8] For women, the lifetime prevalences were 99% for all headache, 25% for migraine, and 88% for tension-type headache. The 1-year period prevalence of migraine was 6% in men and 16% in women; the 1-year period prevalences of tension-type headache were 63% and 86% in men and women, respectively.

In the USA, the first American Migraine Study, based on data collected in 1989, used questionnaires mailed to 15 000 households selected to be representative of the US population.[9] Migraine diagnoses were based on the IHS criteria but headache duration and the lifetime number of previous migraine attacks were not considered. Migraine prevalence was 17.6% for women and 6% for men, in the same range as the estimates of Rasmussen *et al*.[8] A follow-up study, the American Migraine Study II, used virtually identical methodology 10 years later and demonstrated very similar prevalence estimates.[5,13]

In France, Henry and co-workers reported that the prevalence of IHS migraine was 11.9% in women and 4.0% in men.[10] In this study, diagnoses were assigned based on lay interviews using a validated algorithm. For the group that included 'borderline migraine', prevalence estimates were 17.6% for females and 6.1% for males, remarkably close to the findings of Stewart *et al*. A number of other recent studies in Western Europe and North America have examined the prevalence of migraine.[11,12,23,25]

Sociodemographic variables

Sociodemographic variables, including age, gender, education, income, and geography, influence migraine prevalence. Before puberty, migraine prevalence is higher in boys than in girls. As adolescence approaches, incidence and prevalence increase more rapidly in girls than in boys.[20,26–32] Overall, prevalence increases throughout childhood and early adult life until approximately age 40, after which it declines (Fig. 1.1).[1,2,9,13] These dramatic age effects account for some of the variation in prevalence estimates from previous studies.[1]

The female to male migraine prevalence ratio also varies with age.[1,9,13] The onset of hormonal changes associated with menses may contribute to this variation.[33] However, hormonal factors cannot be the sole cause; differences persist to age 70 and beyond, well beyond the time during which cyclical hormonal changes can be considered a factor.[9,13,33]

The relationship between migraine prevalence and socio-economic status is uncertain. In physician- and clinic-based studies, migraine appears to be associated with high intelligence and social class. In his studies of children, Bille did not find an association between migraine prevalence and intelligence.[26,27] Similarly, in adults, epidemiological studies do not support a relationship between occupation and migraine prevalence.[34] In both of the American Migraine Studies I and II, migraine

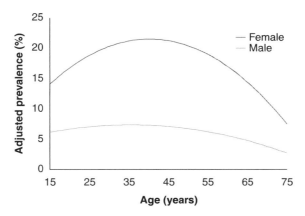

Fig. 1.1 Adjusted prevalence of migraine by age from a meta-analysis of studies using IHS criteria. (From ref. 1.)

prevalence was inversely related to income[9,13] (that is, migraine prevalence fell as household income increased). This inverse relationship between migraine and socio-economic status was confirmed in another US study based on members of a managed care organization[35] and in the National Health Interview Study.[36] In the latter study, migraine prevalence was highest in low-income groups. Prevalence was lowest for middle-income groups and began to rise in the high-income group. Since this study relied on self-reported migraine and migraine awareness rises with income, differential ascertainment by income may account for this relationship in higher-income groups.

Population studies show that individuals from high-income groups are much more likely to report a medical diagnosis of migraine than are those with lower income.[5,22] Perhaps, in the doctor's office migraine appears to be a disease of persons with high income because high-income individuals seek care. As Waters suggested, people from higher-income households are more likely to consult physicians and are therefore disproportionately included in clinic-based studies.[34]

The higher prevalence in the lower socio-economic groups may be a consequence of a circumstance associated with low income and migraine, such as poor diet, poor medical care, or stress.[1,9,13] It may also reflect social selection; that is, migraineurs may have lower incomes because migraine interferes with educational and occupational function, causing a loss of income or of the ability to rise from a low-income group. The relationship of migraine and socio-economic status requires further study. Since migraine prevalence appears unrelated to social class in a number of studies from Europe and elsewhere, it may be influenced by patterns of medical consulting behaviour and access to medical care in different countries.[2,8,11,12,37]

Migraine prevalence also varies by race and geography. In the USA, it is highest in Caucasians, intermediate in African Americans, and lowest in Asian Americans.[1] Similarly, prevalence is highest in North and South America, lower in Africa, and

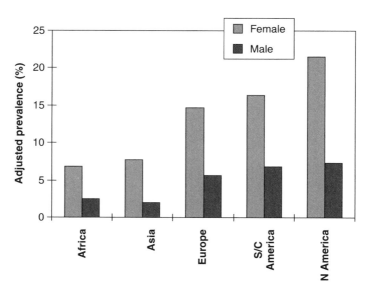

Fig. 1.2 Adjusted prevalence of migraine by geographic area and gender in a meta-analysis of studies using IHS criteria. (From ref. 1.)

often lowest in studies from Asia (Fig. 1.2).[1] The influence of reporting bias on these findings cannot be excluded.

The preponderance of evidence suggests that migraine prevalence has been stable over the last decade. According to the US Centers for Disease Control, self-diagnosed migraine prevalence in the USA increased by 60%, from 25.8/1000 to 41/1000 persons, between 1981 and 1989.[38] Medical records from Olmstead County also suggest that prevalence is increasing.[21] The stability of prevalence in studies in the USA over the past decade does not support the view that prevalence is increasing.[9,13] We have suggested instead that the demonstrable increases in medical consultation and diagnosis may have caused an apparent rather than a real increase.[5,22,39]

Comorbidity of migraine

The term 'comorbidity', coined by Feinstein, is now widely used to refer to the greater than coincidental association of two conditions in the same individual.[4,40] Migraine is associated with a number of neurological and psychiatric disorders, including stroke, epilepsy, depression, and anxiety disorders. Understanding the comorbidity of migraine is potentially important from a number of different perspectives.[4] First, comorbidity has implications for diagnosis. Migraine overlaps in symptom profile with several of the conditions comorbid with it. For example, both migraine and epilepsy can cause transient alterations of consciousness as well as headache. This problem of differential diagnosis is well known. Less well known is the problem of concomitant diagnosis. When two conditions are comorbid, the presence of migraine should increase, not reduce, the index of suspicion for disorders such as epilepsy, depression, and anxiety disorders. Secondly, comorbid conditions may impose therapeutic limitations, but may also create therapeutic opportunities. When migraine and depression occur together, an antidepressant may successfully treat both conditions. When migraine and epilepsy occur together, the anti-migraine anti-epileptic agent, divalproex sodium, may prevent attacks of both migraine and epilepsy. Thirdly, the study of comorbidity may provide epidemiological clues to the fundamental mechanisms of migraine. Finally, the presence of comorbidity may lead to overestimates of the burden of disease. Migraine sufferers may utilize health-care resources not only because of migraine but also because of comorbid depression.

Impact of migraine

Migraine is a public health problem of enormous scope that has an impact on both the individual sufferer and on society.[2,5,9,13] The American Migraine Study II estimates that 28 million US residents have severe migraine headaches.[13] Nearly one in four US households have someone with migraine.[13] Twenty-five per cent of women in the USA who have migraine experience four or more severe attacks a month; 35% experience one to four severe attacks a month; 38% experience one, or less than one, severe attack a month.[13] Similar frequency patterns were observed for men.[13]

In the American Migraine Study II, 92% of women and 89% of men with severe migraine had some headache-related disability.[13] About half were severely disabled or needed bed rest.[19] In addition to the attack-related disability, many migraineurs live in fear, knowing that at any time an attack could disrupt their ability to work, care for their families, or meet social obligations.

Migraine has an enormous impact on society. Recent US studies have evaluated both the indirect costs of migraine as well as the direct costs.[41–43] Indirect costs include the aggregate effects of migraine on productivity at work (paid employment), on household work, and on other roles. The largest components of indirect costs are the productivity losses, which take the form of absenteeism and reduced productivity while at work. Hu *et al.* estimated that productivity losses due to migraine cost American employers 13 billion US dollars per year.[41] These issues have been recently reviewed in more detail elsewhere.[41–43]

Migraine's impact on health-care utilization is marked as well. The National Ambulatory Medical Care Survey, conducted from 1976 to 1977, found that 4% of all visits to physicians' offices (over 10 million visits a year) were for headache.[44] Migraine also results in major utilization of emergency rooms and urgent care centres.[5,45] Vast amounts of prescription and over-the-counter (OTC) medications are taken for headache disorders. OTC sales of pain medication (for all conditions) were estimated to be US$3.2 billion in 1999, and headache accounts for about one-third of OTC analgesic use (Consumer Healthcare Products Association, OTC Sales Statistics—1995–1999, A.C. Neilsen, April 2000). Gross sales for the triptans in the USA are about US$1 billion per year.

Migraine is a lifelong disorder. Bille followed a cohort of children with severe migraine for up to 37 years.[26,27] As young adults, 62% were migraine-free for more than 2 years, but only 40% continued to be migraine-free after 30 years, suggesting that migraine is often a lifelong disorder. For 15 years, Fry collected information on migraine patients in his general practice in Kent.[46] His data showed a tendency for the severity and frequency of attacks to decrease as the patients got older. After 15 years, 32% of the men and 42% of the women no longer had migraine attacks. Waters noted a similar decrease in migraine prevalence.[16,34]

There is a subgroup of migraine sufferers afflicted with a syndrome in which attacks increase in frequency over a number of years until a pattern of daily or near-daily headache evolves.[34,47–50] In subspeciality clinics, about 80% of patients with this disorder are overusing acute headache medication. Medication overuse is believed to contribute to the accelerating pattern of pain through a mechanism that has been termed 'rebound headache'. When the cycle of medication overuse is broken, the headaches often improve.[50] However, in subspeciality clinics, this process of acceleration occurs without medication overuse in about 20% of patients, suggesting that there is a subgroup of migraine sufferers with a progressive condition. The classification of these patients remains controversial. Within the IHS system, they would usually meet criteria for migraine, for chronic tension-type headache, and, perhaps, medication-induced headaches. The term chronic or transformed migraine is sometimes applied to these patients.[47–50]

Tension-type headache

Estimates of the prevalence of tension-type headache have varied widely. In Western countries, 1-year period prevalence ranges from 28% to 63% in men and from 34% to 86% in women.[8,11,51] This variation is explained, in part, by differences in case definition, sampling methods, and the procedures that were used to elicit histories. For example, some studies classified individuals on the basis of their worst headache type only, while others allowed multiple diagnoses per person. Targeting the worst headache type may lead to underestimating the prevalence of tension-type headache, as individuals with migraine headaches who also experience tension-type headaches usually consider migraine their worst headache type. Few tension-type headache studies have been conducted outside the Western world. Wong et al.[52] found very low prevalences in a study he conducted in mainland China. Several studies reported a prevalence of 2–3% for chronic tension-type headache.[8,51,53]

Tension-type headache is more common in women, with gender ratios ranging from 1.04 to 1.8.[8,51,53] Prevalence peaks between the ages of 20 and 50 years and then declines. Schwartz et al.[51] reported a direct relationship between the prevalence of episodic tension-type headache and education.

Tension-type headaches often interfere with activities of daily living. Eighteen per cent of tension-type headache sufferers had to discontinue normal activity, while 44% experienced some limitation of function. Attacks occur with a mean frequency of 2.9 days a month or 35 days a year: most sufferers have less than one attack a month and about one-third have two or more attacks a month.

Like migraine, tension-type headache is an important disorder of middle life, striking individuals early in life and continuing to affect them through their peak productive years. All migraineurs and 60% of tension-type headache patients have a diminished capacity for work or other activities. Despite prominent disability, nearly 50% of migraineurs and more than 80% of tension-type headache patients have never consulted their general practitioner because of headache.

In a Danish study, 43% of employed migraineurs and 12% of employed tension-type headache sufferers missed one or more days of work because of headache.[53] Migraine caused at least one day of missed work in 5%, while tension-type headache caused a day of missed work in 9%. Annually, per 1000 employed persons, 270 lost work days were due to migraine and 820 were due to tension-type headache.[53]

Individuals with frequent episodic tension-type headache may be at increased risk for chronic tension-type headache. When migraine and tension-type headache coexist, tension-type headache may be more frequent and more severe than it is in individuals who do not have migraine. The process whereby headache frequency increases and an episodic disorder becomes chronic is sometimes referred to as transformation or chronification. Overuse of ergotamine and/or analgesics is often found in such patients who consult tertiary referral centres. If analgesics are not withdrawn, these patients may be refractory to prophylactic therapy and have a very poor prognosis.

Though tension-type headache is often attributed to external factors, recent studies support a role for familial aggregation of chronic tension-type headache. Russell and co-workers examined the family relative risk of chronic tension-type headache in first-degree relatives and in spouses. Over 1 year, the relative risk was 3.2 in first-degree relatives and 1.23 in spouses.[54,55] These findings support a role for genetic factors as spouses share some environmental but not genetic risk factors. Complex segregation analysis suggests multifactorial inheritance for chronic tension-type headache.[54,55]

Conclusion

Using the IHS criteria, large population-based epidemiological studies from most regions of the world have shed light on the descriptive epidemiology and burden of headache. While migraine is a remarkably common cause of temporary disability, many migraineurs, even those with disabling headache, have never consulted a physician for the problem. Prevalence is highest in women, in persons between the ages of 25 and 55 years, and, at least in the USA, in individuals from low-income households. Nonetheless, prevalence is high in groups other than these high-risk groups. Migraine prevalence may be increasing in the USA, but this has not been proven. Longitudinal studies are required to better determine the incidence and natural history of migraine as well as the life course of comorbid conditions.

Tension-type headache is much more common than migraine and less disabling from the perspective of individual headache attacks or individual sufferers. Its burden is very substantial because of its prevalence. The burden of headache is a target for clinical and public health interventions designed to reduce the societal burden of disease.

References

1. Scher AI, Stewart WF, Lipton RB. Migraine and headache: a meta-analytic approach. In *Epidemiology of pain* (ed. Crombie IK). Seattle: IASP Press, 1999: 159–70.
2. Rasmussen BK. Epidemiology of headache. *Cephalalgia* 1995; **15**: 45–68.
3. Lipton RB, Amatniek JC, Ferrari MD, *et al*. Migraine: identifying and removing barriers to care. *Neurology* 1994; **44** (Suppl. 6): 56–62.
4. Lipton RB, Silberstein SD. Why study the comorbidity of migraine. *Neurology* 1994; **44** (7): 4–5.
5. Lipton RB, Diamond S, Reed M, Diamond ML, Stewart WF. Migraine diagnosis and treatment: results from the American Migraine Study II. *Headache* 2001; **41**: 638–45.
6. Stang PE, Osterhaus JT, Celentano DD. Migraine: patterns of health care use. *Neurology* 1994; **44** (Suppl. 4): 47–55.
7. Headache Classification Committee of the International Headache Society. Classification and diagnostic criteria for headache disorders, cranial neuralgias, and facial pain. *Cephalalgia* 1988; **8** (Suppl. 7): 1–96.
8. Rasmussen BK, Jensen R, Schroll M, Olesen J. Epidemiology of headache in a general population—a prevalence study. *J Clin Epidemiol* 1991; **44**: 1147–57.
9. Stewart WF, Lipton RB, Celentano DD, Reed ML. Prevalence of migraine headache in the United States. *J Am Med Assoc* 1992; **267**: 64–9.
10. Henry P, Michel P, Brochet B, *et al*. A nationwide survey of migraine in France: prevalence and clinical features in adults. *Cephalalgia* 1992; **12**: 229–37.
11. Göbel H, Petersen-Braun M, Soyka D. The epidemiology of headache in Germany: a nationwide survey of a representative sample on the basis of the headache classification of the International Headache Society. *Cephalalgia* 1994; **14**: 97–106.
12. Launer LJ, Terwindt GM, Ferrari MD. The prevalence and characteristics of migraine in a population-based cohort: the GEM Study. *Neurology* 1999; **53**: 537–42.
13. Lipton RB, Stewart WF, Diamond S, Diamond ML, Reed M. Prevalence and burden of migraine in the United States: data from the American Migraine Study II. *Headache* 2001; **41**: 646–57.
14. Featherstone HJ. Migraine and muscle contraction headaches: a continuum. *Headache* 1985; **24**: 194–8.
15. Raskin NH. *Headache* (2nd edn). New York: Churchill-Livingstone, 1988.
16. Waters WE. *Headache*, Series in Clinical Epidemiology. Littleton, Massachusetts: PSG Co. Inc., 1986.
17. Waters WE. Headache and migraine in general practitioners, the migraine headache and dixarit. Proceedings of a symposium held at Churchill College. Cambridge: Boehringer Ingelheim Brachnell, 1972.
18. Celentano DD, Stewart WF, Linet MS. The relationship of headache symptoms with severity and duration of attacks. *J Clin Epidemiol* 1990; **43**: 983–94.
19. Lipton RB, Stewart WF, Cady R, Hall C, O'Quinn S, Kuhn T, Gutterman D. Sumatriptan for the range of headaches in migraine sufferers: results of the Spectrum Study. *Headache* 2000; **40**: 783–91.

20. Stewart WF, Linet MS, Celentano DD, Van Natta M, Ziegler D. Age and sex-specific incidence rates of migraine with and without visual aura. *Am J Epidemiol* 1993; **34**: 1111–20.
21. Stang PE, Yanagihara T, Swanson JW, *et al*. Incidence of migraine headaches: a population-based study in Olmstead County, Minnesota. *Neurology* 1992; **42**: 1657–62.
22. Lipton RB, Stewart WF, Celentano DD, Reed ML. Undiagnosed migraine: a comparison of symptom-based and self-reported physician diagnosis. *Arch Intern Med* 1992; **152**: 1273–8.
23. Lipton, R.B., Hamelsky, S.W., Stewart, W.F. Epidemiology and impact of headache. In *Wolff's headache and other head pain*, 7th edn, (ed Silberstein SD, Lipton RB, Dalessio DJ). New York: Oxford University Press, 2001: 85–107.
24. Stewart WF, Simon D, Shechter A, Lipton RB. Population variation in migraine prevalence: a meta-analysis. *J Clin Epidemiol* 1995; **48**: 269–80.
25. Rasmussen BK. Epidemiology of headache. *Cephalalgia* 2001; **21** (7): 774–7.
26. Bille B. Migraine in school children. *Acta Paediatr Scand* 1962; **51** (Suppl. 136): 1–151.
27. Bille B. Migraine in children: prevalence, clinical features, and a 30-year follow up. In *Migraine and other headaches* (ed. Ferrari MD, Lataste X). New Jersey: Parthenon, 1989.
28. Sillanpaa M. Prevalence of migraine and other headache in Finnish children starting school. *Headache* 1976; **15**: 288–90.
29. Sillanpaa M. Prevalence of headache in prepuberty. *Headache* 1983; **23**: 10–14.
30. Sillanpaa M. Changes in the prevalence of migraine and other headaches during the first seven school years. *Headache* 1983; **23**: 15–19.
31. Sillanpaa M, Piekkala P, Kero P. Prevalence of headache at preschool age in an unselected child population. *Cephalalgia* 1991; **11**: 239–42.
32. Sillanpaa M. Headache in children. In *Headache classification and epidemiology* (ed. Olesen J). New York: Raven Press, 1994: 273–81.
33. Silberstein SD, Merriam GR. Sex hormones and headache. In *Blue Books of Practical Neurology: Headache* (ed. Goadsby P, Silberstein SD). Boston: Butterworth Heinemann, 1997: 143–76.
34. Waters WE. Migraine: intelligence, social class, and familial prevalence. *Br Med J* 1971; **2**: 77–81.
35. Stang PE, Sternfeld B, Sidney S. Migraine headache in a pre-paid health plan: ascertainment, demographics, physiological and behavioral factors. *Headache* 1996; **36**: 69–76.
36. Stang PE, Osterhaus JT. Impact of migraine in the United States: data from the National Health Interview Survey. *Headache* 1993; **33**: 29–35.
37. D'Alessandro R, Benassi G, Lenzi PL, *et al*. Epidemiology of headache in the Republic of San Marino. *J Neurol Neurosurg Psychiatry* 1988; **51**: 21–7.
38. *Morbidity and Mortality Weekly Report*. Prevalence of chronic migraine headaches—United States, 1980–89. *Morbid Mortal Wkly Rep* 1991; **40**: 331–8.
39. Lipton RB, Stewart WF, Simon D. Medical consultation for migraine: results from the American Migraine Study. *Headache* 1998; **38**: 87–96.
40. Feinstein AR. The pretherapeutic classification of comorbidity in chronic disease. *J Chron Dis* 1970; **23**: 455–68.
41. Hu XH, Markson LE, Lipton RB, Stewart WF, Berger ML. Burden of migraine in the United States: disability and economic costs. *Arch Intern Med* 1999; **159**: 813–18.
42. Osterhaus JT, Gutterman DL, Plachetka JR. Health care resources and lost labor costs of migraine headaches in the United States. *PharmacoEconomics* 1992; **2**: 67–76.
43. Holmes WF, MacGregor A, Dodick D. Migraine-related disability: impact and implications for sufferers' lives and clinical issues. *Neurology* 2001; **56** (Suppl. 1): S13–S19.
44. National Center for Health Statistics. *Vital and health statistics of the United States*, D.H.E.W., PHS Publication No. 53, Advance data. Hyattsville, Maryland: National Center for Health Statistics, 1979.

45. Celentano DD, Stewart WF, Lipton RB, Reed ML. Medication use and disability among migraineurs: a national probability sample. *Headache* 1992; **32**: 223–8.

46. Fry J. *Profiles of disease*. Edinburgh: Livingstone, 1966.

47. Mathew NT, Stubits E, Nigam MP. Transformation of episodic migraine into daily headache: analysis of factors. *Headache* 1982; **22**: 66–8.

48. Mathew NT, Reuveni U, Perez F. Transformed or evolutive migraine. *Headache* 1987; **27**: 102–6.

49. Silberstein SD, Lipton RB, Solomon S, Mathew NT. Classification of daily and near daily headaches. Proposed revisions to the IHS criteria. *Headache* 1994; **34**: 1–7.

50. Silberstein SD, Silberstein JR. Chronic daily headache: long-term prognosis following inpatient treatment with repetitive IV DHE. *Headache* 1992; **32**: 439– 45.

51. Schwartz BS, Stewart WF, Simon D, Lipton RB. Epidemiology of tension-type headache. *J Am Med Assoc* 1998; **279**: 381–3.

52. Wong TW, Wong KS, Yu TS, Kay R. Prevalence of migraine and other headaches in Hong Kong. *Neuroepidemiology* 1995; **14**: 82–91.

53. Rasmussen BK, Jensen R, Olesen J. Impact of headache on sickness absence and utilization of medical services: a Danish population study. *J Epidemiol Commun Hlth* 1992; **46**: 443–6.

54. Russell MB, Iselius L, Ostergaard S, *et al*. Inheritance of chronic tension-type headache investigated by complex segregation analysis. *Hum Genet* 1998; **102**: 138–40.

55. Ostergaard S, Russell MB, Berndtsen E, *et al*. Comparison of first-degree relatives and spouses of people with chronic tension headache. *Br Med J* 1998; **314**: 1092–3.

2 Measuring headache disability

Ann I. Scher, Richard B. Lipton, and Walter F. Stewart

Why measure disability?

Headaches interfere with the activities of everyday life for the majority of migraine sufferers.[1] We use the term disability to describe this effect, although the terminology for pain-related activity limitations varies. For physicians and patients alike, disability may conjure images of wheelchairs, and even patients who frequently miss work due to migraine may not consider themselves disabled. Nonetheless, migraine is a major cause of temporary disability and the term serves to emphasize the severe impact of the disorder.

The degree of headache-related disability experienced with attacks varies considerably from person to person and attack to attack. For example, in the American Migraine Study II,[1] a population-based survey of over 13 000 households, about half of migraine sufferers (49%) required bed rest or were severely impaired, 40% reported only some impairment, and 11% reported no disability with their severe headaches. Severe headaches occurred infrequently (< 1/month) for 38% of the sample. However, a similar proportion (28%) experienced severe headaches once a week or more.

On average, migraine sufferers miss about 2–4 days of work per year due to migraine. Approximately five additional days per year are lost due to reduced productivity while at work with a headache (Table 2.1). These figures represent the work loss experienced by the typical migraine sufferer in the population. Work loss is much higher for those migraine sufferers who present for treatment—perhaps three times as high.[2] In fact, the most disabled 20% of employed migraine sufferers account for 77% of all work loss due to migraine.[3] Not surprisingly, headache-related disability is directly related to the cost of headache treatment. That is, more disabled patients have greater medical costs than less disabled patients.[4] Because the most disabled headache sufferers experience the most work loss, potential productivity gains are greatest for this group. Therefore, disability-based treatment may be cost-effective.

While only about half of migraine sufferers are under a physician's care, those who consult are often not accurately diagnosed or are treated suboptimally. Accurate headache diagnosis and measurement of headache-related disability can help in reducing some of the barriers that keep these individuals from optimal treatment.

Table 2.1   Yearly lost workdays and reduced productivity due to migraine reported in 10 recent surveys*

Ref.	Country	Source	LWD[†]	LWDE[‡]	LWD+LWDE	Comment
33	UK	General population	1.9	4.4	6.3	
34	US	General population	3.1	16.6	18.8	Based on migraine sufferers with at least 6 attacks per year
35	US	General population	3.2	4.9	8.1	
36	US	General population	3.8 (males)			'Severe' headache used as screening question. Includes lost work of homemakers
			8.3 (females)			
37	UK	General population	2.7	15.4	15.8	Based on migraine sufferers with at least 6 attacks per year
38	Netherlands	General population	4.2	8.9	13.1	
3	US	General population	2.8	5.6	8.4	3-month diary study 81% female
39	UK	Hospital employees	2.0	5.5	7.5	
40	Spain	Employees of 11 large companies	0.8 (males) 1.1 (females)		6.3 (males) 9.5 (females)	
2	US	Clinical trial participants	14.8	25.7	40.5	

*Adapted from ref. 41.
[†]LWD, Lost work days (in 1 year).
[‡]LWDE, Lost work day equivalents (in 1 year): the equivalent number of days lost due to reduced productivity while at work.

Empirical information on disability may motivate individuals to seek care as well as lead clinicians to a greater appreciation of the impact that headache is having on the patient's life. This was demonstrated in a recent survey of physicians with an interest in headache.[5,6] In this survey, a patient case history was presented both with and without disability information. Disability information included details such as lost work, leisure activities, and reduced productivity due to headache. Without disability information, that is, with information based on headache characteristics alone, this patient was rated as having 'severe' or 'very severe' headache by 57% of the physicians. With disability data, 89% of the physicians rated this patient as having 'severe' or 'very severe' headaches. Disability information can also identify those patients who may need more aggressive treatment. In the same study, the perceived need for immediate migraine-specific therapy increased from 53% to 79% when disability information was included in the patient's case history. Similarly, a recommendation for follow-up treatment also increased (from 78% to 90%).[5,6]

Finally, disability information provides researchers with tools to stratify patients in clinical trials as well as an outcome against which the efficacy of treatment can be measured.[7]

Strategies for headache-specific disability measurement

A number of questionnaires have been developed for quantifying headache-related disability. Uniform measurement may improve clinician–patient communication and provide a basis for following patients over time in outcome studies and a foundation for stratified care. Any measure needs to be assessed for validity and reliability in the populations of intended use before its use is recommended in practice. The validity of a measurement is 'an expression of the degree to which a measurement measures what it purports to measure'.[8] There are a number of ways in which the validity of a measurement instrument can be assessed, some of which are listed in Table 2.2. Content (or face) validity refers to the extent to which the measure incorporates the domain of the phenomenon under study.[8] The domain of headache disability, for example, might include lost work, reduced productivity, family impact, and effects on social life. Construct validity refers to the extent to which the measure fits into a theoretical model of the phenomenon under measurement. Finally, the instrument would have discriminant validity if, for example, it reliably differentiated between individuals with different headache diagnoses, assuming that disability is different for, say, individuals with migraine than for individuals with episodic tension-type headache.

There are also several forms of reliability. Test–test reliability, perhaps the most important measure, refers to the degree of agreement that the measure has when administered on two separate occasions. If a measure has low test–retest reliability, it is unlikely to be useful in practice. Internal consistency refers to the extent to which the component items of the measurement instrument are related to one another.

A number of such tools have been developed to measure headache-specific disability.[9–13] Three of these tools are described below: the Headache Disability Inventory (HDI), the Headache Impact Test (HIT), and the Migraine Disability Assessment (MIDAS).

Headache Disability Inventory

The Headache Disability Inventory (HDI) was developed by Jacobson, Ramadan, and others at the Henry Ford Hospital.[12] This 25-item questionnaire (Fig. 2.1)

Table 2.2 Research and clinical practice criteria for evaluating clinical measures for headache severity*

Criteria	Analysis
Research criteria	
Internal consistency	The extent to which the items comprising the measure are related to each other
Reliability	Stability and reproducibility of results when the instrument is administered twice to the same person (test–retest)
Content validity	Correlation between the instrument-based measure and a 'gold standard' measure
Construct validity	The extent to which an instrument measures what it purports to measure and fits into a theoretical scheme about the variable of interest
Discriminant validity	The extent to which an instrument distinguished two conditions known to be different
External validity	The extent to which the instrument-based measure is related to other measures
Sensitivity to change	Instrument detects real change over time, such as improvement in outcome in response to effective therapy
Clinical practice criteria	
Face validity	Judgement that the measure meets individuals' conceptions, for example, by selecting items deemed to be important to the disease sufferer or physician
Ease of use	The instrument should be simple to apply
Ease of scoring	The instrument should be simple to score
Intuitively meaningful	The instrument should correlate with physicians' judgements of illness severity and treatment need

*Taken from ref. 42.

consists of 13 questions pertaining to emotional aspects of headache disability (for example, 'No one understands the effect that my headaches have on my life') and 12 questions related to functional disability (for example, 'I am concerned that I am paying penalties at work or at home because of my headaches'). The questionnaire was administered in pencil and paper format, with responses scored on a 3-point scale: yes (4 points), sometimes (2 points), and no (0 points). Headache frequency and headache severity were also assessed.

Various validity tests were performed on a sample of about 100 patients consecutively seen at a headache clinic. An attempt was made to measure the construct validity of this instrument by determining the degree to which the HDI correlated with headache severity (mild, moderate, severe), headache frequency (≤1/month, 2–3 month, 4+ month), and headache type (migraine with aura, migraine without aura, chronic tension headache). The HDI total score as well as functional and emotional subscores were found to be significantly correlated to headache severity. No age or gender differences were found—that is, the correlation of the HDI with headache severity was for men and women and in various age groups. However, the HDI

HEADACHE DISABILITY INVENTORY

INSTRUCTIONS: Please CIRCLE the correct response:

1. I have headache: (1) 1 per month (2) more than 1 but less than 4 per month (3) more than one per week
2. My headache is: (1) mild (2) moderate (3) severe

Please read carefully: The purpose of the scale is to identify difficulties that you may be experiencing because of your headache. Please check off 'YES', 'SOMETIMES', or 'NO' to each item. Answer each question as it pertains to your headache only.

YES   SOMETIMES   NO

E1. Because of my headaches I feel handicapped.
E2. Because of my headaches I feel restricted in performing my routine daily activities.
E3. No one understands the effect my headaches have on my life.
E4. I restrict my recreational activities (eg. sports, hobbies) because of my headaches.
E5. My headaches make me angry.
E6. Sometimes I feel that I am going to lose control because of my headaches.
E7. Because of my headaches I am less likely to socialize.
E8. My spouse (significant other), or family and friends have no idea what I am going through because of my headaches.
E9. My headaches are so bad that I feel that I am going to go insane.
E10. My outlook on the world is affected by my headaches.
E11. I am afraid to go outside when I feel that a headache is starting.
E12. I feel desperate because of my headaches.
E13. I am concerned that I am paying penalties at work or at home because of my headaches.
E14. My headaches place stress on my relationships with family or friends.
F15. I avoid being around people when I have a headache.
F16. I believe my headaches are making it difficult for me to achieve my goals in life.
F17. I am unable to think clearly because of my headaches.
F18. I get tense (eg, muscle tension) because of my headaches.
F19. I do not enjoy social gatherings because of my headaches.
F20. I feel irritable because of my headaches.
F21. I avoid traveling because of my headaches.
F22. My headaches make me feel confused.
F23. My headaches make me feel frustrated.
F24. I find it difficult to read because of my headaches.
F25. I find it difficult to focus my attention away from my headaches and on other things.

Fig. 2.1 Headache Disability Instrument. (Adapted from ref. 12.)

did not differentiate among patients with different levels of headache frequency nor different headache types. This may be due, in part, to the fact that this instrument was tested on a sample of patients who were consulting a subspeciality clinic. Although details of this particular sample were not provided, patients attending such clinics tend to have severe headaches,[14–19] making discrimination among diagnostic groups more challenging. Therefore, it is possible that most of this group of patients fell into the '4+' headaches per month category and that there was not sufficient variability in the frequency scale to validate against the HDI. Similarly, the unexpected and counterintuitive finding that headache disability (as measured by the HDI) was not different by headache type, may also be due to the patient mix seen at subspeciality clinics. For example, there were no patients with episodic tension-type headache in this sample.

Test–retest reliability was measured on a subset of the original sample ($n=77$) by administering the HDI via telephone 6 months after the original test. There was generally a strong correlation for the overall score as well as the subscales. A similar test with shorter follow-up was done on a sample of 42 patients.[20] Based on these results, the authors felt that a change of 29 points (6 months) or 16 points (1 week) in the total HDI score could be used to assess the efficacy of headache management. This change would correspond to, for example, a one-level change in 15 of the 25 items (for example, from 'yes' to 'sometimes' or from 'sometimes' to 'no') in order to assess efficacy at 6 months.

Headache Impact Test

The Headache Impact Test (HIT) is available in an internet-based version and as a six-question paper version (Fig. 2.2). The internet version is currently available at two sites: www.headachetest.com, a site maintained by GlaxoSmithKline and www.amihealthy.com, a site maintained by the commercial developer of the test, QualityMetric. Details of the development of the HIT have been presented in abstracts and a journal supplement.[21–23]

Briefly, the HIT content was initially composed from four headache-specific questionnaires: the HDI (described above), the Headache Impact Questionnaire (HImQ),[9] MIDAS (described below), and the Migraine-Specific Quality of Life Questionnaire (MSQ).[10,11] The questions were supplemented with others suggested by a panel of consulting headache specialists.

A population-based sample of individuals who had experienced a headache in the past month ($n=1016$) was interviewed over the telephone. Subjects were given all 53 items from the four instruments as well as 13 questions used to classify the participants by headache diagnosis (migraine, non-migraine) and severity (mild, moderate, severe). In addition, a subset ($n=300$) of this population was contacted after 3 months for a follow-up interview, the purpose of which was to measure the responsiveness of the instrument to changes in headache disability over time. Standard psychometric measures were performed (content validity, internal consistency, reliability, etc.) and validated against headache diagnosis and severity. The HIT was

HIT-6™

(VERSION 1.0)

This questionnaire was designed to help you describe and communicate the way you feel and what you cannot do because of headaches.

To complete, please circle one answer for each question.

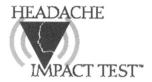

HEADACHE

IMPACT TEST™

1 When you have headaches, how often is the pain severe?

| Never | Rarely | Sometimes | Very Often | Always |

2 How often do headaches limit your ability to do usual daily activities including household work, work, school, or social activities?

| Never | Rarely | Sometimes | Very Often | Always |

3 When you have a headache, how often do you wish you could lie down?

| Never | Rarely | Sometimes | Very Often | Always |

4 In the past 4 weeks, how often have you felt too tired to do work or daily activities because of your headaches?

| Never | Rarely | Sometimes | Very Often | Always |

5 In the past 4 weeks, how often have you felt fed up or irritated because of your headaches?

| Never | Rarely | Sometimes | Very Often | Always |

6 In the past 4 weeks, how often did headaches limit your ability to concentrate on work or daily activities?

| Never | Rarely | Sometimes | Very Often | Always |

COLUMN 1 (6 points each) + COLUMN 2 (8 points each) + COLUMN 3 (10 points each) + COLUMN 4 (11 points each) + COLUMN 5 (13 points each)

To score, add points for answers in each column.

Please share your HIT-6 results with your doctor.

Total Score

Higher scores indicate greater impact on your life.

Score range is 36-78.

Fig. 2.2   Headache Impact Test, paper version. (Courtesy of GlaxoSmithKline.)

calibrated to have a mean of 50 and standard deviation of 10, with a score of 50 representing the average score for a representative US headache population. Each one-point change in score represents a change corresponding to one-tenth of a standard deviation. Thus, a relatively small change in numerical score (for example, from 58 to 51) represents an improvement from the 75th percentile to the 50th percentile.[24]

The dynamic internet-based version of the HIT essentially re-estimates the total HIT score after each question based on the responses to the questions thus far presented. The program chooses the next question to present based on a model that estimates the question that will be most informative as to the final HIT score. For the purposes of this process, the 'gold standard' is a score estimated from the entire item pool. When the desired level of precision is reached, the questioning stops. Generally, the program converges after five or fewer questions.[22] Convergence tends to be faster for severe or migraine headache sufferers than for those with mild headaches. In addition to the adaptive version, a six-item paper version was developed for use in clinical practice. This version was found to correlate well with the internet version, and is available in 23 languages.

MIDAS

The MIDAS questionnaire consists of five disability questions encompassing three domains of activity: work or school; leisure activities; or household work (Fig. 2.3). Internet versions can be found on http://www.midas-migraine.net/us/ (AstraZeneca), at http://www.achenet.org/your/midas.php (American Headache Society), and at http://www.migraines.org (Magnum: Migraine Awareness Group). The psychometric properties and clinical application of the MIDAS questionnaire have been well studied, and reported in multiple publications to date.[7,13,25–29]

Responses are expressed in intuitively meaningful units—units of missed days due to headache in school or paid work, leisure activities, or household work during the last 3 months. In addition to complete days missed, days with reduced productivity (defined as at least 50% reduction) are also captured. Four MIDAS clinical disability grades are defined: grade I (score 0–5), little or none; grade II, score 6–10, mild; grade III, score 11–20, moderate; and grade IV, score 21+, severe.

The MIDAS questionnaire has demonstrated internal consistency and test–retest reliability in two population-based samples, one in the USA ($n=97$) and one in the UK ($n=100$).[13,27] The study participants were randomly selected members of the general population who satisfied diagnostic criteria for migraine in a telephone-based interview. Two interviews were conducted over an interval of about 3 weeks. The test–retest reliability of the total MIDAS score over the 3-week period was found to be around 0.8 for both the USA and UK tests using the Spearman and Pearson correlation coefficients. The Cronbach alpha measure of internal consistency was also high for a questionnaire with relatively few items, at 0.76 for the USA and 0.73 for the UK.

The MIDAS questionnaire was also validated against daily measures of activity limitations recorded in a headache diary.[29] In this study, a population-based sample

This form can help you and your doctor improve the management of your headaches

Do You Suffer From

headaches?

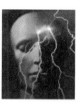

MIDAS QUESTIONNAIRE

INSTRUCTIONS: Please answer the following questions about ALL your headaches you have had over the last 3 months. Write your answer in the box next to each question. Write zero if you did not do the activity in the last 3 months.

1 On how many days in the last 3 months did you miss work or school because of your headaches? ___ days

2 How many days in the last 3 months was your productivity at work or school reduced by half or more because of your headaches? *(Do not include days you counted in question 1 where you missed work or school)* ___ days

3 On how many days in the last 3 months did you not do household work because of your headaches? ___ days

4 How many days in the last 3 months was your productivity in household work reduced by half or more because of your headaches? *(Do not include days you counted in question 3 where you did not do household work)* ___ days

5 On how many days in the last 3 months did you miss family, social or leisure activities because of your headaches? ___ days

TOTAL ___ days

A On how many days in the last 3 months did you have a headache? *(If a headache lasted more than 1 day, count each day)* ___ days

B On a scale of 0-10, on average how painful were these headaches? *(Where 0 = no pain at all, and 10 = pain as bad as it can be)* ___

©Innovative Medical Research 1997

Once you have filled in the questionnaire, add up the total number of days from questions 1-5 (ignore A and B).

Grading system for the MIDAS Questionnaire:

Grade	Definition	Score
I	Little or no disability	0-5
II	Mild disability	6-10
III	Moderate disability	11-20
IV	Severe disability	21+

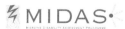

MIGRAINE DISABILITY ASSESSMENT PROGRAMME

The MIDAS programme is sponsored by

Fig. 2.3   MIDAS questionnaire, ©Innovative Medical Research.

of 148 migraine sufferers kept a diary over a 3-month period in which they recorded detailed information on headache features as well as activity limitations in work, household chores, and non-work activities (social, family, and leisure activities). At the end of this 3-month period, the MIDAS questionnaire was completed and scored. This score was compared against a diary-based MIDAS score. Overall, the diary-based MIDAS score correlated well with the MIDAS questionnaire. However, while the MIDAS questions relating to missed days or work, leisure activities, or household work correlated well with the diary data, the MIDAS values for greater than 50% reduced productivity tended to be higher than the diary-based MIDAS score.

In another validation study, the MIDAS questionnaire was evaluated by 49 primary and specialty care physicians for face (construct) validity and clinical utility.[30] Twelve case histories were presented to the physicians, who were unaware of the MIDAS scores. The twelve case histories were systematically sampled (by MIDAS score) from the individuals in the diary study (previous paragraph). Information from the medical record and 90-day diary was summarized and presented as a medical history. A summary of headache features as well as demographic characteristics (age, sex, occupation) were also included in the patient history. Based on this information, the physicians then graded each case for pain level, disability, and need for medical care without access to MIDAS scores. In general, the physician ratings of pain intensity, disability, and need for treatment correlated with the MIDAS score.

After completing the case histories, the physicians were presented with the rationale behind the MIDAS questionnaire and the scoring procedure. Most (89%) found the questionnaire to be 'very easy', 'easy', or 'not difficult' to complete.

Clinical application

Disability tools can play several important roles in the clinical management of headache disorders. First, they can help legitimize the disease by demonstrating the aggregate burden headache causes. Secondly, these measures can facilitate doctor–patient communication regarding headache-related disability. Thirdly, these measures can facilitate treatment decisions. Because migraine and other headache disorders vary in severity, diagnosis alone does not provide enough information to facilitate wise treatment decisions. Treatment guidelines for migraine recommend 'stratified care' approaches. Using stratified, care, treatment is selected based both on diagnosis and severity of illness. Of the disability measures discussed herein, only MIDAS has been used in clinical trials. The Disability and Strategies of Care (DISC) study demonstrated that, when treatment was selected based on MIDAS grade, clinical outcomes improved relative to those of conventional step-care strategies.[7] Finally, disability tools can be used to measure the benefits of medical care. Several studies have shown that MIDAS scores improve during the course of effective clinical treatment.[31,32]

References

1. Lipton RB, Stewart WF, Diamond S, Diamond ML, Reed ML. Prevalence and burden of migraine in the United States: data from the American Migraine Study II. *Headache* 2001; **41**: 646–57.
2. Osterhaus JT, Gutterman DL, Plachetka JR. Healthcare resource and lost labour costs of migraine headache in the US. *PharmacoEconomics* 1992; **2**: 67–76.
3. von Korff M, Stewart WF, Simon DJ, Lipton RB. Migraine and reduced work performance: a population-based diary study. *Neurology* 1998; **50**: 1741–5.
4. von Korff M, Stewart WF, Lipton RB. Assessing headache severity. New directions. *Neurology* 1994; **44**: S40–S46.
5. Holmes WF, MacGregor EA, Sawyer JP, Lipton RB. Information about migraine disability influences physicians' perceptions of illness severity and treatment needs. *Headache* 2001; **41**: 343–50.
6. Holmes WF, MacGregor EA, Dodick D. Migraine-related disability: impact and implications for sufferers' lives and clinical issues. *Neurology* 2001; **56**: S13–S19.
7. Lipton RB, Stewart WF, Stone AM, Lainez MJ, Sawyer JP. Stratified care vs step care strategies for migraine: the Disability in Strategies of Care (DISC) study: a randomized trial. *J Am Med Assoc* 2000; **284**: 2599–605.
8. Last JM, Abramson JH, Friedman GD, Porta M, Spasoff RA, Thuriaux M (ed.). *A dictionary of epidemiology*, 3rd edn. New York: Oxford University Press, 1995.
9. Stewart WF, Lipton RB, Simon D, Liberman J, von Korff M. Validity of an illness severity measure for headache in a population sample of migraine sufferers. *Pain* 1999; **79**: 291–301.
10. Jhingran P, Osterhaus JT, Miller DW, Lee JT, Kirchdoerfer L. Development and valid-ation of the Migraine-Specific Quality of Life Questionnaire. *Headache* 1998; **38**: 295–302.
11. Martin BC, Pathak DS, Sharfman MI, *et al.* Validity and reliability of the migraine-specific quality of life questionnaire (MSQ Version 2.1). *Headache* 2000; **40**: 204–15.
12. Jacobson GP, Ramadan NM, Aggarwal SK, Newman CW. The Henry Ford Hospital Headache Disability Inventory (HDI). *Neurology* 1994; **44**: 837–42.
13. Stewart WF, Lipton RB, Dowson AJ, Sawyer J. Development and testing of the Migraine Disability Assessment (MIDAS) Questionnaire to assess headache-related disability. *Neurology* 2001; **56**: S20–S28.
14. Mathew NT, Reuveni U, Perez F. Transformed or evolutive migraine. *Headache* 1987; **27**: 102–6.
15. Silberstein SD, Lipton RB, Sliwinski M. Classification of daily and near-daily headaches: field trial of revised IHS criteria. *Neurology* 1996; **47**: 871–5.
16. Manzoni GC, Granella F, Sandrini G, Cavallini A, Zanferrari C, Nappi G. Classification of chronic daily headache by International Headache Society criteria: limits and new proposals. *Cephalalgia* 1995; **15**: 37–43.
17. Sandrini G, Manzoni GC, Zanferrari C, Nappi G. An epidemiological approach to the nosography of chronic daily headache. *Cephalalgia* 1993; **13** (Suppl. 12): 72–7.
18. Rothrock J, Patel M, Lyden P, Jackson C. Demographic and clinical characteristics of patients with episodic migraine versus chronic daily headache. *Cephalalgia* 1996; **16**: 44–9.
19. Saper JR. Daily chronic headache [review; 28 refs]. *Neurol Clin* 1990; **8**: 891–901.
20. Jacobson GP, Ramadan NM, Norris L, Newman CW. Headache disability inventory (HDI): short-term test–retest reliability and spouse perceptions. *Headache* 1995; **35**: 534–9.
21. Ware JEJ, Bjorner JB, Kosinski M. Practical implications of item response theory and computerized adaptive testing: a brief summary of ongoing studies of widely used headache impact scales. *Med Care* 2000; **38**: II73–II182.
22. Ware JEJ, Bjorner JB, Dahlöf C, *et al.* Development of the Headache Impact Test (HIT) using item response theory (IRT). Headache World 2000 [abstract].

23. Kosinski M, Bjorner JB, Bayliss MS, Ware JEJ. Measuring the impact of migraine and severe headache with the Headache Impact Test (HIT) using item response theory (IRT) to score widely-used measures of headache impact. American Academy of Neurology 2000 [abstract].

24. Dahlöf C, Dewey J, Tepper S, *et al*. Comparability of Headache Impact Test (HIT) and HIT-6 scoring. 10th Congress of the International Headache Society, 2001 [abstract].

25. Stewart WF, Lipton RB, Kolodner K, Liberman J, Sawyer J. Reliability of the migraine disability assessment score in a population-based sample of headache sufferers. *Cephalalgia* 1999; **19**: 107–14.

26. Sawyer J, Edmeads J, Lipton RB. Clinical utility of a new instrument assessing migraine disability: the Migraine Disability Assessment (MIDAS) questionnaire [abstract]. *Neurology* 1998; **50**: A433–A434.

27. Stewart WF, Lipton RB, Whyte J, *et al*. An international study to assess reliability of the Migraine Disability Assessment (MIDAS) score. *Neurology* 1999; **53**: 988.

28. Edmeads J, Lainez JM, Brandes JL, Schoenen J, Freitag F. Potential of the Migraine Disability Assessment (MIDAS) Questionnaire as a public health initiative and in clinical practice. *Neurology* 2001; **56**: S29–S34.

29. Stewart WF, Lipton RB, Kolodner KB, Sawyer J, Lee C, Liberman JN. Validity of the Migraine Disability Assessment (MIDAS) score in comparison to a diary-based measure in a population sample of migraine sufferers. *Pain* 2000; **88**: 41–52.

30. Lipton RB, Stewart WF, Sawyer J, Edmeads JG. Clinical utility of an instrument assessing migraine disability: the Migraine Disability Assessment (MIDAS) questionnaire. *Headache* 2001; **41**: 854–61.

31. Freitag F, Diamond S, Lyss H, Diamond ML, Urban G, Pepper B. MIDAS as a healthcare utilization tool in the challenging patient [abstract]. *Cephalalgia* 2000; **40**: 365–6.

32. Mathew NT, Villarreal S, Kailasam J. Improvement in headache related disability in chronic daily headache—treatment outcome assessed by MIDAS [abstract]. *Headache* 2000; **40**: 420.

33. Cull RE, Wells NEJ, Miocevich ML. The economic cost of migraine. *Br J Med Econ* 1992; **2**: 103–15.

34. Lipton RB, Scher AI, Kolodner K, Liberman J, Steiner T, Stewart WF. Migraine in the United States: epidemiology and patterns of health care use. *Neurology* 2002; **58**: 885–94.

35. Schwartz BS, Stewart WF, Lipton RB. Lost workdays and decreased work effectiveness associated with headache in the workplace. *J Occup Environ Med* 1997; **39**: 320–7.

36. Stewart WF, Lipton RB, Simon D. Work-related disability: results from the American Migraine Study. *Cephalalgia* 1996; **16**: 231–8.

37. Steiner TJ, Scher A I, Stewart WF, Kolodner K, Liberman J, Lipton RB. The prevalence of adult migraine in England and its relationships to major sociodemographic characteristics. Unpublished work.

38. van Roijen L, Essink-Bot M, Koopmanschap MA, Michel BC, Rutten FFH. Societal perspective on the burden of migraine in The Netherlands. *PharmacoEconomics* 1995; **7**: 170–9.

39. Clarke CE, MacMillan L, Sondhi S, Wells NE. Economic and social impact of migraine. *Quart J Med*. 1996; **89**: 77–84.

40. Lainez JM, Titus F, Cobaleda S, Leton E. Socioeconomic impact of migraine [abstract]. *Funct Neurol* 1996; **11**: 133.

41. Scher AI, Lipton RB, Stewart WF. An epidemiological perspective on the impact of migraine on a personal and societal level. In *Migraine: a neuroinflammatory disease?* (ed. Spierings ELH, Sanchez del Rio M). Basel: Birkhauser Verlag, 2002.

42. Lipton RB, *et al*. Migraine: diagnosis and assessment of disability. *Rev Contemp Pharmacother* 2000; **11**: 63–73.

3 Benefits of treatment on headache disability—a personal view on selected data

Carl G.H. Dahlöf

Introduction

Migraine is a highly prevalent chronic disease that typically affects the sufferers during their most productive years.[1–5] Migraine causes disruption of work, chores, and leisure activities, affects social and family life, produces suffering and emotional stress, and impairs health-related quality of life.[3,6–9] In addition to the disability perceived during the migraine attack, it seems that some impairment is also experienced between attacks.[10–12] The unpredictability of migraine and anxiety regarding the potential occurrence of future attacks may contribute to this interictal (between attack) impact. When a population-based sample of migraine sufferers in Sweden ($N=423$) was asked about 'back to normal functioning', 43%, 43%, and 9% (no reply from 4%) reported that they were 'completely', 'more or less', and 'not', respectively, recovered between the attacks.[13]

Almost all, if not all, migraineurs take medications, whether non-prescription or prescription, in an attempt to relieve the most debilitating symptoms of the migraine attack—pain, nausea, and phono- and photophobia.[2,13] The success of medications and other treatments dictates the extent of the sufferer's immediate disability, which may range from beginning to resume activities within hours to being immobilized in bed for days, arising only with the urge to vomit. Irrespective of the treatment used, total recovery still seems to follow the natural duration of the attack.

Disability

Disability can be defined as being disabled, incapacitated, debilitated, rendered inoperative, or put out of action but also has connotations of a lesser well-being/quality of life. Notwithstanding, the word 'disability' means different things to different people. Some associate the word with specific medical conditions, while others think of difficulties in performing tasks of everyday living. The former World Health Organization (WHO) definition of disability, 'In the context of health experience, a disability is any restriction or lack (resulting from an impairment) of ability to perform an activity in the manner or within the range considered normal for a human being', has recently been changed. WHO has now released a new version of the International Classification of Functioning and Disability (Beta-2 version of ICIDH-2) for field trials.[14] The overall aim of the ICIDH-2 classification is to provide a unified and standard language and framework for the description of human functioning and disability as an important component of health. The classification covers any disturbance in terms of 'functional states' associated with health conditions at body, individual, and society levels. ICIDH-2 organizes information according to three dimensions: body level; individual level; and society level. A list of environmental factors forms part of the classification. Environmental factors have an impact on all three dimensions and are organized from the individual's most immediate environment to the general environment. ICIDH-2 is a multipurpose classification designed to serve various disciplines and different sectors. This new definition minimizes the focus on negative handicaps while emphasizing the importance of functional status by incorporating health-related issues and environmental factors.

It is practically impossible to communicate the pain, anguish, and other symptoms of the migraine attack to a person who has never had migraine. Here is how a woman with migraine (42 years old) describes it. 'The pain is terribly severe and feels as though my left eye will pop out and my entire left upper and lower jaw ache as though I had toothache. My arms feel like lead and I have difficulty remembering what I am doing. I feel sick and when I stand up it is worse and I sometimes vomit.' The former Swedish Minister for Health and Social Affairs, Margot Wallström, said the following about her migraine in an interview, 'There were nightmare situations in my job when I had to force myself to get up on to the platform and deliver a speech in spite of having a throbbing headache and vomiting repeatedly both before and afterwards.' In addition, 'It easily becomes a vicious circle. I worry about having an attack, especially when I have an important meeting coming up, and an attack then often comes without my being able to control it. I sometimes work myself up into a real panic.'

A survey of migraineurs in Sweden ($N=741$) who are presently using a triptan to treat their attacks demonstrated that 65% rest in a dark room in about 60% of their attacks and about 25% use a 'wet and cold towel' in 40% of their attacks (C. Dahlöf, unpublished observations). When a population-based sample of migraine sufferers in Sweden ($N=423$) was asked which the migraine symptom they perceived as the worst, a majority (69%) claimed that pain was the most debilitating symptom.[13] The same population was also asked to rank what they value most in life by choosing from three of ten alternatives. At the top of the list were family life, work performance, good economic status, and leisure activities/meaningful time off, which were reported by 65%, 40%, 33%, and 29%, respectively.[13] The impact of migraine on their favourite activities is demonstrated in Fig. 3.1. The survey of migraineurs mentioned above ($N=741$) demonstrated that subjective disability impact correlates with attack duration (Fig. 3.2) (C. Dahlöf, unpublished observations).

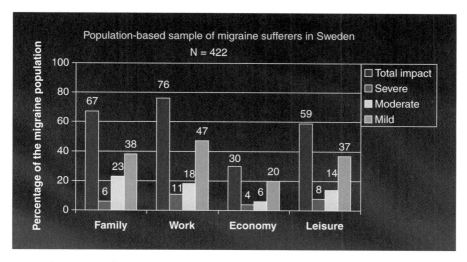

Fig. 3.1   The impact of migraine on the top ranked life activities—family life, work performance, good economic status, and leisure—in a population-based sample of migraine sufferers in Sweden (*N*=423). (See ref. 13.)

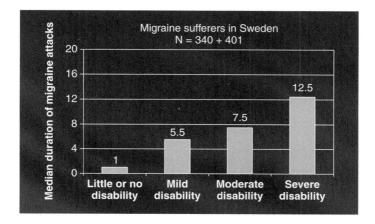

Fig. 3.2   The correlation between median duration of migraine attacks and subjectively rated severity of disability in a migraine population (*N*=741).

It seems, that most migraine disability is suffered at home. A survey of a subset of migraineurs (*N*=76) at Gothenburg Migraine Clinic (GMC) demonstrated that on average they had 98 days with migraine per year yet only 6 days of absenteeism per year due to migraine (C. Dahlöf, personal communication). These data suggest that, while migraineurs are present at work, school, etc. during many of their attacks, they are there with reduced functional status—a scenario often described as 'presenteeism'.

Assessment of disability

Relief of headache pain has repeatedly been reported to be the most important goal to achieve in the acute treatment of migraine attack symptoms.[9,13] If the contributing factors for migraine disability are restricted to the pain, nausea, and phono- and photophobia that the sufferers perceive during the attack from the start to 2–4 hours after treatment, there is sufficient evidence from randomized, controlled clinical trials that the disability induced by migraine attacks can effectively be reduced by treatment of the attack (Figs 3.3 and 3.4).[15,16] Using preventive migraine therapies should lessen migraine disability by reducing attack frequency.

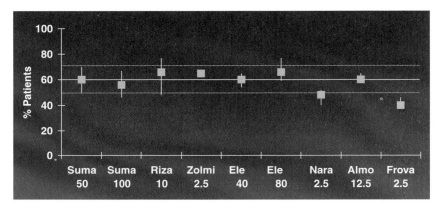

Fig. 3.3 Comparison of the 2-hour pain relief rates for each triptan with respect to means and ranges of results obtained in placebo-controlled trials. (See ref. 16.)

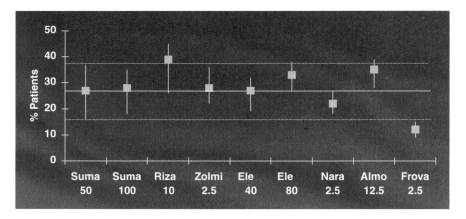

Fig. 3.4 Comparison of the 2-hour pain-free rates for each triptan with respect to means and ranges of results obtained in placebo-controlled trials. (See ref. 16.)

Migraine is debilitating because it obstructs family obligations and social plans, results in absenteeism from work, while also impairing the ability to perform normal tasks at home, school, or in the workplace.[6-9,11] The full impact of migraine extends, however, beyond the obvious disability associated with work, family, and social functioning, to influencing energy levels, the ability to think and reason, as well as contributing to emotional distress and stability. Clinicians, researchers, and patients need a short, yet comprehensive, easy-to-score measure for use in clinical practice and clinical trials. Quantification of the impact of migraine on functional status offers an opportunity to facilitate physician–patient communication and improve patient care. Use of instruments as measures of outcomes to systematically quantify improvement makes intuitive sense, but such studies have yet to be published.

There are a number of validated instruments that have been developed to quantify disability: the Headache Disability Inventory (HDI),[17,18] the Headache Impact Questionnaire (HImQ),[19,20] the Migraine Disability Assessment Questionnaire (MIDAS),[21-23] and the Headache Impact Test (HIT; see Chapter 13, this book). These use different distinctive approaches to measurement. Along with the idea of using objective measurements only came the concept of restriction of disability meaning minutes, hours, or days during which work, school, home activities were missed/affected by 50% or more (that is, MIDAS and HImQ). Although restriction of activities from a time perspective has, on the face of it, a high validity, research in other therapeutic areas has suggested that it may be a challenge for patients to accurately recall time missed beyond 2–4 weeks.

A prospective, observational study without control group assessed the outcomes of migraineurs in a mixed-model staff/independent practice association managed care organization for patients previously diagnosed as having migraine who received their first prescription for sumatriptan.[24] Data collected included medical as well as pharmacy claims and patient surveys to measure changes in satisfaction, health-related quality of life, workplace productivity, and non-workplace activity after sumatriptan therapy was initiated. A total of 178 patients completed the study. Results obtained from 178 patients showed significant decreases in the mean number of migraine-related physician office visits, emergency department visits, and medical procedures in the 6 months after sumatriptan therapy compared with the 6 months before sumatriptan was used ($p<0.05$).[24] There were also improvements in patient satisfaction and significant reductions in time lost from workplace productivity and non-workplace activity.

Unfortunately, there is very limited double-blind and controlled prospective data on the effects of headache therapy on disability in this respect. A prospective sequential multinational (five countries) study concurrently evaluated the effects of subcutaneous sumatriptan on clinical parameters, health-related quality of life (HRQoL) measures, workplace productivity, and patient satisfaction.[12] Patients ($N=58$, aged 18 to 65 years) diagnosed with moderate to severe migraine treated their symptoms for 24 weeks with subcutaneous sumatriptan after a 12-week period of treating symptoms with their customary (non-sumatriptan) therapy. Patients used diary cards to record information concerning the effects of migraine on workplace productivity and non-workplace activity time. The average workplace productivity time lost was 23.4 hours per patient during 12 weeks of customary therapy, compared with 7.2 and 5.8 hours per patient during the first and second 12-week periods of sumatriptan therapy, respectively. An average of 9.3 hours of non-workplace activity time was lost per patient during the customary therapy phase, compared with 3.2 and 2.8 hours during the first and second 12-week periods of sumatriptan therapy, respectively. Treatment of migraine with subcutaneous sumatriptan compared with customary therapy was associated with an average gain per patient of approximately 16 hours of workplace productivity time and 6 hours of non-workplace activity time, over a 3-month period.[12]

In a phase III, multinational, randomized clinical trial, 692 patients treated a migraine attack with eletriptan 40 mg or 80 mg or placebo.[25] Patients responded to a questionnaire seeking information concerning the amount of time lost from usual activities during the attack. Time loss assessments were made 24 hours after the last dose taken and recorded in a diary. Patients receiving either dose of the active compound were unable to perform their usual activities for a median period of 4 hours compared with the 9 hours experienced by those taking placebo. This difference was highly statistically significant ($p < 0.001$).[25] The time saving associated with eletriptan usage reflected the differences in efficacy findings in the clinical component of the study.

A standard method where the migraine patient is instructed to wait for the headache pain to become moderate or severe before treatment has been used in most clinical trials addressing the efficacy of active drugs in the acute treatment of migraine. The concern is that this approach delays the administration of treatment, which *per se* may have impact on several of the applied efficacy parameters, that is, relief of symptoms, headache recurrence, consistency of response, etc. This is in contrast to a scenario where the patient would be allowed to start treating the migraine attack at a mild degree of severity, which in many cases would more appropriately reflect their normal behaviour. In the latter case, a good response to active treatment would be defined as relief from mild headache pain to no pain or inhibition of a development in headache pain intensity from mild to moderate and/or severe. It is generally believed and has also been demonstrated in subpopulations of migraineurs that initiating treatment while pain is mild may be more cost-effective than delaying treatment until pain has become moderate to severe.[26,27] Return to normal functioning has been evaluated by means of retrospective analyses of three studies where headaches were treated during mild pain. A higher number of attacks treated early with sumatriptan 50 or 100 mg were associated with normal function 4 hours after dosing compared with placebo (70% and 93% versus 46%, respectively).[28]

Functional impairment is a dimension of HRQoL and improvements in HRQoL have been demonstrated with migraine therapy—through both education and medication—but similar improvements in disability have not yet been published.[8,24,29]

Assessing disability in clinical practice

The Migraine Disability Assessment (MIDAS) questionnaire is a brief, self-administered questionnaire designed to quantify headache-related disability.[21–23] Headache sufferers answer five questions, noting the number of days in the past 3 months of activity limitations due to migraine. The MIDAS score is the sum of missed work or school days, missed household chore days, and missed non-work activity days, and days at work or school plus days of household chores where productivity was reduced by half or more in the last 3 months. The MIDAS scores are then categorized by disability level: little or no disability (0–5); mild disability (6–10); moderate disability (11–20); and severe disability (20+).

MIDAS was recently used to assess disability in a group of 69 referred headache patients at the GMC. The purpose of this pilot study was to evaluate headache management at GMC by means of MIDAS. According to the diagnosis obtained at first visit at GMC (baseline), the group consisted of 30 migraineurs, 2 patients with tension-type headaches, and 37 with both migraine and tension-type headache. The MIDAS questionnaire was completed by the patients on three occasions, 3 months apart—before coming to GMC, at their first visit (baseline), and at follow-up, respectively. Divided into the different MIDAS grades of severity, 5.6%, 7.9%, 18.0%, and 68.5% had little or no, mild, moderate, and severe disability at pre-visit, respectively. Table 3.1 and Fig. 3.5 detail MIDAS scores at pre-visit, baseline, and follow-up, respectively. No major changes were observed in the MIDAS scoring between the three assessment periods, that is, the patients did not change disability

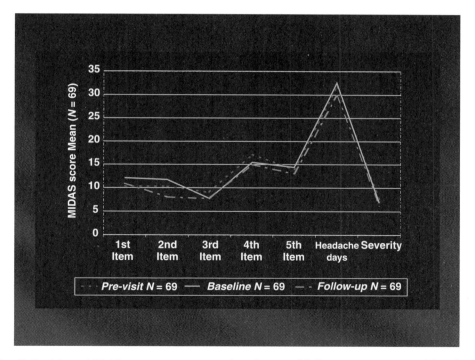

Fig. 3.5 Mean MIDAS scoring at pre-visit, baseline, and follow-up in a group of headache patients ($N=69$).

Table 3.1 MIDAS scores at pre-visit, baseline, and follow-up in a GMC study of referred headache patients ($N=69$)

	Response (range) to MIDAS question number					Total score (range)	No. of headache days (range)	Pain intensity (range)
	1	2	3	4	5			
Pre-visit	10.4 (0–92)	10.4 (0–60)	9.0 (0–85)	17.2 (0–90)	14.0 (0–92)	55.4 (3–274)	31.7 (2–92)	7.7 (4–10)
Baseline	12.1 (0–91)	11.8 (0–90)	7.8 (0–70)	15.5 (0–91)	14.4 (0–91)	59.9 (0–273)	32.5 (1–90)	6.9 (3–10)
Follow-up	11.0 (0–90)	8.1 (0–50)	7.7 (0–90)	15.0 (0–90)	13.1 (0–90)	52.8 (0–270)	29.8 (1–92)	6.4 (2–10)

categories. This occurred despite the fact that more than half (59%) of the studied headache patients claimed that the medication always or sometimes helped to relieve their symptoms.

If correct, the apparent discrepancy between patient's subjective judgement and the information obtained by MIDAS is curious and deserves further study to determine the factors influencing changing disability score. MIDAS assessments reflect disability during the last 3 months and it may be difficult for the headache patient to remember and provide correct information for anything that is beyond a fortnight away, especially in the absence of a diary. Sometimes two or three of the five MIDAS questions were not applicable and accordingly not filled in by the headache sufferers. Missing data for questions 1 to 5 ranged between 9% and 17% of the questionnaires filled in. This may result in a reduction of the sensitivity of MIDAS for picking up changes over time. MIDAS may also be more sensitive to detecting changes over time induced by preventive therapy (reduction in days) than improvements made by acute attack therapies (reduction in symptom intensity).

MIDAS is, in my opinion, a validated instrument that is simple to use and has been demonstrated to improve communication between patients and health-care professionals regarding migraine disability but it is perhaps not sensitive enough to be used as an outcome measure tool. In any case, further research studies using a prospective research design to examine the sensitivity of MIDAS and other disability tools in detecting longitudinal changes in headache impact are warranted. In addition, further research is needed to obtain data clarify what is a meaningful change on these disability tools from the perspective of the clinician.

Natural course of the migraine attack

Several years ago clinical features of 750 patients seen with an acute migraine attack at the Copenhagen Acute Headache Clinic were analysed.[30] In 47%, pain was pulsating, in 42% pressing, and in 11% pain was of other types. Unilateral pain was seen in 56% and bilateral in 44%. In patients with severe pain the pain was significantly more often pulsating. After detailed questioning of 50 patients with uncomplicated migraine, Blau introduced the term 'complete migraine' including five phases—the prodrome, the aura, the headache phase, the resolution phase, and the recovery phase (postdrome), respectively.[31] In another study, systematic prospective records of aura symptoms were obtained from 50 patients, who filled in report forms during the aura phase of two migraine attacks. The pattern of the various aura symptoms was remarkably constant during two attacks.[32] Visual aura was recorded by 94% of the patients, somatosensory aura symptoms by 40%, motor disturbances by 18%, and speech difficulties by 20%. Existing International Headache Society (IHS) criteria for the diagnosis of headache do not indicate which clinical features are most important in establishing or excluding primary headache diagnoses.[33] According to a comprehensive review by Smetana the features most predictive of migraine, when compared with tension-type headache, are nausea, photophobia, phonophobia, and exacerbation by physical activity.[34]

   Several recent surveys among migraineurs indicate that the absolute vast majority (>95%) use medications acutely, whether non-prescription or prescription, in order to relieve the symptoms of the migraine attack.[2,13] Accordingly, there is almost no information available on the natural course of the migraine attack since very few migraine sufferers will experience a debilitating migraine attack without any treatment. As a consequence of this, it can sometimes be difficult to interpret the observations made after the attack medication has been administered. Diagnosing migraine according to the IHS criteria may be inaccurate since the attack characteristics, due to treatment, do not fulfil the requirements for migraine without aura, etc.[33] Instead, too many patients will be diagnosed as having migrainous headache (IHS 1.7). In addition, how does one differentiate between treatment-induced effects and spontaneous relief of symptoms? Further, which of the adverse events are more likely to be related to the pathophysiological mechanisms of the migraine attack than caused by the treatment? For these reasons, a prospective study with detailed documentation of the dynamics of the whole migraine attack without any influence of pharmacotherapy seemed sensible and 'A Natural History of the Migraine Attack' study is presently ongoing at GMC, Sweden. The primary objective of this study is to evaluate the natural course of the migraine attack without pharmacological intervention (the migraineurs may rest or sleep) using a newly developed diary. A further objective is to compare the obtained information intraindividually with an attack treated with a triptan. Obviously, it would be very interesting to include treatment with placebo in order to find out how that compares to no treatment at all, but I do not think it would be feasible. In particular, in the recently revised version of the Declaraon of Helsinki, it is stated that the use of placebo in clinical trials is only acceptable when no proven treatment exists for the studied disease.[35]

   The Ethics Review Committee at the Sahlgren's University hospital has approved the present study protocol. Patients signed consent forms affirming a complete understanding of the study's purpose, the procedures involved, and the potential benefits and risks of participating in the study. Male and female subjects aged between 18 and 65 years were invited to participate if they could meet the IHS diagnostic criteria for migraine, with or without aura, and could reasonably expect to suffer between 2 and 4 acute attacks of migraine each month. The migraineurs use a newly developed diary that addresses the time and intensity of the following symptoms: aura, pain, photo- and phonophobia, nausea, and vomiting. The intensity of each of the symptoms is graded on a visual analogue scale from 0 (none) to 10 (unbearable). In addition to the descriptive information obtained in the diary, the area under curve (AUC) for duration and intensity of each symptom is calculated by means of an electronic digitizer (Fig. 3.6). This essential information is collected over 3 days from three separate attacks. The first is a 'practice attack' which the migraineurs treat as usual, the second is an attack without any medication at all, and the third attack is treated early during the headache phase with a triptan.

   Since the start of the study (1999) we have asked more than 300 individuals with migraine to participate but so far only 30 have felt that they could manage to bear the symptoms of a migraine attack without any treatment and have volunteered. Despite the fact that almost 3 years have passed since we started, only 0.5% of the

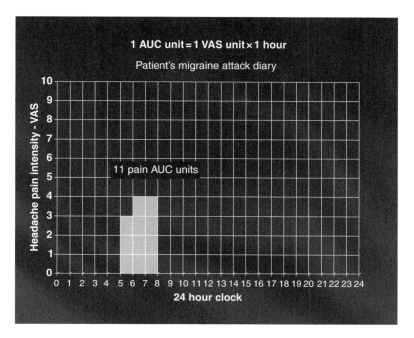

Fig. 3.6 Illustration of the pain intensity over time diary and an example of a given pain in area under curve (AUC) units. VAS, Visual analogue scale.

migraineurs ($N=12$, 10 women and 2 men) have been able to provide us with information on non-treated attacks. All these individuals claim that this was about the most horrible experience they had ever had, and that they would be most reluctant to go through it again. The recruitment failure to this study and the experiences that the migraineurs had during their non-treated attacks impressively indicate how extraordinarily debilitating the migraine attack generally is. In fact, it provides more extraordinary information on migraine disability than the data so far obtained by specific impact measures.

Although the information obtained on non-treated attacks is very limited (12 migraineurs and 36 attacks), the preliminary results are very interesting. In a very remarkable way the results from non-treated attacks demonstrate how debilitating the migraine attack is to the individual and how good triptans are in relieving the symptoms. Especially when looking at the parameter pain intensity over time (PIT-AUC) it was demonstrated that treatment with a triptan reduced the PIT-AUC by 77–96% (mean 87%) over the assessment period of 3 days (Fig. 3.7). The attack duration was 30–67 hours without treatment and 5–45 hours when using a triptan. On the other hand, if the observation period was limited to 2 hours only, no differences in the calculated PIT-AUC could be demonstrated (Fig. 3.8). It seems that the AUC of the associated symptoms closely go in parallel with the pain AUC. Similar results, with respect to percentage values, were obtained when total (pain, nausea, vomiting, phono- and photophobia) AUC units were calculated (Fig. 3.9).

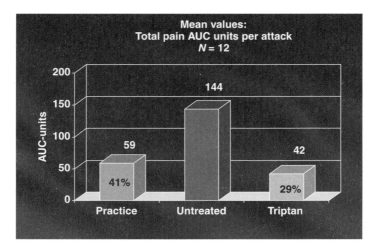

Fig. 3.7   Comparison of the mean value of pain AUC units over 3 days for a 'practice attack' with usual treatment, an attack without any medication at all, and a third attack that was treated early during the headache phase with a triptan (N=12).

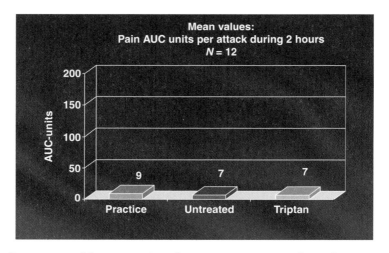

Fig. 3.8   Comparison of the mean value of pain AUC units over 2 hours for a 'practice attack' with usual treatment, an attack without any medication at all, and a third attack that was treated early during the headache phase with a triptan (N=12).

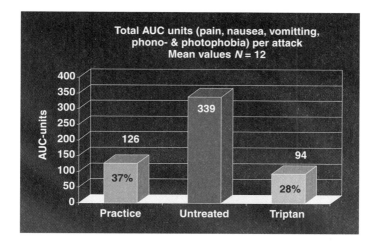

Fig. 3.9 Comparison of the mean value of total (pain, nausea, vomiting, and phono- and photophobia) AUC units over 3 days for a 'practice attack' with usual treatment, an attack without any medication at all, and a third attack that was treated early during the headache phase with a triptan (N=12).

Conclusion

It has been convincingly demonstrated that migraine attacks cause suffering and emotional stress and disruption of work, chores, and leisure activities, affect social and family life, impair health-related quality of life, and increase the use of health care resources. Despite this, it has been difficult to demonstrate substantial benefits of migraine therapy on headache disability. One reason may be that only a fraction of the whole migraine attack has been assessed in most studies. Another possibility is that the effect of triptans always has been compared using active controls. Further, currently available assessment tools may not be sensitive enough in demonstrating change over time. More prospective information on the natural history of migraine attacks would be extremely useful to all within the migraine research field, not least the migraineurs. This type of information would significantly help us to communicate the seriousness of migraine to those who still may be in doubt with respect to the consequences migraine may have. The information so far obtained does demonstrate the severe impact migraine has on the individual.

References

1. Lipton RB, Stewart WF. Migraine in the United States: a review of epidemiology and health care use. *Neurology* 1993; **43** (6, Suppl. 3): S6–10.
2. Lipton RB, Stewart WF, Diamond S, Diamond ML, Reed M. Prevalence and burden of migraine in the United States: data from the American Migraine Study II. *Headache* 2001; **41** (7): 646–57.

3. Mannix LK. Epidemiology and impact of primary headache disorders. *Med Clin North Am* 2001; **85** (4): 887–95.
4. Rasmussen BK. Epidemiology and socio-economic impact of headache. *Cephalalgia* 1999; **25** (2): 20–3.
5. Dahlöf C, Linde M. One-year prevalence of migraine in Sweden: a population-based study in adults. *Cephalalgia* 2001; **21** (6): 664–71.
6. Osterhaus JT, Townsend RJ, Gandek B, Ware JE, Jr. Measuring the functional status and well-being of patients with migraine headache. *Headache* 1994; **34** (6): 337–43.
7. Dahlöf CG, Solomon GD. The burden of migraine to the individual sufferer: a review. *Eur J Neurol* 1998; **5** (6): 525–33.
8. Solomon GD, Dahlöf C. Impact of headache on the individual sufferer. In *The headaches*, 2nd edn (ed. Olesen J, Tfelt-Hansen P, Welch KMA). Philadelphia: Lippincott Williams & Wilkins, 2000: 25–31.
9. Lipton RB, Stewart WF, Reed M, Diamond S. Migraine's impact today. Burden of illness, patterns of care. *Postgrad Med* 2001; **109** (1): 38–40.
10. Dahlöf CG, Dimenäs E. Migraine patients experience poorer subjective well-being/quality of life even between attacks. *Cephalalgia* 1995; **15** (1): 31–6.
11. Lipton RB, Hamelsky SW, Kolodner KB, Steiner TJ, Stewart WF. Migraine, quality of life, and depression: a population-based case-control study. *Neurology* 2000; **55** (5): 629–35.
12. Cortelli P, Dahlöf C, Bouchard J, Heywood J, Jansen JP, Pham S, *et al.* A multinational investigation of the impact of subcutaneous sumatriptan. III: Workplace productivity and non-workplace activity. *PharmacoEconomics* 1997; **1**: 35–42.
13. Dahlöf C, Linde M. Attitudes and impact of disease in Swedish migraineurs. *Cephalalgia* 2002; submitted.
14. http://www.who.int/icidh. 2002.
15. Ferrari MD, Loder E, McCarroll KA, Lines CR. Meta-analysis of rizatriptan efficacy in randomized controlled clinical trials. *Cephalalgia* 2001; **21** (2): 129–36.
16. Dahlöf CGH, Dodick D, Dowson AJ, Pascual J. How does almotriptan compare to other triptans? A review of data from placebo-controlled clinical trials. *Headache* 2002; **42** (2): 99–113.
17. Jacobson GP, Ramadan NM, Aggarwal SK, Newman CW. The Henry Ford Hospital Headache Disability Inventory (HDI). *Neurology* 1994; **44** (5): 837–42.
18. Jacobson GP, Ramadan NM, Norris L, Newman CW. Headache disability inventory (HDI): short-term test–retest reliability and spouse perceptions. *Headache* 1995; **35** (9): 534–9.
19. Stewart WF, Lipton RB, Simon D, Von Korff M, Liberman J. Reliability of an illness severity measure for headache in a population sample of migraine sufferers. *Cephalalgia* 1998; **18** (1): 44–51.
20. Stewart WF, Lipton RB, Simon D, Liberman J, Von Korff M. Validity of an illness severity measure for headache in a population sample of migraine sufferers. *Pain* 1999; **79** (2–3): 291–301.
21. Stewart WF, Lipton RB, Kolodner K, Liberman J, Sawyer J. Reliability of the migraine disability assessment score in a population-based sample of headache sufferers. *Cephalalgia* 1999; **19** (2): 107–14.
22. Stewart WF, Lipton RB, Kolodner KB, Sawyer J, Lee C, Liberman JN. Validity of the Migraine Disability Assessment (MIDAS) score in comparison to a diary-based measure in a population sample of migraine sufferers. *Pain* 2000; **88** (1): 41–52.
23. Stewart WF, Lipton RB, Dowson AJ, Sawyer J. Development and testing of the Migraine Disability Assessment (MIDAS) questionnaire to assess headache-related disability. *Neurology* 2001; **56** (6, Suppl. 1): S20–8.

24. Lofland JH, Johnson NE, Batenhorst AS, Nash DB. Changes in resource use and outcomes for patients with migraine treated with sumatriptan: a managed care perspective. *Arch Intern Med* 1999; **159** (8): 857–63.

25. Wells NE, Steiner TJ. Effectiveness of eletriptan in reducing time loss caused by migraine attacks. *PharmacoEconomics* 2000; **18** (6): 557–66.

26. Dahlöf C. Sumatriptan: pharmacological basis and clinical results. *Curr Med Res Opin* 2001; **17**: in press.

27. Cady RK, Sheftell F, Lipton RB, Kwong WJ, O'Quinn S. Economic implications of early treatment of migraine with sumatriptan tablets. *Clin Ther* 2001; **23** (2): 284–91.

28. Cady RK, Sheftell F, Lipton RB, O'Quinn S, Pharmd, Jones M, *et al*. Effect of early intervention with sumatriptan on migraine pain: retrospective analyses of data from three clinical trials. *Clin Ther* 2000; **22** (9): 1035–48.

29. Dahlöf C, Bouchard J, Cortelli P, Heywood J, Jansen JP, Pham S, *et al*. A multinational investigation of the impact of subcutaneous sumatriptan. II: Health-related quality of life. *PharmacoEconomics* 1997; **1**: 24–34.

30. Olesen J. Some clinical features of the acute migraine attack. An analysis of 750 patients. *Headache* 1978; **18** (5): 268–71.

31. Blau JN. Migraine prodromes separated from the aura: complete migraine. *Br Med J* 1980; **281** (6241): 658–60.

32. Jensen K, Tfelt-Hansen P, Lauritzen M, Olesen J. Classic migraine. A prospective recording of symptoms. *Acta Neurol Scand* 1986; **73** (4): 359–62.

33. Headache Classification Committee of the International Headache Society. Classification and diagnostic criteria for headache disorders, cranial neuralgias, and facial pain. *Cephalalgia* 1988; **8** (Suppl. 7): 1–96.

34. Smetana GW. The diagnostic value of historical features in primary headache syndromes: a comprehensive review. *Arch Intern Med* 2000; **160** (18): 2729–37.

35. World Medical Association Declaration of Helsinki. Adopted by the 52nd WMA General Assembly E, Scotland, October 2000. (Accessed 8 November, 2001, at http://www.wma.net/e/policy/17-c_e.html).

4
Comparing disability and psychological factors in migraine and transformed migraine

J.E. Magnusson and W.J. Becker

Introduction

Diagnosis of a headache disorder is typically based upon criteria of symptoms and characteristics. At present, the most widely used diagnostic criteria are those of the International Headache Society (IHS);[1] however, not all headaches fit well into these established criteria. For example, it has been observed that some patients who initially meet all migraine diagnostic criteria experience increasing headache frequency over time and eventually develop chronic daily headache.[2,3] This evolution from intermittent to chronic daily headaches is the basis of the 'transformed migraine' classification of Silberstein et al.[4] who state that transformed migraine (TM) is characterized by episodic migraine that then 'transforms' into a more frequent, and often less intense, headache. Although analgesic overuse may be associated with this migraine transformation,[2,3,5] some patients with this syndrome do not improve despite terminating their analgesic overuse.[6] Also, some patients appear to develop TM in the absence of analgesic overuse.[3] It is therefore unclear what mechanism(s) produce the transformation from intermittent to persistent headache.

The classification of TM is not accepted by all,[7] and there are those who feel that many of these patients are best classified as patients with migraine attacks and chronic tension-type headache attacks. The purpose of the present study was therefore to compare two groups of patients, one group with IHS migraine and one group with TM,[4] on measures of depression, pain-related anxiety, and headache-related disability in order to determine the similarities and/or differences of these two headache diagnoses.

Methods

Procedures

All new patients referred to the University of Calgary Headache Research Clinic completed headache diaries and the following assessment measures prior to their initial appointment: Beck Depression Inventory (BDI);[8] Pain Anxiety Symptom Scale (PASS);[9] Headache Disability Inventory (HDI);[10] and headache diaries. Headache diaries documented headache intensity using a 0–10 scale (10 being the 'worst pain imaginable') for three segments of the day (morning, afternoon, and evening–night). Any calendar day with a headache intensity score of greater than zero in one of the daily segments was considered a day with headache. Headache frequency was measured as days with headache per month. Headache intensity for a day with headache was determined by averaging the pain intensity values in the three segments of each calendar day with headache (including zeros).

Patients

Entry criteria for this study included a diagnosis of migraine or TM. Patients with migraine were diagnosed according to IHS diagnostic criteria and patients with migraine who had headache on more than 15 days a month were diagnosed with TM according to the criteria of Silberstein et al.[4] Patients who had been given a diagnosis of other headache types (that is, tension-type headache) in addition to migraine were excluded. Also excluded were patients who, for any reason, had not completed all the questionnaires or kept headache diaries.

Data analysis and results

Using the t-test for independent groups, migraine and TM patients were compared on measures of mean number of headache days per month, mean headache intensity on headache days, depression, anxiety, and disability.

Of the 121 patients who completed all questionnaires, 87 met study entry criteria—50 with migraine and 37 with TM. The majority of these patients were women. A significant difference was found between intermittent migraine and TM patients on the number of days with headache ($p < 0.001$) but not mean headache intensity ($p > 0.01$). Patients with TM had, on average, more than three times as many days with headache per month than patients with intermittent migraine (26.92 for TM and 9.22 for migraine). The two groups only differed slightly in terms of headache intensity (3.1 for migraine and 3.9 for TM). No significant differences were found between patients with intermittent migraine and TM patients on measures of mean depression, pain-related anxiety, or headache-related disability (see Fig. 4.1).

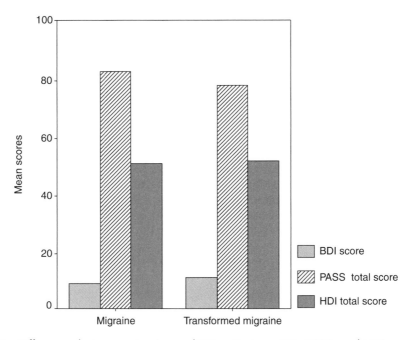

Fig. 4.1 Differences between migraine and TM patients on BDI, PASS, and HDI scores.

Conclusions

The classification of patients with migraine who develop chronic daily headache is controversial, with some classifying such patients as 'transformed migraine'. To investigate similarities and/or differences between these diagnoses, we compared patients with intermittent migraine attacks and patients with transformed migraine in terms of mean headache intensity on days with headache, depression, pain-related anxiety, and headache-related disability. Patients classified clinically as also having tension-type headache were excluded. Despite differences in the number of headache days per month and headache intensity, patients with intermittent migraine and patients with TM show many similarities in terms of depression, pain-related anxiety, and headache-related disability. Our results support the concept that these two headache groups are closely related and may be part of the same diagnostic category.

Acknowledgements

This work was supported by Pfizer Canada Inc. We also gratefully acknowledge the contributions of Constance Riess and Anila Umar who tabulated and entered much of the data.

References

1. Headache Classification Committee of the International Headache Society. Classification and diagnostic criteria for headache disorders, cranial neuralgias, and facial pain. *Cephalalgia* 1988; **8** (Suppl. 7): 1–96.
2. Mathew NT. Drug-induced headache. *Neurol Clin* 1990; **8** (4): 903–13.
3. Mathew NT. Transformed migraine. *Cephalalgia* 1993; **13** (Suppl. 12): 78–83.
4. Silberstein SD, Lipton RB, Sliwinski M. Classification of daily and near-daily headaches: Field trial of revised IHS criteria. *Neurology* 1996; **47**: 871–5.
5. Silberstein SD, Lipton RB, Solomon S, Mathew NT. Classification of daily and near-daily headaches: proposed revisions to the IHS criteria. *Headache* 1994; **34**: 1–7.
6. Silberstein SD, Silberstein JR. Chronic daily headache: long-term prognosis following inpatient treatment with repetitive IV DHE. *Headache* 1992; **32**: 439–45.
7. Olesen J, Rasmussen BK. The International Headache Society classification of chronic daily and near-daily headaches: a critique of the criticism. *Cephalalgia* 1996; **16** (6): 407–11.
8. Beck AT. *The Beck Depression Inventory*, The Psychology Corporation. San Antonio, Texas: Harcourt Brace, 1993.
9. McCracken LM, Gross RT. The Pain Anxiety Symptoms Scale (PASS) and the assessment of emotional responses to pain. In *Innovations in clinical practice*, Vol. 14 (ed. Vandecreek L, Knapp S, Jackson TL). Sarasota: Professional Resource Press, 1995.
10. Jacobson, GP, Ramadan NM, Aggarwal SK, Newman CW. The Henry Ford Hospital Headache Disability Inventory (HDI). *Neurology* 1994; **44**: 837–42.

5 Cognitive efficiency following migraine therapy

Kathleen Farmer, Roger K. Cady, Dennis Reeves,
and Joseph Bleiberg

Clinical trials have shown that triptan tablets are efficacious agents in the acute treatment of migraine. Other studies have demonstrated that during an acute episode of migraine there are significant restrictions on a migraineur's cognitive efficiency, which recovers after administration of a 5-HT_1 agonist.[1–3] But the question remains, would cognitive recovery occur as well when using a non-specific analgesic for migraine compared to a migraine-specific medication? The primary objective of this study was to evaluate and compare the effects of a butalbital agent (combination of 325 mg aspirin, 40 mg caffeine, 50 mg butalbital; 2 tablets) and rizatriptan (10 mg) on the recovery of cognitive efficiency among migraineurs.

Methods

Subjects

Men and women aged 18 to 65 years with a diagnosis of migraine with or without aura using the International Headache Society (IHS) criteria (1.1 and 1.2)[4] were eligible for study participation. Subjects were required to have at least a 1-year history of migraine with onset prior to age 50 years. Patients who had experienced one to six moderate-to-severe migraine attacks that affected usual daily activities in the 2 months prior to study enrolment participated in the study.

There were 33 individuals, 29 women and 4 men, who were enrolled. Of these, 27 treated 51 headaches. Their ages ranged from 22 to 66 years with a mean age of 39 years. No subjects had a history of prior head trauma or brain injury.

Measures

The Headache Care Center-Automated Neuropsychological Assessment Metrics (HCC-ANAM), a computerized neuropsychological assessment battery, measured cognitive function under three conditions: migraine-free; untreated migraine; and following rizatriptan (10 mg) or butalbital–aspirin–caffeine (2 tablets). This battery consisted of four subtests, which included simple reaction time (SRT), continuous performance test (CPT), matching to sample (MTS), and mathematical processing (MATH).[5] The HCC-ANAM was administered by an IBM-compatible computer using a keyboard or mouse as the response device.

Simple reaction time

Simple reaction time is a classical visuomotor response time test that measures the speed and the ability to detect a stimulus. As a simple stimulus (*) appears on the computer screen, the subject presses a mouse button as quickly as possible each time the stimulus appears.

Continuous performance test

The CPT is a continuous letter comparison task. A randomized sequence of upper-case letters, A through Z, is presented one at a time on the centre of the computer screen. The subject presses one button if the letter on the screen matches the letter that immediately preceded it; a different button if the letter on the screen is different than the immediately preceding letter. The CPT was designed to assess components of memory, attention, efficiency, and consistency.

Matching to sample

MTS is a measure of visuospatial skills and short-term memory. A design is presented in the centre of the screen for 3 seconds, followed by a screen that contains two designs. The subject matches one of the two designs with the sample by pressing the appropriate button.

Mathematical processing

Arithmetic problems are presented in the middle of the screen. Working from left to right, the subject solves the addition and subtraction and decides if the answer is greater or less than the number 5.

Procedures

After receiving institutional board approval to conduct the study at the Headache Care Center in Springfield, Missouri, USA, the subjects completed written informed consent prior to study enrolment. Participants were screened in the clinic while migraine-free and provided medical and migraine histories as well as concurrent medication use. Each received a physical examination including vital signs. Subjects completed the HCC-ANAM three times and were instructed to return to the clinic for treatment of their next moderate-to-severe headache.

Subjects returned to the clinic during an acute migraine (visit 2) and updated their medical history and concurrent medication use. Vital signs were performed. The HCC-ANAM was administered twice prior to taking medication.

In this cross-over design, subjects were randomized into either a rizatriptan first group or a butalbital agent first group. After taking the medication, the subjects were administered the HCC-ANAM at 30, 60, and 120 minutes posttreatment. Non-responders were given rescue medication at 120 minutes postadministration of study drug.

Subjects returned to the clinic during another acute migraine (visit 3) and updated their medical history and concurrent medication use. Vital signs were performed. The HCC-ANAM was administered twice prior to taking the medication (either rizatriptan, 10 mg, or butalbital–aspirin–caffeine, 2 tablets) that they had not taken at visit 2. After taking the medication, the subject was administered the HCC-ANAM at 30, 60, and 120 minutes posttreatment. Non-responders were given rescue medication at 120 minutes postadministration of study drug.

Results

Of the 51 headaches treated in the clinic, 61% (31) were rated as moderate head pain, 10% (5) were rated as moderately severe (2.5/3.0), and 29% (15) were reported as severe head pain. On average, subjects self-rated their cognitive effectiveness during untreated migraine (pre-dose) as being only 58% of their normal level of cognitive function.

Objectively, findings of HCC-ANAM showed a significant drop in mental efficiency comparing scores without migraine to those during an untreated migraine. The 1X3 analyses of variance for each individual measure of cognitive function were significantly different for three of the 4 subtests at $p < 0.01$. Post-hoc paired t-tests showed that overall mental efficiency was significantly impaired during untreated migraine compared to baseline (migraine-free) for the cognitive function tests of SRT, CPT, and MATH; the drop was not significant for MTS.

Mental efficiency showed recovery following successful treatment of an acute attack of migraine with either rizatriptan or butalbital–aspirin–caffeine. The 1X3 analyses of variance of changes in performance for each subtest across three trials at 30, 60, and 120 minutes indicated that rizatriptan produced statistically significant recovery in performance of tests to measure SRT ($p < 0.01$), CPT ($p < 0.001$), MTS ($p < 0.01$), and MATH ($p \sim 0.001$). The mental efficiency in those subjects treating with butalbital–aspirin–caffeine, showed numerical improvement but not statistically significant improvement for SRT and MATH. Butalbital–aspirin–caffeine produced statisically significant cognitive recovery in MTS ($p < 0.05$) but not as striking as in the rizatriptan group ($p < 0.01$). On CPT, rizatriptan and butalbital–aspirin–caffeine both produced superior recovery, making both equally effective.

Because there were no effects within 30 minutes after administration of the study medication, the 30-minute measurement was collapsed to coincide with the untreated migraine measurement. In this way, the 60-minute measurement

Cognitive Efficiency Following Migraine Therapy

Kathleen Farmer, Psy.D., Roger K. Cady, M.D.
Headache Care Center
Springfield, MO

Dennis Reeves, Ph.D.
U.S. Navy
Camp Pendleton, CA

Joseph Bleiberg, Ph.D.
National Rehabilitation Hospital
Washington, D.C.

Objective

1. To examine measures of cognitive function during acute migraine, before and after treatment with the rizatriptan tablet (10 mg) and a butalbital agent (butalbital-aspirin-caffeine) (2 tablets).
2. To compare the effects of the rizatriptan tablet, a migraine-specific medication, with a butalbital agent (non-specific analgesic) on migraineurs' cognitive efficiency.

Methods

Subjects: 25 migraineurs were enrolled at the Headache Care Center, Springfield, Missouri.

Measures: The Headache Care Center-Automated Neuropsychological Assessment Metrics (HCC-ANAM), a computerized neuropsychological assessment battery, measured cognitive function under three conditions: migraine-free, untreated migraine, and following rizatriptan or butalbital-aspirin-caffeine.

Procedure: In this cross-over design, subjects returned to the clinic to treat two migraines. Subjects were randomized into either a rizatriptan first group or a butalbital agent first group.

Results

1. Cognitive efficiency (Simple Reaction Time, Continuous Performance Test, Matching to Sample, and Mathematical Processing) was adversely affected during migraine compared with migraine-free performance (P<.01).
2. Cognitive function recovered following both rizatriptan (10 mg) and butalbital-aspirin-caffeine (2 tablets).
3. Rizatriptan produced superior recovery of cognitive efficiency on 3 of 4 HCC-ANAM tasks (Simple Reaction Time, Matching to Sample, Mathematical Processing).
4. Rizatriptan is equivalent to butalbital-aspirin-caffeine on recovering cognitive function in the remaining task (Continuous Performance Test).

This study was supported by a Merck Medical School Grant.

Significance of Recovery from Migraine

Changes in Performance/Throughput Across 3 Trials
1-way within ANOVAs

	Rizatriptan Tx 30-60-120 mins	Butalbital-Aspirin-Caffeine Tx 30-60-120 mins
Simple Reaction Time (SRT)	F=6.10,p<.01	F=2.45
Continuous Performance Test (CPT)	F=9.10,p<.001	F=10.15,p<.001
Matching to Sample (MSP)	F=5.40,p<.01	F=3.61,p<.05
Math (MTH)	F=7.22,p<.001	F=0.57

Conclusion:

1. Rizatriptan results in superior recovery for migraine on 3 of 4 HCC-ANAM tasks.
2. Rizatriptan is equivalent to butalbital-aspirin-caffeine on CPT.
3. Migraine-specific medication is superior for recovery of cognitive efficiency compared to a non-specific analgesic.

Cognitive Efficiency Before Migraine and During Migraine

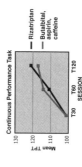

Reaction Time (ms)

400 · 300 · 277 · 200

paired t-tests
366=MSRT M=3.76*
386=FSRT F=2.88*

Throughput # Correct Rs/ms

120 · 119 · 60 · 35 · 35 · 30 · 28 · 25

103=MCPT M=2.86* F=3.38*
99=FCPT
35=MMSP M=1.09 F=1.90
35=FMSP
28=MMATH M=3.52* F=2.18*
25=FMATH

Migraine Free   Migraine

* p<.01
x p<.05

Cognitive Recovery After Migraine Therapy At 60 and 120 Minutes

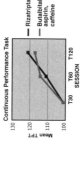

Math

Simple Reaction Time

Matching To Sample

Continuous Performance Task

— Rizatriptan
— Butalbital, aspirin, caffeine

T30 T60 T120
SESSION

Fig. 5.1 Summary of the study assessing cognitive efficiency following migraine therapy.

became the starting point for analyses, which demonstrated clearly the recovery of cognition following administration of either rizatriptan or butalbital–aspirin–caffeine at 60 and 120 minutes postdose (see graphs in Fig. 5.1).

Discussion

The HCC-ANAM is a unique measure of mental efficiency because of its ability to objectively measure and test several levels of cognitive function. This battery of validated neuropsychological tests is a repeated measures test with the performance of each subject compared against his or her own best performance. Consequently, deviations from the baseline are specific to each individual. This adds to the sensitivity of this measure.

Historically, subjective changes have been reported as a consequence of acute migraine. The question has been, are these non-specific changes related to pain or are they a consequence of the migraine process? Earlier studies using the HCC-ANAM to measure the performance of migraineurs suggested that marked changes in the four subtests of the HCC-ANAM occur even before the onset of headache. Thus, it would appear that the biology of migraine is responsible for these changes not just the presence of pain.

This study looks at whether triptans are unique in their ability to restore mental efficiency. In this study butalbital–aspirin–caffeine was selected as an analgesic to compare to rizatriptan because of its pharmacological composition. Caffeine is known pharmacologically to aid in mental efficiency and butalbital may assist cognitive function through inhibition of anxiety.

Conclusions

The significance of a drop in efficiency over four levels of cognition has been confirmed by this study. Two agents of recovery were compared in this study. Even though both an analgesic and a migraine-specific medication begin the process of cognitive recovery, the speed is slower with an oral medication, compared to injection and nasal spray. In addition, migraine-specific medication produces a significant change toward recovery of cognitive efficiency compared to a non-specific analgesic in three of the four levels of thinking, specifically, simple reaction time, matching to sample, and math. These agents were equivalent on the continuous performance test, which measures focus, attention, and concentration.

References

1. Farmer K, Cady R, Bleiberg J, Reeves D. Sumatriptan nasal spray and cognitive function during migraine: results of an open-label study. *Headache* 2001; **41**: 377–84.
2. Farmer K, Cady R, Bleiberg J, Reeves D. A pilot study to measure cognitive efficiency during migraine. *Headache* 2000; **40**: 657–61.

3. Meyer JS, Thornby J, Crawford K, Rauch GM. Reversible cognitive decline accompanies migraine and cluster headache. *Headache* 2000; **40**: 638–46.
4. Headache Classification Committee of the International Headache Society (1988). Classification and diagnostic criteria for headache disorders, cranial neuralgias and facial pain. *Cephalalgia* 1988; **8** (Suppl. 7): 1–96.
5. Reeves D, Kane R, Winter K, Raynsford K, Pancella T. *Automated Neuropsychological Assessment Metrics (ANAM): test administrators guide version 1.0*. San Diego: National Cognition Recovery Foundation, 1994.

6 Comparative evolution of MIDAS score after monotherapy with triptans

S. Harmoussi-Peioglou, A. Dimitriadis, and G. Vlachogianni

Introduction

In migraine therapy, clinicians and doctors have a large spectrum of treatment choices based mainly on empirical evidence. Treatment guidelines have been imposed to systematize strategies, in order to avoid empirical methods. The main target of optimal migraine care is to introduce treatment strategies, reducing the disability and relieving the pain as early as possible. Three different acute treatment strategies have been suggested for migraine: step care across attacks; step care within attacks; and stratified care.[1]

The results from previous studies support the use of stratified care as the more effective treatment strategy compared with traditional step care approaches. In stratified care the initial treatment is based on the patient's needs, measuring the headache-related disability. To improve the recognition of headache-related disability the MIDAS (Migraine Disability Assessment) questionnaire was developed. MIDAS is based, in part, on the Headache Impact Questionnaire (HImQ). Like the HImQ the MIDAS questionnaire gives information on disability in terms of missed days at paid work, school, household work; family or social activity, and leisure.[2–4]

The MIDAS questionnaire is simple and flexible enough to measure the broad variation in headache experience among and within migraine patients. Among individuals migraine may be moderate to severe and result in a range of intensity of pain and disability. Also headache varies within individuals from attack to attack in pain intensity, duration, disability, and associated symptoms. The MIDAS questionnaire includes five questions regarding days of activity limitation the previous 3-month period, including limitations in paid work, household work, and non-work energy (social life, family life, and leisure).[2,3,5]

The MIDAS questionnaire is a tool to assess the severity of migraine and categorizes patients in four grades for stratifying assessment and treatment needs (Table 6.1).

Table 6.1 The grading system of the MIDAS questionnaire

Grade	Midas score	Disability	Medical needs	Treatment
I	0–5	No–little	Low	Simple analgesic
II	6–10	Mild	Moderate	Combination treatments; prophylaxis
III	11–20	Moderate	High	Triptans; analgesics; prophylaxis
IV	21+	Severe	High	Triptans; analgesics; prophylaxis

Results

The charts of 85 migraineurs who were on monotherapy with triptans were reviewed. Patients were taking Sumatriptan (Su), Naratriptan (N), Zolmitriptan (Z), or Rizatriptan (R). The main demographic data are summarized in Table 6.2. Triptans were given to all of them in the context of a stratified care regime and all had evaluation of MIDAS score before starting therapy. For 54 patients (63.5%) only one triptan was used. Two triptans were needed for 22 patients (26%) while 8 patients took 3 and 1 patient 4 triptans (10.5%).

Changes of grading before and after 3 months on treatment were evaluated for:

(1) the totality of patients;
(2) patients starting with Sumatriptan (Su) compared to those starting with all others triptans (N+Z+R);

Table 6.2 Principal demographic data for the groups of patients studied

	Number	Male/female	Median age in years (range)	Mean headache duration in months (range)
All patients	85	11/74	42 (16–63)	20.8 (3–52)
With aura (Au +)	25	2/23	40 (20–63)	20.9 (5–46)
Without aura (Au –)	60	9/51	41 (16–61)	20.7 (3–52)
Analgesic abusers (Ab +)	17	3/14	45 (19–58)	24.7 (3–52)
Non abusers (Ab –)	68	8/60	40 (16–63)	19.8 (3–46)
Started with Sumatriptan (Su)	59	10/49	41 (16–63)	20.5 (3–46)
Started with other triptans (N+Z+R)	26	1/25	40 (19–61)	21.5 (5–52)
Remained on Sumatriptan	36	6/30	47 (16–63)	19.1 (3–46)
Changed to other triptan	23	4/19	40 (27–55)	22.6 (5–41)
With only 1 triptan	54	7/47	45 (16–63)	19.5 (3–52)
With more triptans	31	4/27	41 (22–55)	23.1 (5–41)

(3) patients starting and remaining on sumatriptan (Su → Su) compared to those who changed to other triptans (Su → N+Z+R. Side-effects and non-response were the main causes for changes of treatment;
(4) patients with aura (Au+) to those without (Au−);
(5) patients abusing analgesic drugs (Ab+) to the non-abusers (Ab−);
(6) patients who remained on one triptan (Tr1) compared to those who used more than one (Tr>1).

For statistical evaluation the comparison of changes was done using the χ^2 test (Yates correction). Given the small numbers of patients in each group, we evaluated the changes adding grades I and II and grades III and IV.

The majority of patients (91.3%) treated with triptans initially had MIDAS scores of grade III and IV. An impressive change of grading towards grades I and II (from 8.9% to 75.2%) was observed after 3 months treatment (Fig. 6.1)

Almost the same initial profile was seen for all groups studied and in each group the change of grading after treatment was significant ($p < 0.001$). Patients who were on N+Z+R showed a worse response than those who received Su (grade I and II 68.1% versus 84.2%), even though this was not significant.

Patients who did not respond to Su and changed to N+Z+R had a worse initial grading than those who remained on Su (grades III and IV 100% versus 86.1%; $p < 0.01$). Their grading after treatment was also less favourable with 47.9% of them graded III and IV compared to 16.7% of those remained on Su ($p < 0.01$).

Patients with aura showed no difference in grading from those without aura. Changes of MIDAS score after treatment were almost the same for both groups (Table 6.3). Migraineurs abusing analgesics had a worse initial MIDAS score with 88.2% belonging to grade IV, compared to 61.8% of the others (Table 6.3). After

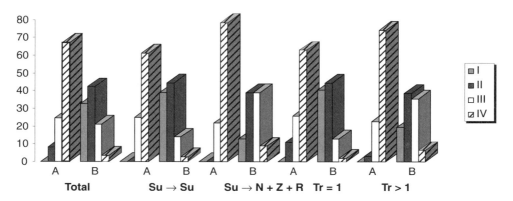

Fig. 6.1 Percentage distribution of patients according to MIDAS score (I, II, III, IV) before (A) and after 3 months on treatment (B). Total, all patients; Su → Su, patients who remained on Sumatriptan; Su → N+Z+R, patients who changed to another triptan; Tr = 1, patient treated with only one triptan; Tr > 1, patient treated with more than one triptan.

Table 6.3 Percentage distribution and statistical valuation of the MIDAS scoring for all studied groups before (A) and after 3 months on treatment (B)

Patient group*	Number		Percentage of patients in MIDAS group[†]							
	A	B	I(A)	I (B)	II (A)	II (B)	III (A)	III (B)	IV(A)	IV(B)
All patients	85	85	—	32.9	8.2	42.3	24.7	21.2	67.1	3.6
Su	59	38	—	39.5	8.5	44.7	23.7	13.1	67.8	2.7
NZR	26	47	—	27.7	7.7	40.4	26.9	27.7	65.4	4.2
Su→Su[‡]	36	36	—	38.9	13.9	44.4	25.0	13.9	61.1	2.8
Su→NZR[‡]	23	23	—	13	—	39.1	21.7	39.1	78.3	8.8
Tr=1[§]	54	54	—	40.7	11.1	44.4	25.9	13	63	1.9
Tr>1[§]	31	31	—	19.3	3.2	38.7	22.6	35.5	74.2	6.5
Au+	25	25	—	44	12	40	40	12	48	4
Au−	60	60	—	28.3	6.7	43.3	18.3	25	75	3.4
Ab+[¶]	17	17	—	17.6	11.8	47.1	—	23.5	88.2	11.8
Ab−[¶]	68	68	—	36.8	7.3	41.2	30.9	20.6	61.8	1.4

*Su, treatment started with Sumatriptan; NZR, treatment started with other triptan; Su Su, patient remained on sumatriptan; Su NZR, patient changed to other triptan; Tr = 1, patient treated with only one triptan; Tr > 1, patient treated with more than one triptan; Au+, migraine with aura; Au−, migraine without aura; Ab+, analgesic abuser; Ab−, analgesic non-abuser.
[†]$p < 0.001$ for differences between A and B for all groups.
[‡]$p < 0.01$ for differences between Su → Su and Su → NZR at both A and B.
[§]$p < 0.001$ for differences between Tr = 1 and Tr > 1 at B.
[¶]$p < 0.05$ for differences between Ab+ and Ab− at A.

3 months the abusers showed a less favourable improvement of MIDAS scoring than the others with 64.7% graded I and II against 78% (p, not significant).

Patients who used only one triptan had almost the same profile before treatment as those using multiple triptans. They had a significantly better grading after treatment ($p < 0.001$) than those who used multiple triptans (grade I and II, 85.1% versus 58%).

Discussion

Stratified care with MIDAS score is considered as the best system for evaluating and treating patients.[1] Most of our patients stratified to the triptan regimen had the highest MIDAS score. Treatment with triptans was proved quite effective as is seen by the impressive scoring change of grading after treatment. It is extremely interesting that 63.5% of patients who remained on one triptan, irrespective of which one, had a good response. Patients for whom a change of triptan was needed had a worse outcome, even though their initial MIDAS score profile was almost the same as that of those who remained on one triptan. Regardless of the manner in which we tried to group our patients (according to the drug used, the existence or not of aura, drug abuse, etc.), their initial MIDAS grading was the same and its change was significant after treatment.

The group of analgesic abusers was the only one who at the initial scoring showed a difference, though not significant, from the compared group of non-abusers. Their response was also the least favourable of all the groups studied. Thus, it can be suggested that patients abusing analgesic drugs and with a higher MIDAS score are more resistant to treatment with triptans. In our experience a significant percentage of the patients with high MIDAS score, especially those with known drug abuse, dropped out of follow-up.

In conclusion, patients who needed triptans almost always are those with the highest MIDAS score. The evolution of MIDAS score after a short period of treatment can help to distinguish patients who will respond to triptans from non-responders.

References

1. Lipton RB, Stewart WF, Stone AM, *et al*. Stratified care vs step care strategies for migraine. The disability in strategies of care (DISC) study: a randomized trial. *J Am Med Assoc* 2000; **284**: 2599–605.
2. Stewart WF, Lipton RB, Kolodner KB, *et al*. (2000). Validity of the Migraine Disability Assessment (MIDAS) score in comparison to a diary-based measure in a population sample of migraine sufferers. *Pain* 2000; **88**: 41–52.
3. Stewart WF, Lipton RB, Whyte J, *et al*. (1999). An international study to assess reliability of the Migraine Disability Assessment (MIDAS) score. *Neurology* 1999; **53**: 989–94.
4. Stewart WF, Lipton RB, Kolodner K, *et al*. (1999). Reliability of the migraine disability assessment score in a population-based sample of headache sufferers. *Cephalalgia* 1999; **19**: 107–14.
5. Lipton RB, Stewart WF, Sawyer J. (2000). Stratified care is a more effective migraine treatment strategy than stepped care: results of a randomized clinical trial. *Neurology* 2000; **54**: A14.

7 Disability-adjusted life years (DALYs) and MIDAS in Japan

F. Sakai, H. Igarashi, and M. Iigaya

....

Disability-adjusted life years (DALYs)

A nationwide survey of migraine in Japan was undertaken to investigate the prevalence and the burden of migraine in Japan.[1]

Method

In order to obtain a representative sample of the Japanese population by telephone interview, we used a combination of a random sampling method and a quota method. The quota method was used by Henry *et al.*[2] in a nationwide survey of migraine in France. It is an epidemiological sampling method by which a group of people representative of the national population is selected. In our study a total of 38 779 telephone calls were made in order to obtain a representative sample of 4029 subjects strictly satisfying an even distribution with regard to gender, age, and district of residence.

Among the 4029 representative subjects interviewed by telephone, 2738 (68%) had experienced headache in their life and 2241 (55.6%) had experienced recurrent headaches in the past year.

The questionnaire on headache comprised 40 questions for the purpose of establishing the diagnosis of headache according to the International Headache Society (IHS) criteria[3] and for investigating migraine-related problems such as family history, triggering factors, the awareness of being a 'headache sufferer' or having migraine, doctor attendance, medication, and influences on daily and social activity and work life.

Results

The overall prevalence of migraine in Japan in the past year was 8.4% of the population. Figure 7.1 shows the prevalence of chronic headaches found by our questionnaire. The overall prevalence of migraine was 3.6% in men and 13.0% in

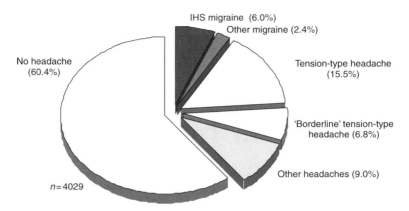

Fig. 7.1 Prevalence of primary headache in Japan. The overall prevalence of migraine was 8.4%. The prevalence of migraine strictly meeting IHS criteria was 6.0%. The prevalence of additional migraine that did not meet the IHS criteria in terms of number of attacks and duration of pain was 2.4%. The 'additional' migraine satisfied all the other migraine characteristics and was considered to be migraine.

women. The ratio of women to men was 3.6. The highest prevalence of migraine was in women in their 30s, in whom one in five suffered migraine.

Our question on the severity of migraine graded according to the degree of influence on functional daily activity revealed that 4% of migraine sufferers always required bed rest, 30% frequently required bed rest with severely impaired daily activity, 40% suffered from moderate impairment of daily activity, 21% suffered from only minor impairment of daily activity, and 5% had no impairment (Fig. 7.2 and Table 7.1). As many as 74.2% complained that migraine headache impaired their daily activity significantly.

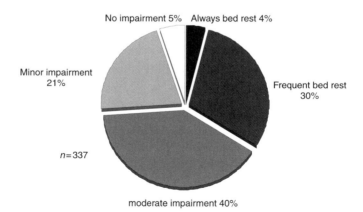

Fig 7.2 Influence of migraine on functional daily activity: results of the nationwide Japanese survey reported in this chapter.

Table 7.1 Severity of migraine graded in terms of daily activity and disability in social activity

	Percentage of questionnaire respondents reporting		
	Severe	Moderate	Mild or none
Severity of migraine*	34.0	40.0	26.0
Disability in social activity†	4.5	27.5	68.0

*Severity of migraine: severe, requiring bed rest always or frequently; moderate, moderate impairment of daily activity; mild or none, mild or no impairment of daily activity.
†Disability in social activity: severe, cancelling work or appointments always or frequently; moderate, moderate impairment of social activity; slight or none, slight or no impairment of social activity.

Disability-adjusted life years (DALYs) in migraineurs were calculated to be reduced by 2.3 years during the age range 20–40 years.

Conclusions

In our study, the severity of migraine, in terms of DALYs of headache, was significantly high. However, a large number of migraine sufferers reported that they still work during headache attacks producing considerable disability.

MIDAS

Previous studies have demonstrated that the English language MIDAS (Migraine Disability Assessment) questionnaire is highly reliable and valid.[4] For MIDAS to be useful in countries where English is not the principal language, and to enable comparison of international data, translation of the questionnaire and subsequent testing for reliability and validity are necessary.

We organized a study to assess the test–retest reliability and validity of a Japanese translation of the MIDAS questionnaire amongst a sample of Japanese headache sufferers, and to prove its conceptual and linguistic equivalence to the original version.

Method

Patients attending the Kitasato University or an allied clinic and reporting six or more primary headaches per year were eligible for study entry. For the reliability testing, participants completed the MIDAS questionnaire on two occasions, 2 weeks apart. To assess the validity of the questionnaire, patients were also invited to participate in a diary study, where the similarities in responses between a prospective 90-day diary and a third MIDAS questionnaire completed at the end of this 90-day period were examined.

Table 7.2 Summary of MIDAS data from the test–retest reliability study of the Japanese MIDAS questionnaire

MIDAS question	Baseline		Retest			Spearman's correlation	Pearson's correlation
	Mean (SD)	Median	Mean (SD)	Median			
1 On how many days in the last 3 months did you miss work or school because of your headaches? (n=99)	2.2 (7.0)	0.0	2.9 (8.2)	0.0		0.74*	0.88*
2 On how many days in the last 3 months was your productivity at work or school reduced by half or more because of your headaches? (n=98)	5.1 (9.0)	1.0	5.3 (7.8)	1.0		0.80*	0.54
3 On how many days in the last 3 months did you not do household work because of your headaches? (n=99)	3.6 (4.8)	2.0	3.9 (5.0)	2.0		0.76*	0.63*
4 On how many days in the last 3 months was your productivity in household work reduced by half or more because of your headaches? (n=99)	5.6 (6.4)	3.0	5.7 (6.2)	3.0		0.73*	0.69*
5 On how many days in the last 3 months did you miss family, social, or leisure activities because of your headaches? (n=99)	3.5 (5.0)	2.0	4.2 (6.2)	2.0		0.59	0.77*
A On how many days in the last 3 months did you have any headache? (n=99)	30.9 (28.2)	20.0	31.7 (28.9)	18.0		0.87*	0.90*
B On a scale of 0–10, on average how painful were these headaches? (n=99)	5.7 (1.8)	6.0	5.6 (1.9)	5.0		0.66*	0.61
Total MIDAS score (n=99)	19.7 (20.1)	12.5	21.7 (22.1)	14.0		0.83*	0.82*

*p<0.0001.

Results

A total of 101 patients aged between 20 and >60 years were recruited (81 women and 20 men). Ninety-eight of these (79 women and 19 men) participated in the diary study. At baseline, headache impact was low in 46% of patients, intermediate in 22%, and high in 32%. Test–retest Spearman's correlations for individual items ranged from 0.59 to 0.80. The test–retest Pearson's coefficient of the overall MIDAS score was 0.82. Spearman's correlation coefficients between the individual MIDAS questions and the diary-based measures ranged from 0.35 to 0.89. These results are summarized in Table 7.2.

Conclusions

The reliability and validity of the Japanese MIDAS questionnaire are comparable with the original English version and it may be used for evaluating migraine disability.[5]

References

1. Sakai F, Igarashi H. Prevalence of migraine in Japan: a nationwide survey. *Cephalalgia* 1997; **17**: 15–22.
2. Henry P, *et al.* The GRIM. A nationwide survey of migraine in France: prevalence and clinical features in adults. *Cephalalgia* 1992; **12**: 229–37.
3. Stewart WF, Lipton RB, Whyte J, *et al.* An international study to assess reliability of the Migraine Disability Assessment (MIDAS) score. *Neurology* 1999; **53** (5): 988–94.
4. Lipton RB, Stewart WF, Stone AM, *et al.* Stratified care is more effective than step care strategies for migraine: results of the Disability in Strategies of Care (DISC) study. *J Am Med Assoc* 2000; **284**: 2599–605.
5. Headache Classification Committee of the International Headache Society. Classification and diagnostic criteria for headache disorders, cranial neuralgias and facial pain. *Cephalalgia* 1988; **8** (Suppl. 7): 1–96.

8 Disability in German headache sufferers: evaluation of a German headache disability inventory

Stefan Evers, Birgit Bauer, Ingrid Gralow, and Ingo W. Husstedt

Introduction

Pain-related impairment or disability is a very important factor for the quality of life in pain patients and crucial for evaluation of therapy. There are only very few German inventories to assess the chronic disability of pain patients, for example, the German version of the Pain Disability Index (PDI)[1] and the Multidimensional Pain Inventory (MPI).[2] With respect to headache, there is a specific English scale available describing the individual pain experience;[3] the reliability of this scale is, however, poor.[4] Furthermore, there is a specific inventory for the quality of life in headache patients evaluating a period of 4 weeks[5] and a migraine-specific questionnaire for the quality of life.[6] Acute impairment by headache attacks has been a focus of interest in recent years, in particular for migraine.[7,8] These scales show a high validity and are an appropriate measure of treatment success in single attacks.[9] However, there are no German versions of these scales.

In the English language, Jacobson et al.[4,10] developed a headache disability inventory (HDI) in order to assess the subjective impairment by chronic headache disorders both on the emotional and on the functional level. Scores for the two subscales and a total score can be calculated. This English version has a high internal consistency and validity. It needs very little time and can thus be applied both in the clinical and in the scientific context. We developed and tested a German version of the HDI called 'Inventar zur Beeinträchtigung durch Kopfschmerzen' (IBK).

Patients and methods

We enrolled 94 consecutive unselected patients admitted to the headache out-patient clinic of the Department of Neurology, University of Münster, Germany. Headache diagnosis was made according to the criteria of the International Headache Society (IHS); all criteria for a particular diagnosis had to be fulfilled. Duration of the chronic headache disorder had to be at least 5 years, the time of assessment had to be in a period with high probability of headache attacks (for example, to be within a bout for cluster headache patients). The inventory had to be filled out in a headache-free state (except for the patients with chronic tension-type headache). Patients with drug-induced headache, with a symptomatic headache, or with a neurological or psychiatric disease were excluded.

After obtaining written permission from the authors, the items of the HDI[4] were translated into German and then checked by four physicians experienced in pain therapy. The IBK consists of 25 items that can be answered by 'yes' (4 points), 'sometimes' (2 points), or 'no' (0 points). Thus, a high total score means a high impairment. We also divided the scale of 25 items into the subscales, emotion (13 items) and function (12 items). Patients were also asked to rate the average frequency of their headaches (1, <1 per month; 2, 1–4 per month; 3, >4 per month) and the average intensity (1, mild; 2, moderate; 3, severe).

The patients filled out the IBK at the beginning of their appointment. They were then instructed to treat their headaches according to the recommendations of the German Migraine and Headache Society. After 3 months, the IBK was sent to the patients for a follow-up in order to examine the test–retest reliability. Sixty-four patients could be evaluated for follow-up (68%). The demographic and clinical data of the patients are presented in Table 8.1.

Data are presented as percentages or as arithmetic means with simple standard deviation. We applied non-parametric tests (Wilcoxon test, Kruskal–Wallis analysis

Table 8.1 Demographic and clinical data of the patients (n=94). Data are presented as arithmetic mean ± simple standard deviation

Diagnosis	Sex Female	Male	Age (years)	Frequency (days per month)	Duration of disease (years)
Migraine with aura (n=14)	10	4	47±12	3.7±2.3	17±10
Migraine without aura (n=17)	13	4	32±7	6.9±4.7	15±8
Cluster headache (n=15)	3	12	43±9	21.9±9.0	13±8
Episodic tension-type headache (n=9)	7	2	43±17	10.5±8.7	11±13
Chronic tension-type headache (n=12)	4	8	40±10	20.3±10.4	12±8
Combined headache (n=27)	22	5	39±12	7.2±3.0	18±11
Total sample (n=94)	59	35	40±12	10.2±8.6	15±10

with multiple-range-test, and Mann–Whitney U-test). Correlation between the scales was analysed using the Spearman rank-correlation coefficient. The internal consistency was measured by Cronbach's alpha. The significance level was set at $p=0.05$.

Results

Reliability

As a measure for the homogeneity and internal consistency, we calculated Cronbach's alpha for every single item and obtained values between 0.890 and 0.903. The total Cronbach's alpha was 0.903. The mean score for the total scale was 57.3±20.1, for the subscale emotion 30.8±11.2, and for the subscale function 26.4±9.8. The correlation between the two subscales was $r=0.84$ ($p<0.0001$). Cronbach's alpha for the retest was 0.926. The total score of the retest was 54.3±23.3, for the subscale emotion 28.4±12.6, and for the subscale function 26.0±11.0. The results of the retest were lower than the results of the first test. This difference was only significant for the subscale emotion ($p<0.038$). The test–retest reliability for the total score was $r=0.87$ ($p<0.0001$), for the subscale emotion $r=0.81$ ($p<0.0001$), and for the subscale function $r=0.83$ ($p<0.0001$).

Analysis of the different scores

In Table 8.2, the different scores are presented separately for the different headache disorders. Kruskal–Wallis analysis of the total score obtained $p<0.190$. In the multiple-range test, there was a significant difference between cluster headache and migraine ($p<0.05$) both for the total scale and for the subscales. However, there were no significant differences between the different types of migraine and tension-type headache.

Table 8.2 Total scores and subscores (presented as arithmetic mean±simple standard deviation of the first test in 94 headache patients. For statistical analysis see text

	Total score (maximum 100)	Score of subscale	
		Emotion (maximum 52)	Function (maximum 48)
Migraine with aura (n=14)	49.0±20.7	26.1±11.4	22.9±9.7
Migraine without aura (n=17)	54.6±19.6	30.4±11.3	24.2±9.8
Cluster headache (n=15)	65.2±22.6	35.2±12.3	30.0±11.0
Episodic tension-type headache (n=9)	48.7±11.3	26.0±7.9	22.7±5.3
Chronic tension-type headache (n=12)	60.8±20.4	32.7±9.7	28.2±11.2
Combined headache (n=27)	60.0±18.0	31.9±10.5	28.2±8.2
Total sample (n=94)	57.3±20.1	30.8±11.2	26.4±9.8

Table 8.3 Arithmetic mean ± simple standard deviation and correlation coefficients of the different scores with sex, age, headache intensity, headache frequency, and duration of disease

		Score of subscale	
	Total score (maximum 100)	Emotion (maximum 52)	Function (maximum 48)
Sex			
Female (n=59)	55.9±18.7	30.1±11.8	25.8±8.8
Male (n=35)	59.5±22.2*	32.1±12.8†	27.4±11.2†
Age (years)	r=0.09 (p=0.4‡)	r=−0.03 (p=0.8‡)	r=0.05 (p<0.7‡)
Intensity			
Mild (n=2)	48.0±12.0	24.0±8.0	24.0±4.0
Moderate (n=29)	44.6±14.0	24.4±8.6	20.2±7.2
Severe (n=63)	63.0±21.0§	34.1±11.5¶	29.1±10.1‖
Frequency (days per month)	r=0.41 (p<0.0003‡)	r=0.42 (p<0.0003‡)	r=0.36 (p<0.002
Duration of disease (years)	r=0.15 (p=0.2‡)	r=0.13 (p<0.3‡)	r=0.14 (p<0.2‡)

*p=0.5; Mann–Whitney U-test.
†p<0.5; Mann–Whitney U-test.
‡Spearman rank-correlation coefficient.
§p<0.0003; Kruskal–Wallis analysis.
¶p<0.002; Kruskal–Wallis analysis.
‖p<0.0004; Kruskal–Wallis analysis.

There were highly significant correlation coefficients between the different scores and clinical data of the patients. The most important correlation coefficients are presented in Table 8.3. For the total score ($p<0.0003$), for the score of function ($p<0.0004$), and for the score of emotion ($p<0.002$), there were significant differences between the different intensities of pain. We obtained significantly higher scores for the severe headache intensities as compared to the moderate or mild intensity. No difference could be found between moderate and mild intensity. The frequency of headaches per month was significantly correlated with the total score ($r=0.41$; $p<0.0003$) and the scores for the subscales function ($r=0.36$; $p<0.002$) and emotion ($r=0.42$; $p<0.0003$). No significant correlation could be found between the different scores and the duration of disease, age, and sex.

Discussion

The IBK shows a high internal consistency and a high test–retest reliability that is comparable to that of the English original version. In agreement with the English version, a significant relation between the sex and age of the patients and the different scores could not be observed. The intensity of the headache and the frequency per month show a high correlation with the scores. This finding emphasizes the validity of the inventory.

The English version only differentiated between migraine and chronic tension-type headache without observing any significant differences. We also did not observe significant differences between migraine and tension-type headache. Cluster headache patients, however, showed significantly higher scores than migraine patients. This finding suggests that cluster headache, at least during the bout, leads to a higher impairment than other headache types. This agrees with previous observations on higher pain disability and higher impairment of social functions as measured by the short form (SF)-36 in cluster headache patients.[11]

In summary, the IBK shows very good results in the evaluation of its test criteria and can thus be regarded as an appropriate measure to assess the disability caused by chronic headache disorders. It needs only very little time to fill out the questionnaire and it can be interpreted very easily by summing up the scores. Therefore, we suggest the use of this inventory for the evaluation of headache treatment in addition to measuring the conventional parameters such as headache frequency and intensity.

References

1. Dillmann U, Nilges P, Saile H, Gerbershagen HU. Behinderungseinschätzung bei chronischen Schmerzpatienten. *Schmerz* 1994; **8**: 100–10.
2. Flor H, Rudy TE, Birbaumer N, Streit B, Schugens MM. Zur Anwendbarkeit des West Haven-Yale Multidimensional Pain Inventory im deutschen Sprachraum. *Schmerz* 1990; **4**: 82–7.
3. Hunter M. The Headache Scale: a new approach to the assessment of headache pain based on pain descriptions. *Pain* 1983; **16**: 361–73.
4. Jacobson GP, Ramadan NM, Aggarwal SK, Newman CW. The Henry Ford Hospital Headache Disability Inventory (HDI). *Neurology* 1994; **44**: 837–42.
5. Babiak LM, Miller DW, MacMillan JH, Sprang G. Migraine-specific quality of life: a comparison of U.S. and Canadian results. *Qual Life Res* 1994; **3**: 58.
6. Wagner TH, Patrick DL, Galer BS, Berzon RA. A new instrument to assess the long-term quality of life effects from migraine: development and psychometric testing of the MSQOL. *Headache* 1996; **36**: 484–92.
7. Hartmaier SL, Santanello NC, Epstein RS, Silberstein SD. Development of a brief 24-hour migraine-specific quality of life questionnaire. *Headache* 1995; **35**: 320–9.
8. Santanello NC, Hartmaier SL, Epstein RS, Silberstein SD. Validation of a new quality of life questionnaire for acute migraine headache. *Headache* 1995; **35**: 330–7.
9. Santanello NC, Polis AB, Hartmaier SB, Kramer MS, Block GA, Silberstein SD. Improvement in migraine-specific quality of life in a clinical trial of rizatriptan. *Cephalalgia* 1997; **17**: 867–72.
10. Jacobson GP, Ramadan NM, Norris L, Newman CW. Headache Disability Inventory (HDI): short-term test–retest reliability and spouse perception. *Headache* 1995; **35**: 534–9.
11. Solomon GD, Skobieranda FG, Gragg LA. Does quality of life differ among headache diagnoses? Analysis using the Medical Outcomes Study Instrument. *Headache* 1994; **34**: 143–7.

9 MIDAS as a tool for monitoring the benefits of treatment strategies over time

S. Chauvet and E.A. MacGregor

Introduction

The Migraine Disability Assessment (MIDAS) tool[1] quantifies the impact headaches have on the lives of patients, highlighting their disabilities in three activity domains:

- paid or school work;
- household work;
- family or leisure activities.

The MIDAS score is the sum of the response to five disability questions. Two additional questions (questions A and B) provide the physician with further information of clinical relevance (number of days with headache and pain intensity), but these are not included in the actual MIDAS score. One of the advantages of MIDAS is that it is scored in clinically meaningful units (days missed from activities) and therefore can be included in the physicians' assessment of severity and impact of illness.

To date, clinical testing has demonstrated that the MIDAS questionnaire shows high internal consistency, reliability, accuracy, and validity.[1–3] To be a fully useful assessment tool in clinical practice, however, MIDAS should show sensitivity to change in response to appropriate management strategies or treatment. This chapter presents initial and 3-month follow-up data for a population of patients attending the City of London Migraine Clinic as part of an ongoing study with the following objectives:

- to monitor changes in migraine-related disability over time;
- to evaluate the utility of MIDAS as a clinical measure to assess patient benefit in response to appropriate migraine management strategies in a specialist care setting.

Methods

Patients with an established diagnosis of migraine completed both an initial (during or just prior to their first visit to the clinic) and follow-up MIDAS questionnaire (3 months after the first visit) (Fig. 9.1). The first questionnaire was reviewed with the physician during the consultation to ensure that it had been correctly completed and to record patients' comments on the disability questions. The total MIDAS score was also discussed. The consultation was conducted routinely with a history obtained and physical examination, followed by recommendations for migraine management. After 3 months, a second MIDAS questionnaire was completed. The results of this second questionnaire were then used as a basis for discussion with patients on their progress. Patients were also asked whether there had been a relevant improvement or deterioration in their condition. These discussions were used to identify any further treatment and migraine management needs.

Results

Participants were all females whose ages ranged from 30 to 55 years, with the exception of two teenagers. A total of 52 migraine sufferers completed both initial and follow-up MIDAS questionnaires.

At entry, the median number of days with headache over the 3 previous months (MIDAS question A) was 18 (range 4 to 60) and the median headache intensity (0–10 scale, MIDAS question B) was 8 (range 4 to 10) (Table 9.1). Median entry MIDAS score was 25 (range 6 to 88), with 0, 7, 13, and 32 patients having MIDAS grades I (minimal/infrequent disability), II (mild/ infrequent disability), III (moderate disability), and IV (severe disability), respectively (Fig. 9.2).

At the 3-month follow-up visit, the median number of days with headache over the 3 previous months was 15 (range 0 to 44) and median headache intensity was 7 (range 0 to 10) (Table 9.1). The median MIDAS score had reduced to 19 (range 0 to 112), with 7, 6, 15, and 24 patients having MIDAS grades I, II, III, and IV, respectively (Fig. 9.2).

The change in MIDAS score, over a period of 3 months, showed an approximately 25% decrease in the level of disability experienced by migraine patients following a prescribed course of treatment or recommended migraine management strategy. The median number of days with headache showed a smaller decrease over this period (from 18 to 15, a 17% reduction), although the maximum value reduced

Table 9.1   Median values for MIDAS questions and MIDAS score

Question	1	2	3	4	5	MIDAS score	A	B
Initial	1	2	6	5	4	25	18	8
Follow-up	0	3	4	3	3	19	15	7

This form can help you and your doctor improve the management of your headaches

Do You Suffer From

headaches?

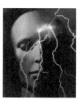

MIDAS QUESTIONNAIRE

INSTRUCTIONS: Please answer the following questions about ALL your headaches you have had over the last 3 months. Write your answer in the box next to each question. Write zero if you did not do the activity in the last 3 months.

1 On how many days in the last 3 months did you miss work or school because of your headaches?   days

2 How many days in the last 3 months was your productivity at work or school reduced by half or more because of your headaches? *(Do not include days you counted in question 1 where you missed work or school)*   days

3 On how many days in the last 3 months did you not do household work because of your headaches?   days

4 How many days in the last 3 months was your productivity in household work reduced by half or more because of your headaches? *(Do not include days you counted in question 3 where you did not do household work)*   days

5 On how many days in the last 3 months did you miss family, social or leisure activities because of your headaches?   days

TOTAL   days

A On how many days in the last 3 months did you have a headache? *(If a headache lasted more than 1 day, count each day)*   days

B On a scale of 0-10, on average how painful were these headaches? *(Where 0 = no pain at all, and 10 = pain as bad as it can be)*

©Innovative Medical Research 1997

Once you have filled in the questionnaire, add up the total number of days from questions 1-5 , Do not include the answers to Questions A and B in the overall score

Grading system for the MIDAS Questionnaire:		
Grade	**Definition**	**Score**
I	Little or no disability	0-5
II	Mild disability	6-10
III	Moderate disability	11-20
IV	Severe disability	21+

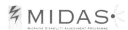

MIGRAINE DISABILITY ASSESSMENT PROGRAMME

The MIDAS programme is sponsored by

Fig. 9.1   MIDAS Questionnaire, ©Innovative Medical Research.

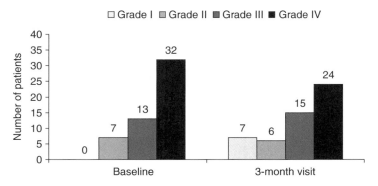

Fig. 9.2 Distribution of MIDAS grades at baseline and 3-month follow-up.

from 60 days to 44 days (that is, a similar 25% reduction). For pain intensity, the reduction in median value was from 8 to 7, a 13% reduction.

Discussion

These results suggest that the MIDAS questionnaire may help in assessing changes in overall migraine-associated disability, as measured by the MIDAS score. An overall reduction of 25% was seen in the MIDAS score following a course of treatment and/or recommendations for migraine management, suggesting that the MIDAS score is a useful tool for measuring disability change in response to migraine management strategies. Per individual, the total MIDAS score was sometimes higher than the number of days affected by headache (question A) if more than one domain of activity was affected on the same day (for example, lost paid work or household work time plus leisure time). This reflects how important it is to discuss with the patient the score in each domain of activity. Overall, the total MIDAS score showed a greater percentage reduction over the 3-month period (25%) versus the reduction in the number of days with headache (17%). This indicates that headache frequency is not in itself an adequate assessment of disability.

Generally, there was good correlation between the changes in MIDAS score and the comments from patients on the changes they felt had occurred between the two consultations. However, in some cases, the change in MIDAS score may underestimate the level of improvement and degree of patient benefit following treatment. For example, one patient had an initial MIDAS score of 8 and a follow-up score of 9 and, yet, during the patient–doctor discussion, reported a substantial improvement and reduction of migraine-related disability. This reflected fewer days lost to headache, but an increase in days with reduced productivity, with the resultant overall MIDAS score remaining unchanged despite a clinical improvement.

From discussions with patients based on their completed MIDAS questionnaire, it was apparent that some individuals altered their lifestyle significantly due to their migraine (for example, working from home, arranging social activities around their attacks). In this study, it was also noted that patient benefit, assessed by the MIDAS questionnaire, was attributable to factors other than relief of migraine *per se*, including management of comorbid conditions with treatments that also have anti-migraine properties (for example, one patient received a prescription of a beta-blocker for hypertension and showed a large improvement in MIDAS score).

Conclusions

Using the MIDAS questionnaire to assess the impact of individualized management strategies, an overall reduction in disability score of almost 25% was seen over a 3-month period. However, comparison of individual question responses may provide increased sensitivity to change, within patients, over time. There was generally a good correlation between the change in MIDAS score and patient reports of improvement in response to treatment, although, for some patients, changes in individual MIDAS question responses may cancel each other out. Again, this highlights the importance of physician–patient communication in the assessment of migraine severity and impact.

The MIDAS questionnaire is a useful aid for facilitating communication between physicians and patients and therefore provides a useful clinical tool to assess the impact of migraine on the lives of sufferers.

References

1. Stewart WF, Lipton RB, Kolodner K, Liberman J, Sawyer J. Reliability of the Migraine Disability Assessment (MIDAS) score in a population-based sample of headache sufferers. *Cephalalgia* 1999; **19**: 107–14.
2. Stewart WF, Lipton RB, Kolodner KB, Sawyer J, Lee C, Liberman JN. Validity of the Migraine Disability Assessment (MIDAS) score in comparison to a diary-based measure in a population sample of migraine sufferers. *Pain* 2000; **88**: 41–52.
3. Stewart WF, Lipton RB, Sawyer J. An international study to assess the reliability of the Migraine Assessment Disability (MIDAS) score. *Neurology* 1999; **52**: 988–94.

10 The MIDAS questionnaire in children and young adolescents with headache: a pilot study

L. Grazzi, D. D'Amico, F. Andrasik, S. Usai, M. Leone,
A. Rigamonti, and G. Bussone

Introduction

Recently, researchers have began to employ standardized methodologies to investigate the global impact of illness in primary headache disorders. This research has been aimed primarily at adult headache sufferers, and marked functional disability and decrease in quality of life have been reported overall. The Migraine Disability Assessment Score (MIDAS) questionnaire is one of the more specific instruments to assess functional disability in headache patients. It is a simple-to-use and a scientifically sound instrument that captures impairment in all activity domains.[1-4] Although it is well validated for adult headache patients, it has not been widely used with children and adolescents.

Recurrent headaches are common in children and adolescents. Without distinguishing the different headache types, recurrent headaches that occur once a week or more often are reported by more than 15% of schoolchildren.[5] Headache affects the individual, the family, and society for young patients too, so the impact of headache in children has been studied in terms of absenteeism from school and medical consumption.

Only a few studies have investigated quality of life as a multidimensional phenomenon in paediatric headache patients and these studies focus on the design of questionnaires for children aged 12 and older.[6] A tool for assessing headache disability in children that accounts for child-specific activities (school, home, and peer interaction) as well as differences among age groups has not yet been developed. We performed this study assessing disability in young headache sufferers, using the MIDAS questionnaire to extend this work to non-English-speaking samples and to complete a previous examination of the psychometric properties of the Italian version.[4]

Material and methods

Seventy-four patients aged 9–16 years completed the study. Forty-four were diagnosed with tension-type headache, 19 with migraine without aura, and 4 with migraine with aura, and 7 patients received diagnosis of tension-type headache combined with migraine. All were diagnosed according to International Headache Society (IHS) criteria.[7] At first consultation, patients were given the MIDAS questionnaire to complete. They were invited to come back to the Headache Centre after 1 month to complete the MIDAS a second time, in order to examine test–retest reliability. No treatment intervention occurred during this period. The Italian translation of MIDAS, which was recently developed by our group using standardized methods, was used.[4] The test–retest reliability of MIDAS scores was evaluated by Spearman's test.

Results and conclusions

The mean MIDAS scores at baseline and at retest after 1 month are reported in Table 10.1. Spearman correlation coefficients were 0.6 for the overall score, and 0.8, 0.4, 0.5, 0.1, 0.7 for individual items 1–5, respectively.

Table 10.1 Mean scores of MIDAS questionnaire at first compilation and at second compilation: test–retest reliability obtained using the Spearman correlation coefficient

MIDAS question*	Score (days in last 3 months)		Spearman correlation coefficient
	Baseline	1 month later	
1 Study/work missed	3.18	2.21	0.8
2 Study/work productivity reduced by ≥ 50%	6.30	5.94	0.4
3 Household work missed	2.95	1.90	0.5
4 Household work productivity reduced by ≥ 50%	1.99	3.13	0.1
5 Family/social/leisure activities missed	2.95	2.43	0.7
Overall MIDAS score	17.36	15.60	0.6

*The MIDAS questions ask on how many days in the last 3 months the patient has missed (or had his/her productivity reduced by ≥ 50% in) study/work, household work, and family/social/leisure activities.

Our preliminary results showed that young headache sufferers reported some form of disability in all rated activities. Reduction in school performance was the most reported problem. A satisfactory test–retest reliability was found for the overall MIDAS score, as well as for items that investigate total disability in school perform-ance, and family/social/leisure activities. Lower reliability coefficients were found in items pertaining to household work and to partial disability in school performance, which was not unexpected, as impairment in these activities may be more difficult to record. These data suggest that the MIDAS questionnaire can be used in the assessment of disability in young headache patients, although some changes might be required to make it a more suitable instrument for young headache sufferers.

References

1. Stewart WF, Lipton RB, Kolodner K. Reliability of the migraine disability assessment score in a population sample of headache sufferers. *Cephalalgia* 1999; **19**: 107–14.
2. Stewart WF, Lipton RB, Whyte J, *et al*. An international study to assess reliability of the Migraine Disability Assessment (MIDAS) score *Neurology* 1999; **53**: 988–94.
3. D'Amico D, Grazzi L, Usai S, *et al*. Migraine-related disability in different activity domains. *J Neurol* 2001; **248** (Suppl. 2): II/165.
4. D'Amico D, Mosconi P, Genco S, *et al*. Reliability of Italian translation of migraine disability assessment (MIDAS) questionnaire. *Cephalalgia* 1999; **20**: 317.
5. Sillanpaa M. Headache in children. In *Headache classification and epidemiology* (ed. Olesen J). New York: Raven Press, 1994: 273–81.
6. Langeveld JH, Koot HM, Loonen MCB, Hazebroek-Kampschreur AAJM, Passchier J. A quality of life instrument for adolescents with chronic headache. *Cephalalgia* 1996; **16**: 183.
7. Headache Classification Committee of the International Headache Society. Classification and diagnostic criteria for headache disorders, cranial neuralgias and facial pain. *Cephalalgia* 1988; **8** (Suppl. 7): 1–96.

11 Relationship between disability and quality of life in migraine

D. D'Amico, S. Usai, A. Solari, L. Grazzi, M. Leone,
A. Rigamonti, and G. Bussone

Introduction

It is well known that migraine has a negative influence on patients' lives. Over the last decade standardized instruments to assess health-related quality of life (HRQoL) have been used in migraineurs. Lower scores than in the general population—and in other chronic conditions—have been found in migraineurs using HRQOL generic tools such as the 'short forms' SF-36 and SF-20.[1–3] A specific tool to assess headache-related disability has been developed and validated, namely, the Migraine Disability Assessment Score (MIDAS) questionnaire.[4] The MIDAS score is obtained as the sum of the scores to five questions regarding the extent to which headaches interfere with daily activities. From this score, each patient is assigned to one of four MIDAS disability grades: scores from 0 to 5 correspond to grade I (little or no disability); scores 6–10 to grade II (mild/infrequent disability); scores 11–20 to grade III (moderate disability); and a score of 21 or over to grade IV (severe disability).

The main aims of our study were to evaluate the impact of migraine in a group of patients attending our headache centre who completed SF-36 and MIDAS questionnaires and to determine whether MIDAS disability grades correlated with HRQoL scores in these patients.

Materials and methods

Sixty-eight patients with an International Headache Society (IHS) diagnosis of migraine without aura[5] were studied. They were 52 women and 16 men of mean age 38.52 years (range 17–69); the mean illness duration was 21.18 years (range 1–50). Patients completed the SF-36 and MIDAS questionnaires during a consultation at the headache centre. The validated Italian versions of both questionnaires were used.[6–7] The Student t-test with Bonferroni correction was used to compare the SF-36 scores of the patients with Italian normative data. The correlation between MIDAS disability grades and SF-36 scores was assessed by the Kruskal–Wallis test, again with the Bonferroni correction.

Results

Migraine patients' mean scores were numerically lower than those in the Italian general population for all components (scales) of the SF-36, suggesting poorer QoL. Scores were significantly lower than normal for the categories, 'role functioning–physical', 'bodily pain', 'social functioning' ($p < 0.0001$), and 'role functioning–emotional' ($p = 0.02$) (Table 11.1). Patients' mean MIDAS disability score was 23.47 (SD 16.36; range 0–65). The distribution of MIDAS disability grades was as follows: grade I+grade II, 19 patients (27.9%); grade III, 18 patients (26.5%); grade IV, 31 patients (45.6%). A significant correlation between increasing MIDAS disability grade and decreasing SF-36 score was found for the following SF-36 scales: role functioning–physical, bodily pain ($p = 0.002$), social functioning ($p = 0.03$), and role functioning–emotional ($p = 0.03$) (Fig. 11.1).

Conclusion

Our results confirm that migraine patients attending a headache centre are markedly impaired, as reported by previous studies.[1–3,8] MIDAS grades reflect disability in all

Table 11.1   SF-36 scores in 68 patients with migraine without aura and differences from Italian normative data (Student's t-test with Bonferroni correction)

SF-36 categories	SF-36 scores		
	Patients with migraine without aura (mean ± SD)	Italian normative data (mean ± SD)	p-value*
Physical functioning	88.60 ± 15.33	84.46 ± 23.18	NS
Role functioning–physical	44.48 ± 36.35	78.21 ± 35.93	0.0001
Bodily pain	50.29 ± 8.09	73.67 ± 27.65	0.0001
General health	63.45 ± 21.30	65.22 ± 22.18	NS
Vitality	59.85 ± 11.62	61.89 ± 20.69	NS
Social functioning	59.19 ± 17.62	77.43 ± 23.34	0.0001
Role functioning–emotional	63.23 ± 37.82	76.16 ± 37.25	0.02
Mental health	65.89 ± 17.90	66.59 ± 20.89	NS

*NS, Not significant.

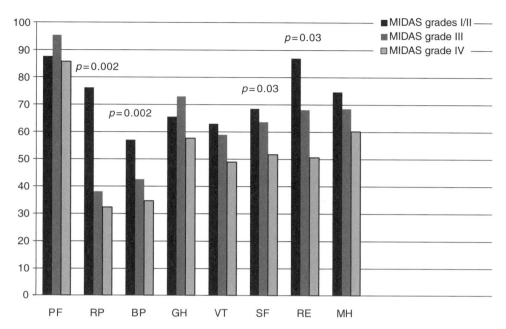

Fig. 11.1 Correlations between MIDAS disability grades and scores on individual SF-36 categories in 68 migraine patients (Kruskal–Wallis test with Bonferroni correction). SF-36 categories: PF, physical functioning; RP, role functioning–physical; BP, bodily pain; GH, general health; VT, vitality; SF, social functioning; RE, role functioning–emotional; MH, mental health.

activities (lost days in paid work or study, household work, family/social/leisure activities plus productivity reduced by $> 50\%$ in paid work, study, and household activities). We found that increasing disability (as reflected by higher MIDAS disability grade) correlated with the SF-36 scales that assess the extent to which physical health, emotional state, and pain interfere with functioning in several domains (including impairment in workplace productivity, in household duties, and in social activities. This confirms the ability of the MIDAS questionnaire to detect the functional status of migraine patients and suggests it may be an ideal short instrument for capturing migraine-related functional disability. In this context it is important to emphasize that MIDAS is brief, easy to complete by the patient, and simple to score by the examiner; furthermore, the disability grades are intuitive. By contrast, most HRQoL instruments take considerably more time to complete, are much more complicated to score, and produce percentile scores that are not immediately interpretable.

MIDAS therefore presents itself as an optimal tool for assessing the impact of migraine on patients' daily activities, both in clinical practice and in clinical trials.

References

1. Solomon GD, Skobieranda FG, Gragg LA. Quality of life and well being of headache patients: measurement by the Medical Outcomes Study instrument. *Headache* 1993; **33**: 351–8.
2. Osterhaus JT, Townsend RJ, Gandeck B, Ware JE. Measuring the functional status and well-being of patients with migraine headache. *Headache* 1994; **34**: 337–43.
3. Terwindt GM, Ferrari MD, Tijhuis M, *et al*. The impact of migraine on quality of life in the general population. *Neurology* 2000; **55**: 624–9.
4. Stewart WF, Lipton RB, Kolodner K, Liberman J, Sawyer J. Reliability of the migraine disability assessment score in a population sample of headache sufferers. *Cephalalgia* 1999; **19**: 107–14.
5. Headache Classification Committee of the International Headache Society. Classification and diagnostic criteria for headache disorders, cranial neuralgias and facial pain. *Cephalalgia* 1988; **8** (Suppl. 7): 1–96.
6. Apolone G, Mosconi P. The Italian SF-36 health survey: translation, validation and norming. *J Clin Epidemiol* 1998; **51** (11): 1025–36.
7. D'Amico D, Mosconi P, Genco S, *et al*. The Migraine Disability Assessment (MIDAS) questionnaire: translation and reliability of Italian version. *Cephalalgia* 2001; **21**: 947–52.
8. D'Amico D, Grazzi L, Usai S, *et al*. Migraine-related disability in different activities domains. *J Neurol* 2001; **248** (Suppl. 2): II/165.

12 Migraine in France in 2000: epidemiological data

P. Henry, J.P. Auray, G. Duru, G. Chazot, J.F. Dartigues,
M. Lantéri-Minet, C. Lucas, A. Pradalier,
A. El Hasnaoui, and A.F. Gaudin

Introduction

Ten years ago, a French national epidemiology study on migraine was presented at the Migraine Trust (1990). It was the first such study to cover an entire country.[1] The study provided data on the burden of migraine disease in terms of individual repercussions and quality of life, as well as on migraine's global economic and social impact.

The goal of the present study was to estimate the evolution of epidemiological data since the last study, and to assess the impact of a new class of medication (triptan drugs) on the disease management and social repercussions of migraine headache. In this work we will analyse new epidemiological data, comparing it to the data obtained in 1989.

Method

The survey was carried out by ISL, a national polling institute. A nationwide, representative sample of 10 585 subjects in France aged 15 years and older was constituted according to the quota method. The French population was stratified by gender, age, occupational category, and place of residence.

Data collection

The study was carried out by means of two successive home interviews. Persons suffering from headache were selected during the first interview, or screening. They were then contacted for a second interview, which lasted 90 minutes. During the second interview, a validated questionnaire for diagnosing migraine disease (Table 12.1) was administered along with a global questionnaire. This questionnaire

Table 12.1   The standardized diagnostic questionnaire

Q. 31   Are you subject to headaches?
Q. 32   Do you suffer from headaches every day?
Q. 33   Do your headaches come as periodic attacks, with intervals
          between during which you do not suffer from headaches?
Q. 34   How long do your headaches usually last without medication?
          1. less than 4 hours
          2. between 4 and 72 hours
          3. more than 72 hours
          4. don't know
Q. 35   How long do your headaches usually last with medication?
          1. less than 4 hours
          2. between 4 and 72 hours
          3. more than 72 hours
          4. don't know
Q. 36   Where is your headache usually located?
          1. strictly unilateral
          2. alternately right or left
          3. don't know
Q. 37   Are your headaches pulsating?
Q. 38   Do your headaches inhibit daily activity?
Q. 39   Do your headaches get worse with usual physical activity?
Q. 40   Are your headaches accompanied by nausea or vomiting?
Q. 41   Are your headaches accompanied by photophobia?
Q. 42   Are your headaches accompanied by phonophobia?
Q. 43   Have you had more than four attacks in your life?

was the same as the one used in 1989, with several supplementary questions, notably concerning triptan drugs. Data were gathered on the severity of headaches, quality of life, sociodemographic and economic status, pharmaceutical habits, and use of medical services.

In the screening interview, headache sufferers were detected in the global sample of 10 585 subjects by the question: 'Are you subject to headaches?' Of the 3087 subjects who complained of headaches, 1486 responded to the second interview.

Instruments

The diagnostic instrument used was a validated algorithm based on International Headache Society (IHS) criteria (Fig. 12.1). Its concurrent validity was examined in the 1989 study with a clinical sample, using a neurologist's diagnosis as gold standard. The sensitivity and specificity of the instrument in a population suffering from headache were 86% and 94%, respectively.[2]

Further to critical remarks concerning the 1989 study,[3] we modified our algorithm (Fig. 12.2 and Table 12.2), classifying headache patients into the following categories:

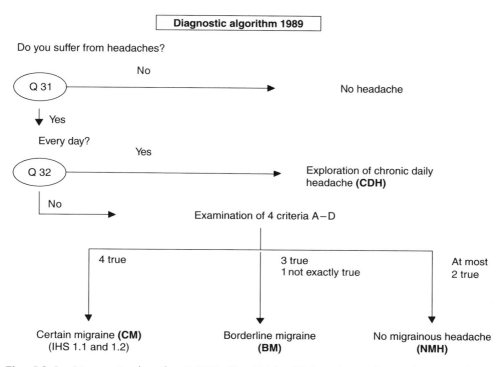

Fig. 12.1   Diagnostic algorithm (1989). (See Tables 12.1 and 12.2 for explanation of questions 31 and 32 and criteria A–D and Table 12.3 for IHS criteria.)

- certain migraine (CM), with or without aura, corresponding strictly to IHS criteria 1.1 and 1.2) (Table 12.3);
- borderline migraine group (BM), corresponding to IHS criteria, but with one criterion that is not quite true (for example, duration of attack <4 hours; only photophobia or phonophobia; fewer than 5 attacks);
- migraine disorder (MD) fulfils all criteria but one (IHS 1.7); MD includes BM, but is broader in range;
- global migraine group M comprises groups CM and MD;
- chronic daily headaches (CDH);
- no migraine headaches (NMH).

Results

Figure 12.3 summarizes the results of applying the algorithm in Fig. 12.2 in terms of numbers of respondents in each category. The global prevalence rate of migraine headache in the French population aged 15 years and over is 8.2% for certain

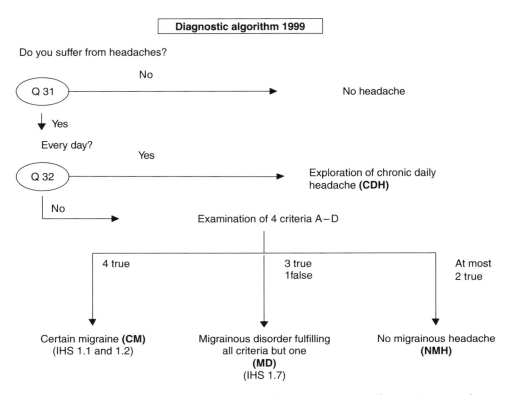

Fig. 12.2 Diagnostic algorithm (1999). (See Tables 12.1 and 12.2 for explanation of questions 31 and 32 and criteria A–D and Table 12.3 for IHS criteria.)

Table 12.2 Criteria A–D*

Criterion A	Answers are 'yes' to Q. 34.2 or to Q. 34.4 *and* Q. 35.2
Criterion B	Answers to at least 2 of the following 4 is 'yes': 1. Q. 36.1 or 36.2 2. Q. 37 3. Q. 38 4. Q. 39
Criterion C	Answer to at least 1 of the following 2 questions is 'yes' 1. Q. 40 2. Q. 41 *and* Q. 42
Criterion D	Answer to Q. 43 is 'yes'

*See Table 12.1 for content of questions Q. 31–Q. 43.

migraine (CM) and 9.1% for migrainous disorder (MD), giving a total of 17.3% for CM and MD combined. Figure 12.4 shows the prevalence of CM and MD adjusted by gender and age group.

Table 12.3   IHS diagnostic criteria (ref. 6)

1.1   Migraine without aura
    A. At least 5 attacks fulfilling B–D
    B. Headache attacks lasting 4–72 hours (untreated or unsuccessfully treated)
    C. Headache has at least two of the following charactersitics:
        1. Unilateral location
        2. Pulsating quality
        3. Moderate or severe intensity (inhibits or prohibits daily activities)
        4. Aggravation by walking upstairs or similiar routine physical activity
    D. During headache at least one of the following:
        1. Nausea and/or vomiting.
        2. Photophobia and phonophobia.
    E. At least one of the following:
        1. History and physical and neurological examinations do not suggest one of the disorders listed in groups 5–11
        2. History and/or physical and/or neurological examinations do suggest such a disorder, but it is ruled out by appropriate investigations
        3. Such a disorder is present, but migraine attacks do not occur for the first time in close temporal relation to the disorder
1.2   Migraine with aura
    A. At least 2 attacks fulfilling B.
    B. At least 3 of the following 4 characteristics:
        1. One or more fully reversible aura symptoms indicating focal cerebral cortical and/or brainstem dysfunction
        2. At least one aura symptom develops gradually over more than 4 minutes or 2 or more symptoms occur in succession
        3. No aura symptom lasts more than 60 minutes. If more than one aura symptom is present, accepted duration is proportionally increased
        4. Headache follows aura with free interval of less than 60 minutes. (It may also begin before or simultaneously with the aura)
    C. At least one of the following:
        1. History and physical and neurological examinations do not suggest one of the disorders listed in groups 5–11
        2. History and/or physical and/or neurological examinations do suggest such a disorder, but it is ruled out by appropriate investigations
        3. Such as disorder is present, but migraine attacks do not occur for the first time in close temporal relation to the disorder
1.7   Migrainous disorder not fulfilling above criteria
    A. Fulfils all criteria but one for one or more forms of migraine (specify type(s))
    B. Does not fulfil criteria for tension-type headache

Discussion

A comparison of prevalence rates for migraine headache in France between 1989 and 1999 seems to show a clear increase in prevalence, rising from 12.1% in 1989 to

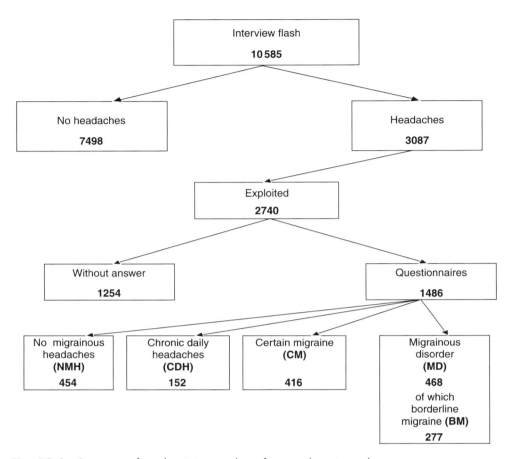

Fig. 12.3 Summary of results giving number of respondents in each category.

17.3% in 1999. In fact, these results are not strictly comparable because the criteria applied to the borderline migraine (BM) group in 1989 were much more restrictive[4] than those applied in 1999 to the migrainous disorder (MD) group (IHS 1.7).

If we compare the results for the certain migraine (CM) group, we find that they are virtually identical (8.1% (1989) versus 8.2% (1999)). However, the borderline migraine (BM) group retained in 1989 represented only 4% of the population, whereas the migrainous disorder (MD) group in 1999 represents 9.1% of our population sample, a considerably higher amount.

In 1989 we showed[2] that the populations CM and BM were comparable on all points and that, together, they could be classified under the heading 'definite migraine'. Does this hold true for the 1999 MD group? It is not certain, and only further investigation would enable us to affirm this. What we have gained in sensitivity we may possibly have lost in specificity.

(a)

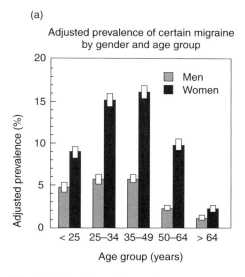

(b)

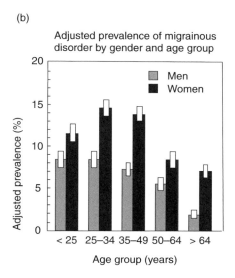

Fig. 12.4 Adjusted prevalence rates according to age and gender for (a) certain migraine and (b) migrainous disorder.

The use of criteria 1.1 and 1.2 of the IHS classification clearly leads to an under-estimation of migraine prevalence; however, doesn't the use of criterion 1.7 lead to an overestimation?

A recent study (the Framig study) carried out in France,[5] strictly based on IHS criteria 1.1 and 1.2, shows a prevalence rate of 12.45%, considerably above that observed in our study for the same criteria. This is partially due to the age difference in the population sample. The Framig study considers a population ranging from 18 to 65 years (age groups in which prevalence is the highest), whereas our 1989 and 1999 studies concern a population aged 15 years and over, with no upper threshold.

Conclusion

The results presented in this work are based on epidemiological data concerning migraine headache in France in 2000. They are only one aspect of a more global study. The other data in the study concerns pharmacoeconomic and quality of life data, and incorporates the appearance of triptan drugs on the reimbursable drug market.

References

1. Henry P, *et al*. Migraine prevalence in France. In *New advances in headache research*, Vol. 2 (ed. Rose C). London: Smith Gordon, 1991; 11–14.
2. Michel P, *et al*. Validity of the IHS criteria for migraine *Neuroepidemiology* 1993; **12**: 51–7.

3. Rasmussen BK, Olesen J. Migraine epidemiology [letter to the editor]. *Cephalagia* 1993; **13**: 216–17.
4. Henry P, *et al*. *Cephalalgia* 1992; **12**: 229–37.
5. Lantéri-Minet M, Lucas C, Leroy L. Etude Framig 99. *Rev Neurol* 2000; **156** (Suppl. 1): 133–4.
6. Headache Classification Committee of the International Headache Society. Classification and diagnostic criteria for headache disorders, cranial neuralgias and facial pain. *Cephalalgia* 1988; **8** (Suppl. 7): 1–96.

13
Validation of the Headache Impact Test™ using patient-reported symptoms and headache severity

J.B. Bjorner, J.E. Ware Jr, M. Kosinski, M. Diamond, S. Tepper, A. Dowson, M.S. Bayliss, and A.S. Batenhorst

Introduction

Many headache sufferers are misdiagnosed and/or undertreated due to communication difficulties between patients and physicians. Research suggests that questionnaires designed to elicit data regarding headache-related impairment or disability may provide a basis to improve patient–physician communication and allow doctors to design the most effective treatment plan. While appropriate for population-based decisions, published tools that measure headache impact and disability often lack the accuracy needed to make clinical decisions for individual patients at different levels of headache severity. Also, these short forms were designed to allow for quick administration and reduce patient and physician burden, but may sacrifice comprehensiveness, precision, and accuracy across the full range of headache impact. To facilitate clinical decision-making, physicians and patients would benefit from a tool that is quick and easy to administer yet provides a precise and easily interpreted score.

The Headache Impact Test (HIT) was developed as an internet-based, dynamic assessment tool using modern psychometric models (namely, item response theory (IRT)). HIT uses computerized administration and IRT models to efficiently and accurately deliver an individually tailored test to the patient.[1] HIT matches questions to each patient's level of impact, estimates a score on a common metric, and evaluates measurement precision and response consistency during the assessment.

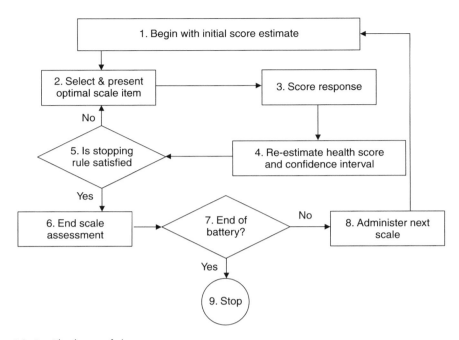

Fig. 13.1 The logic of dynamic assessments.

HIT is the first health assessment tool designed to link the computerized adaptive testing technologies and modern psychometric models used extensively in the educational and psychological testing disciplines in an internet-based application that is available to both patients and physicians at no charge.

HIT was programmed using the DynHA^{TM} engine (Fig. 13.1) and can be accessed via the Internet at www.headachetest.com or www.amIhealthy.com. The administration of HIT consists of five easy steps. HIT first begins with an initial estimate of headache impact based on the response to an item that is asked of all respondents (step 1). This first item is termed the HIT global item. Response to the global item is used to initiate HIT scoring and select the next most informative item from the item pool to administer to the respondent (step 2). At step 3, the response to the item selected and administered in step 2 is scored. At step 4, the scored response in step 3 is used to estimate the HIT score and compute a respondent-specific confidence interval (CI). Finally, in step 5, the computer determines whether the HIT score has been estimated within a predetermined standard of measurement precision based on the CI. Patients also have the option of completing demographic and headache history questions that are used to customize patient and physician reports. Reports were designed by clinicians with input from patients and researchers and include four sections for the patient—'Your score', 'Your progress', 'What your score means', and 'What you should do'—and four sections for the doctor (see Fig. 13.2). Patients also have the option of printing a copy of the questions that they have answered.

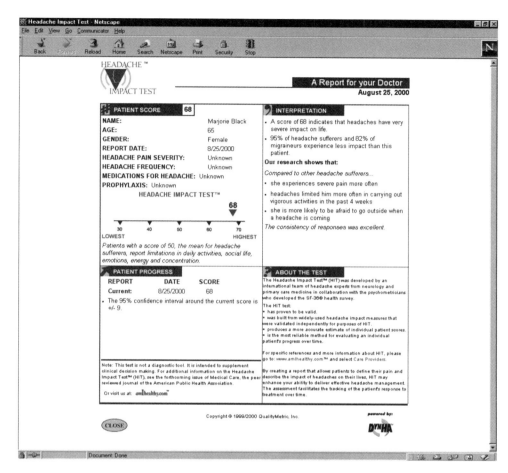

Fig. 13.2   Report chart for the HIT test (doctor's report).

The HIT item pool consists of 55 questions covering relevant areas of headache impact such as pain (frequency/severity), role functioning, social functioning, energy/fatigue, cognition, and emotional distress. The items have been adapted from four published and widely used headache and migraine questionnaires, the Headache Disability Inventory (HDI),[2] the Headache Impact Questionnaire (HImQ),[3] the Migraine Disability Assessment (MIDAS),[4] and the Migraine-Specific Questionnaire (MSQ).[5] One experimental item has been added. Each of the items has been calibrated and scored on a single index of headache impact and then standardized using norm-based methods to achieve a mean score of 50 and a standard deviation of 10. HIT has been designed to cover a full range of impact. Validity has been established using psychometric standards including content of items, item internal consistency, factor analysis of interitem correlations, IRT models, reliability and stability of score and score distributions and range covered, plus clinical criteria of validity and responsiveness to change in severity over time.[6,7]

The objectives of this study were to establish the validity of HIT in discriminating across groups of patients differing in migraine diagnosis and headache severity and symptoms and to establish the validity of HIT in comparison to widely used migraine and headache questionnaires.

Methods

Data were collected via a telephone survey (n=1016). The sampling frame was a randomly generated list of phone numbers from the 48 contiguous states in the USA. Participants were 18 to 65 years of age and had had a headache within the last 4 weeks that was not due to cold, flu, head injury, or hangover.[7] We used data from the baseline study and from a 3-month follow-up. Respondents provided data on all 55 HIT items, plus questions regarding migraine symptoms and headache severity. The HDI, HImQ, MIDAS, and the MSQ questionnaires were scored using the developers' algorithms. Two IRT-based scores were estimated for HIT: HIT-total score (55 items) and HIT-dynamic score (simulated dynamic administration of five or fewer HIT items from the pool of 55 items). Migraine headache cases were identified on the basis of reported symptoms using established diagnostic criteria.[8] Discriminant validity tests (analysis of variance (ANOVA) and relative validity (RV)) were used to evaluate how well each instrument discriminates between groups of respondents differing in headache severity and migraine diagnosis. Responsiveness to change in severity over time was evaluated using six criteria.

(1) On a scale from 1 to 10, where 0 means 'no pain' and 10 means 'pain as bad as it can be', on average how painful were your headaches in the past 4 weeks?
(2) Compared to 3 months ago, are you having fewer or more headaches now?
(3) Compared to 3 months ago, do your headaches bother you more or less?
(4) Compared to 3 months ago, are you more or less limited now in your everyday physical activities because of your headaches?
(5) Compared to 3 months ago, how often do you feel frustrated, irritable, or tense because of your headches?
(6) Compared to 3 months ago how often do headaches now limit your usual daily activities, including housework, work, and/or social activities?

Results

All instruments significantly discriminated across groups differing in migraine diagnosis and level of headache severity ($p < 0.001$, Tables 13.1 and 13.2). The HIT-total scale score was the most valid (RV=1.0) in relation to both migraine diagnosis and headache severity, followed by the HIT-dynamic scale (RV=0.998 and 0.978, respectively). HIT-dynamic scores were valid in responding to changes in headache

Table 13.1 HIT-total and HIT-dynamic scores are most valid in discriminating among patients differing in migraine diagnosis

Scale	Number of items	Migraine diagnosis (mean (SE))		F	RV
		Yes ($n=226$)	No ($n=520$)		
HIT-total	54	60.5 (0.4)	45.1 (0.3)	540.6*	1.000
HIT-dynamic	≤5	59.7 (0.5)	46.0 (0.3)	539.6*	0.998
Other scales[†]					
High	7	55.6 (1.3)	85.1 (0.6)	535.4*	0.990
Medium	8	45.9 (1.3)	18.1 (0.7)	524.4*	0.970
Low	5	21.9 (2.6)	1.0 (0.2)	145.2*	0.268

*$p < 0.001$.
[†]Represents ordering of seven scales from four widely used migraine headache questionnaires.

Table 13.2 HIT-total and HIT-dynamic scores are most valid in discriminating among patients differing in headache severity

Scale	Number of items	Headache severity (mean (SE))			F	RV
		Mild ($n=275$)	Moderate ($n=522$)	Severe ($n=204$)		
HIT-total	54	42.9 (0.5)	51.7 (0.3)	59.6 (0.6)	222.1*	1.000
HIT-dynamic	≤5	44.5 (0.4)	51.1 (0.3)	59.2 (0.6)	217.2*	0.978
Other scales[†]						
High	8	14.6 (0.6)	28.3 (0.7)	46.4 (1.5)	220.4*	0.992
Medium	12	86.4 (1.0)	70.2 (1.0)	48.0 (1.9)	163.5*	0.736
Low	5	1.4 (0.2)	7.7 (0.9)	21.1 (2.7)	49.0*	0.221

*$p < 0.001$.
[†]Represents ordering of seven scales from four widely used migraine headache questionnaires.

severity and impact with respect to HIT-total scores with RV on the six criteria of change ranging from 91% to 97%.

HIT-DynHA is brief yet accurate with 95% of respondents achieving precise scores (95% CI) in five or fewer questions. 98% of those with migraine, 97% with severe headache, 87% with moderate headache, and 61% with mild headache achieved clinical standards of accuracy in five or fewer questions.

Specificity of HIT scores was high for diagnosis of migraine headache. Over 90% of respondents with scores ≥56 had migraine and 78% of respondents with scores <56 did not have migraine according to the study criteria.

Conclusions

The IRT methods and computer software make it feasible to quickly estimate valid and reliable scores of headache impact. HIT was created by adapting questions from widely used headache quality of life, impact, and disability measures that have been independently validated. The scores based on the total pool of items (HIT-total) were most valid in discriminating across groups differing in migraine diagnosis and headache severity. HIT assessments meet standards based on clinical criteria allowing identification of patients most likely to have a migraine diagnosis and reliable estimation of the severity of headache impact. Administration of HIT via the internet using computer-adaptive testing logic significantly reduces respondent burden while maintaining a high standard of measurement validity.

Acknowledgements

The authors gratefully acknowledge the contributions of B. Bowers and J. Carranza Rosenzweig from GlaxoSmithKline, Inc to this chapter.

References

1. Wainer H, Dorans NJ, Flaugher R, *et al*. *Computerized adaptive testing: a primer*. Hillsdale, New Jersey: Lawrence Erlbaum Associates, 1990.
2. Jacobson GP, *et al*. Headache Disability Inventory (HDI): short-term test–retest reliability and spouse perceptions. *Headache* 1995; **35**: 534–9.
3. Stewart WF, Lipton RB, Simon D, *et al*. Validity of an illness severity measure for headache in a population sample of migraine sufferers. *Pain* 1999; **79**: 291–301.
4. Stewart WF, Lipton RB, Whyte J, *et al*. An international study to assess reliability of the Migraine Disability Assessment (MIDAS) score. *Neurology* 1999; **53**: 988–94.
5. Jhingran P, Osterhaus JT, Miller DW, *et al*. Development and validation of the Migraine-Specific Quality of Life Questionnaire. *Headache* 1998; **38**: 295–302.
6. Ware JE Jr, Kosinski M, Bjorner JB, *et al*. *Quality Life Res*, in press.
7. Ware JE Jr, Bjorner JB, Kosinski M. Practical implications of item response theory and computerized adaptive testing. *Med Care* 2000; **38** (Suppl. II): II-72–II-82.
8. Stewart WF, Lipton RB, Celentano DD, *et al*. *J Am Med Assoc* 1992; **267** (1): 64–9.

14
Headache-related disability: discussion summary

T.J. Steiner

It is beyond all doubt that headache disorders are prevalent and ubiquitous and that, in many cases, they are lifelong conditions. Since the International Headache Society clarified the diagnostic criteria for headache disorders[1] and case definitions have been standardized, epidemiological studies of high quality, whilst showing geographical and perhaps culturally determined variations, nonetheless confirm this wherever in the world they have been performed. Can there still be doubts about the scale of disability attributable to headache disorders? And, if so, why is this? These questions of public health go to the heart of the troublesome issue of securing the priority that is due to headache-related health-care services.

Headache disorders are manifestly associated with recognizable burdens, which include personal suffering and impaired quality of life. Their impact extends beyond those immediately affected.[2] In what sense are they disabling, and how much of the total burden of disease attributable to headache is due to disability? People with headache disorders are not in wheelchairs because of them: whatever disability results is not visible in that way. But most migraineurs, for example, seek rest in a quiet, darkened room during most of their attacks, which clearly represents a severe limitation on normal functioning. There is, also, a measurable drop in cognitive efficiency.

Estimates of the financial cost of headache disorders, which is high, relate principally to lost time in gainful employment ('work') or reduced productivity due to impaired working effectiveness.[3–5] These factors tend to dominate discussion of headache-related disability, probably because money is politically persuasive and measures of financial losses are easy to harness in arguments calling for greater investment in better care. But, if that is what is meant by disability, its consequences in developing countries may be quite different from those in the affluent Western world. And this concept of disability is of uncertain meaning for those whose 'work' is caring for others including children, or for the retired and whose activities and functioning are no less interfered with. How does it apply to someone forced to retire early because of headache?

As a first issue, therefore, we must take care to think of headache-related disability in terms that do not diminish it anywhere in the world or for any sector of the population. Nor, since we wish the case for due priority for headache to be presented legitimately, should we magnify it anywhere. The World Health Organization (WHO), who are concerned especially with disability as a summary measure of population health alongside mortality, have recognized headache disorders as a public health concern.[6] They remind us that disability is not independent of baseline function and scope of operation in the environment of the individual: that is to say, the disabling effect of an illness is limited to the range of what a particular person, in his or her own circumstances, *could* and *would* do if well.

This is intuitively reasonable, but it implies that disability cannot readily be predicted from *impairment*, if that term is used to sum up the effects of all of the symptoms of a particular headache disorder experienced by an individual. Whether considering loss of work time, paid or otherwise, or the abandonment of social activity, there is an aspect of *choice*—of behavioural response to impairment—in those things that are or are not done during illness, with various levels of motivation (itself driven by needs) as partial determinants. So what is expressed as disability—things not done that would or should have been done—is far from being objectively determined.

The second issue, to which this leads, is disability measurement. Arguably, what is to be assessed is what *can be* done (and with what difficulty), not what actually *is* done, but this is not at all easy to measure. Of course, much depends on who wants to assess disability and for what purpose. For example, the fact that, on any working day, large numbers of people are absent from work or school because of migraine is a verifiable effect of illness that has consequences of importance to employers and governments. It seems helpful to know that 50% of migraineurs account for more than 80% of work loss, if productivity gains will be greatest through targeting this group for treatment. This depends on the causal link, and expectation that alleviating impairment brings functional recovery hand-in-hand, whereas studies are not yet wholly convincing of this or indicate some lag. Indeed, in individual cases, reported high disability from migraine is predictive of treatment failure with current therapies. This suggests, on the one hand, that disability assessment is important in the initial evaluation of a patient for management purposes and, on the other, that those most disabled may not so easily be brought back to work.

Thirdly, the need to measure headache-related disability has spawned a series of instruments designed for this purpose in individuals. No consensus exists as to whether any of these instruments comes near to meeting a theoretical ideal. They may more accurately claim to measure something or a combination of things that are reasonably correlated with disability. Work underway with some is showing sensitivity to change attributable to treatment, although it is not clear what the 'gold standard' is. The desire for a single, valid, agreed instrument is far from being met.

In populations, estimates rely on assumptions and averages. The WHO approach is based on a judgement of what expected level and duration of disability are attributable to an average episode of a headache disorder (and of some lesser disability between episodes, important where it occurs because it is continuous), which are then multiplied according to average lifetime duration of the disorder from its onset and the average frequency of episodes during that period. Different averages may be applied to milder or more severe forms of the disorder where these are distinguishable. It is crude, but informative provided that the assumptions have legitimacy, and persuasive if they are credible. And so to the fourth issue: the size of the disability burden of migraine world-wide, measured in this way in disability-adjusted life-years, is *greater than that of epilepsy*. Disability burdens attributable to tension-type headache and to frequently recurring headache disorders remain largely unknown, but perhaps an impetus has been unleashed to begin their measurement.

To conclude, it is not wholly agreed what the scope of headache-related disability is, or how to measure the scale of it. It is not certain, when we claim to measure it, that whatever is captured is what is most important to patients. But, when we do measure it in populations, it reflects a very heavy illness burden and that is an important public health issue. It means that not only we but also those in government and elsewhere who influence allocation of health-care resources should want to do something about it, always assuming that headache-related disability is at least to some extent a remediable burden. Finally, this session included some evidence that it is, and that is a political message that should have great impact in our endeavours to move headache disorders up the health-care priority queue.

References

1. Headache Classification Committee of the International Headache Society. Classification and diagnostic criteria for headache disorders, cranial neuralgias and facial pain. *Cephalalgia* 1988; **8** (Suppl. 7): 1–96.
2. Steiner TJ. Headache burdens and bearers. *Funct Neurol* 2000; **15** (Suppl. 3): 219–23.
3. Osterhaus JT, Gutterman DL, Plachetka JR. Healthcare resource and lost labour costs of migraine headache in the US. *PharmacoEconomics* 1992; **2**: 67–76.
4. Stewart WF, Lipton RB, Simon D. Work-related disability: results from the American Migraine Study. *Cephalalgia* 1996; **16**: 231–8.
5. Schwartz BS, Stewart WF, Lipton RB. Lost workdays and decreased work effectiveness associated with headache in the workplace. *J Occup Environm Med* 1997; **39**: 320–7.
6. World Health Organization. *Headache disorders and public health. Education and management implications*. Geneva: WHO, 2000.

Section

II

Patient-centred measures: health-related quality of life

15 Measuring health-related quality of life: general principles

Patrick Henry, Virginie Chrysostome, Philippe Michel, and
Jean François Dartigues

Every one knows the importance of headache-related disability but the disruptive effect of headache is not confined to the duration and intensity of the attack. Between attacks, headache and especially migraine may impart a burden of fear and anxiety to the sufferers, who often report difficulties in interacting with family, friends, or work colleagues. The combination of these factors may lead headache sufferers to modify their behaviour. To appreciate the effects of headache therapy, clinical measures such as frequency, severity, time to relief of pain, and the presence or relief of associated symptoms are important, but, in the primary headache disorders, the traditional outcome measures used in other diseases such as physical markers, biological tests, or diagnostic images are not relevant. Everyone feels that the traditional clinical measures are insufficient to evaluate the real burden of headaches. There are other criteria such as work performance, economic cost, and patient-perceived quality of life (QoL)[1] that seem more appropriate for quantifying headache-related disability.

The concept of health-related quality of life (HRQoL)

In everyday language, the term 'quality of life' is usually used to describe what the individual perceives as positive. However, as the frames of references are different, the meaning of the term may vary widely between individuals.

Since the individual's subjective well-being is a central component of the quality of life concept, it is difficult to give a completely objective definition. The World Health Organization defines QoL as 'The individual's perception of their position in life, in the context of culture and value systems in which they live, and in relation to their goals, expectations, standards and concerns. It is a very wide concept which may be influenced by the person's physical and psychological condition, level of independence, social relationships, environment and personal beliefs.'

Dahlöf[2] in defining HRQoL draws attention to three major factors, well-being, health, and welfare, based on objective and subjective effects. *General well-being* is the expression of the individual's subjective perception and describes a personal evaluation of general well-being in relation to a disorder, treatment, or both. This subjective variable comprises the individual's global judgement of what is positive and negative in his life. A high general well-being does not mean absence of negative events but the preponderance of positive facts. *Health* is the second important factor in HRQoL. Its evaluation is based on objective signs of illness and subjective symptoms that the individual perceives as obvious signs of illness, for example, pain, tiredness, and loss of appetite. *Welfare* is an expression of factors that can be assessed objectively, such as consumption of drugs, consultations, need for ambulance transport, etc. It is also important to appreciate the effect of medical treatment on the patient's quality of life, which is the result of the positive and negative effects of the treatment on each of the three main factors.

In brief, HRQoL represents the net effect of an illness and its consequent therapy on a patient's perception of his ability to live a useful and fulfilling life.

Quality of life measures

To evaluate the HRQoL and to apply the results in various clinical and research settings, standardized instruments were scientifically developed and evaluated with regard to reliability, validity, and sensitivity.[3,4] *Reliability* describes how stable or reproducible the questionnaire is when used for repeated measurements. Reliability issues of internal consistency and test–retest, interrater, and intrarater agreement must be statistically analysed. *Validity* represents the ability of a questionnaire to measure what it is intended to measure. The three main charecteristics of validity are content validity, criterion validity, and construct validity.

◆   Content validity is determined by critical analysis based on explicit criteria of the appropriateness of the HRQoL definition, the relevance of its dimensions, and the semantic content and way of formulating of items in relation to the dimensions used to describe the quality of life.
◆   Criteria validity is determined by comparing the concordance of the results of the studied measurement tool with an external criterion considered as a reference measure.
◆   Construct validity is determined by comparing the concordance of the results of the studied measurement tool with one of other measurements of HRQoL, in the absence of reference.

The *sensitivity* of a questionnaire represents its ability to record changes that are clinically or statistically relevent for the patient and physician.

HRQoL can be measured with generic and/or specific instruments. Generic questionnaires allow comparisons between different populations and diseases, whereas specific questionnaires are designed to study problems associated with only one disease.

Generic HRQoL instruments

These may be used to measure the HRQoL, whatever the health problem of the studied population. At present, at least 11 generic scales have been described: short form (SF)-20, SF-36, NPH (Nottingham Health Profile), EuroQol, Coop/Wonca, MSEP (Minor Symptoms Evaluation Profile), SSAP (Subjective Symptoms Assessment Profile), PGWB (Psychological General Well-Being), QWB (Quality of Well Being Scale), QWB-SA (Quality of Well-Being Scale self-administered), and HFHDI (Henry Ford Headache Disability Inventory). All are written in English. Some have been translated into other languages and validated.[4,5]

The Medical Outcomes Study short form (SF-36) is the most widely used in the world. In the field of headache studies, the SF-36 appears to be a robust instrument with a good reliability, internal consistency, and content validity, and very good discriminative validity and sensitivity. The SF-36 is made up of 36 items that assess: physical functioning (10 items); role functioning (4 items); bodily pain (2 items); general health (5 items); vitality (4 items); social functioning (2 items); emotional state (3 items); mental health (5 items); and health transition (1 item). A major advantage of using the SF-36 in headache evaluation is the wealth of data accumulated with the questionnaire. Data have been obtained from headache patients from the general population, from the workplace, and from patients enrolled in many clinical trials. Three main results will be discussed here:

When SF-36 profiles were compared between patients with migraine and those with other chronic conditions such as arthritis, diabetes, hypertension, and angina, the burden of perceived HRQoL for migrainers was worse in certain domains, not only for pain but also with regard to role functioning, social functioning, mental health, and health perception (ref. 6; see also Chapter 16, this volume). Solomon et al.[7] using the SF-20 showed that each common headache disorder has a relatively specific HRQoL score profile. In the last 10 years, the SF-36 has been used in the evaluation of specific headache treatments, essentially the triptans (for example, see Chapter 21, this volume).

Other health scales used in migraine include the Sickness Index Profile and the Nottingham Health Profile, which measure behaviour and perceived health status. The Psychological Well-Being (PGWB) index assesses changes in the patient's sense of well-being while the Minor Symptoms Evaluation Profile (MSEP) is designed to evaluate subjective central nervous system-related symptoms that might affect a patient's well-being.[5]

These different scales are relevant for studying some aspects of quality of life but their use is not widespread at the moment, so comparative studies are difficult to perform. At the present time, the SF-36 has become the most used and one of the standard measures of the HRQoL in headache populations. However, generic HRQoL instruments may be less useful for measuring changes in the population over time than disease-specific instruments.

Disease-specific instruments

These have been developed to evaluate limitations or restrictions of HRQoL associated with a specific state not usually included in generic surveys. Disease-specific instruments may be more sensitive in evaluating the long-term effects of treatment, in comparing different treatments for a given disease, or in highlighting variations in a patient's perception of HRQoL during the course of a disease. At the present time, there are many headache-specific and especially migraine-specific QoL instruments; many of them were developed under sponsorship by the pharmaceutical industry to evaluate the effects of therapy on quality of life. Here we will only examine general principles. To develop and test headache-specific instruments, three successive steps are usually followed:

(1) identification of items relevant to those with migraine through quantitative interviews;
(2) formation and testing of a draft questionnaire;
(3) development of the final questionnaire and evaluation of its validity, reliability, and feasability.

The existing questionnaires may be classified into different categories:

◆ disability and productivity instruments: MIDAS (Migraine Disability Assessment), MWPLQ (Migraine Work and Productivity Loss Questionnaire), MBQ (Migraine Background Questionnaire), HDI (Henry Ford Hospital Disability Inventory);[8]
◆ HRQoL instruments: MSQoL,[9] QVM (Qualité de Vie et Migraine—only in French);[10]
◆ HRQoL and productivity composite instruments: Migraine-specific Quality of Life Questionnaire (MSQ), HImQ (Headache Impact Questionnaire), and Brief 24 Hour MSQoL.

Most instruments study HRQoL during and between the headache attacks but Santanello *et al.*[11] developed their migraine-specific quality of life questionnaire to assess the quality of life decrease associated with an acute migraine attack in the 24-hour period following headache onset (Brief 24 Hour MSQoL).

Langeveld *et al.*[12] developed the Quality of Life Headache Youth (QLH-Y) questionnaire to assess quality of life in adolescents with chronic headache including migraine.

Characteristics of measures that have been used in recent studies are summarized in Table 15.1. We have chosen to analyse only four questionnaires, which seemed to us to be the most interesting.

The QVM questionnaire[10]

This questionnaire includes 20 items. The feasibility, validity, and reliability of the questionnaire were assessed during a study performed on 107 patients. The study was designed as a test–retest study, the self-assessment questionnaire being filled in

Table 15.1 Headache-specific measures

Instrument (ref. no.)	Number of items	Description*	Internal consistency	Test–retest reliability	Validity			Sensitivity
					Convergent	Content	Discriminative	
QVM (10)	20	4 dimensions: psychological; physical; social; iatrogenic	++	++	++	++	++	+
Brief 24 hour MSQoL (11)	15	5 dimensions: work; social; energy; concerns; symptoms	++	++	+	+++	++	+++
MSQoL (9)	25	General QoL	++	+	+	+++	?	++
QLH-Y (12)	71	6 dimensions: psychological; functional; physical; social; general satisfaction with life; satisfaction with health	++	++	++	++	++	?

*All questionnaires in this table are self-administered.

twice at an interval of 1 week. The filling in time was on average 8 minutes. The items were assessed 'very interesting' or 'interesting' by 94% of the patients, and 'easy' or 'fairly easy' to understand by 96%.

The principal component analysis performed on the whole sample allowed the extraction of four meaningful factors that were in agreement with the predefined structure of the QVM questionnaire. The first axis was a factor of psychological repercussion, the second axis was a factor of functional and somatic repercussion, the third was a factor of social repercussion and the fourth was a factor of disturbance generated by the treatment. The QVM questionnaire allowed the calculation of a global index of life and indices according to the multifactorial structure. The global index was significantly higher for the most severe patients recruited in hospital, which means that the repercussion of migraine on quality of life was greater than for patients of general practitioners. Thus, the measures obtained are sensitive to the severity of migraine. The reliability of the different indices as assessed by the correlation coefficient between the test–retest measures is good. Unfortunately, QVM is a French questionnaire, not translated into English.

The 24 Hour MSQoL questionnaire[11]

This questionnaire was developed to assess QoL in the 24-hour period after an acute migraine attack. The questionnaire has 15 questions across five domains (work functioning, social functioning, energy, concerns, and symptoms). It showed very good internal consistency, construct and discriminant validity, and responsiveness to acute migraine attacks. This questionnaire is a composite evaluation of a patient's day with migraine and of the impact of acute therapy.

The MSQoL questionnaire[9]

This was designed to assess the long-term QoL resulting from migraine. This reliable and validated 25-item questionnaire is probably the most utilized among the specific instruments. Its internal consistency, reproducibility, and construct validity are high. The MSQoL questionnaire measures psychological well-being more than functional status.

The QLH-Y questionnaire[12]

QLH-Y was developed for adolescents between 12 and 18 years of age. It is a 71-item QoL measurement scale. Thirteen subscales were developed to cover the four QoL subdomains: psychological functioning; functional status; physical status; and social functioning. Satisfaction with life in general and satisfaction with health were covered by two visual analogue scales.

Combined use of generic and specific questionnaires

It may be useful to compare general health status, measured for example by the SF-36 or the PGWB, and headache-specific QoL questionnaires.[13] Analysis of the data supplied by the two types of questionnaires, first separately and then jointly, makes it possible to evaluate their relevance and to appreciate the gain of information. For instance, Wagner et al.[9] studied the correlation between the MSQoL measure and other measures with similar constructs. Correlations between the MSQoL and PGWB ranged from 0.42 to 0.54 and those between the MSQoL and SF-36 from 0.32 to 0.53. In general, correlations between the MSQoL and the PGWB were higher than those for the SF-36. Study of correlations suggests that the MSQoL measures something other than functional status, which is probably the global subjective impact of migraine headaches.

Conclusion

We have valid and reliable tools at the moment to evaluate general and headache-specific QoL. These tools are valuable for assessing aspects of the burden of disease on individual headache sufferers. They can be used as an outcome measure in clinical practice or clinical trials. They may be used to identify treatments that optimize outcomes. Nevertheless, no single instrument is at present recognized as the gold standard in headache QoL assessment. Many different QoL instruments are at our disposal and the headache community has to evaluate which outcome measure or measures are most valid to be recommended.

References

1. Solomon GD. Evolution of the measurement of quality of life in migraine. *Neurology* 1997; **48** (Suppl. 3): S10–S15.
2. Dahlöf CGH. Assessment of health-related quality of life in migraine. *Cephalalgia* 1993; **13**: 233–7.
3. Steiner DL, Norman GV. *Health measurement scales*, 2nd edn. Oxford: Oxford University Press, 1995.
4. Last JM. *A dictionary of epidemiology*. Oxford: Oxford University Press, 2001.
5. Solomon GD, Dahlöf CGH (2000). Impact of headache on the individual sufferer. In *The headaches*, 2nd edn (ed. Olesen J, Tfelt-Hansen P, Welch KMA). Philadadelphia: Lippincott-Williams and Wilkins, 2000: 25–31.
6. Osterhaus JT, TownseNd RJ, Gandek B, Ware JE. Measuring the functional status and well-being of patients with migraine headache. *Headache* 1994; **34**: 337–43.
7. Solomon GD, Skobieranda FG, Gragg LA. Does quality of life differ among headache diagnoses? Analysis using the Medical Outcomes Study instrument. *Headache* 1994; **34**: 143–7.
8. Holroyd KA, Penzian DB, Lipchik GL. Behavioral management of headache. In *Wolff's headache and other head pain*, 7th edn (ed. Silberstein SD, Lipton RB, Dalassio DJ). New York: Oxford University Press, 2001: 562–606.
9. Wagner TH, Patrick D, Galer BS, Berzon RA. A new instrument to assess the long-term quality of life effects from migraine: development and psychometric testing of the MSQoL. *Headache* 1996; **36**: 484–92.
10. Richard A, Henry P, Chazot G, *et al*. Qualité de la vie et migraine. Validation du questionnaire QVM en consultation hospitalière et en médecine générale. *Thérapie* 1993; **48**: 89–96.

11. Santanello NC, Hartmaier SL, Epstein RS, Silberstein SD. Validation of a new quality of life questionnaire for acute migraine headache. *Headache* 1995; **35**: 330–7.

12. Langeveld JH., Koot HM, Loonen MCR, Hazebrook-Kampschreur AJM, Passchier J. A quality of life instrument for adolescents with chronic headache. *Cephalalgia* 1996; **16**: 183–96.

13. Michel P, Henry P. Etude de la qualité de vie des migraineux. In *Expertise collective Inserm eds. La migraine. Connaissances descriptives, traitement et prévention*. Paris: Editions Inserm, 1998: 265–74.

16
Effect of headache on quality of life

G.M. Terwindt, M.D. Ferrari, and L.J. Launer

....

Introduction

Both general and disease-specific quality of life (QoL) measurements can be used to evaluate health-related quality of life (HRQoL) in headache patients. General HRQoL measurements can provide a method for comparing the burden of different types of headache. Furthermore, with a general instrument the impact on HRQoL of headache can be compared with that of other diseases. Examples of general instruments are the Medical Outcomes Study Short Form-20 (SF-20) and the Medical Outcomes Study Short Form Health Survey (SF-36). Disease-specific HRQoL questionnaires focus on particular limitations or restrictions associated with a specific disease status and can be very useful as an outcome measure in clinical trials or clinical practice to identify treatments that optimize outcomes.[1,2] Examples of migraine-specific HRQoL instruments are the 24-hour Migraine-specific Quality of Life (24-h MSQoL), the Migraine-Specific Quality of Life (MSQoL) questionnaire, and the Migraine-Specific Quality of Life (MSQ) questionnaire.

HRQoL studies can be performed in patients referred to a headache clinic, but these patients represent a selected group of headache patients. This may not be a problem when studying the effect of specific headache treatments on HRQoL. Population-based studies also identify patients with headache who never see a physician for their headache and, therefore, will give a clearer picture of the effect of headache on HRQoL.

Impact of migraine on HRQoL in the general population

In a large Dutch population-based study we compared the HRQoL of migraineurs and non-migraineurs.[3] The HRQoL of migraineurs was also compared with people from the same cohort with asthma, chronic musculoskeletal pain, and both conditions. Both conditions reportedly have a higher prevalence in migraineurs than in non-migraineurs[4–9] and both affect HRQoL.[10–13] In addition, each condition shares different common characteristics with migraine: asthma is a chronic paroxysmal disorder and chronic musculoskeletal pain is a chronic pain disorder.

Table 16.1 Dimensions of HRQoL in the Medical Outcome Study Short Form RAND-36

Dimension	Abbreviation	Number of items	Definition
Physical functioning	PF	10	Capacity to perform a variety of common physical activities
Social functioning	SF	2	Extent to which health interferes with social activities (previous 4 weeks)
Role limitations (physical)	RP	4	Extent to which physical health interferes with daily activities (previous 4 weeks)
Role limitations (emotional)	RE	3	Extent to which emotional problems interfere with daily activities (previous 4 weeks)
Mental health	MH	5	General mood or affect in previous 4 weeks
Pain	BP	2	Bodily pain in previous 4 weeks
Vitality	VT	4	General energy, level of fatigue in previous 4 weeks
General health perception	GH	5	Overall rating of health in general

To assess HRQoL we used the Dutch version of the RAND-36, a questionnaire developed from the Medical Outcome Study General Health Survey Instrument.[14] The RAND-36 includes 36 items measuring health across eight domains (Table 16.1). Responses to each item within a dimension are combined to generate a score from 0–100, where 100 indicates best functioning.[14] Because the RAND-36 measures the perception of health in the previous 4 weeks, the analysis was based on 620 migraineurs who had active migraine during the last year.

Of the 620 migraineurs who were identified, 396 persons (63.9%) had migraine without aura only, 111 (17.9%) migraine with aura, and 81 (13.1%) attacks of both types. Five per cent could not be classified. The median number of migraine attacks was 12 per year; 25% of migraineurs suffered at least two attacks per month. Among the non-migraineurs, 171 persons (3.2%) were identified with asthma and 1345 persons (25%) with chronic musculoskeletal pain. Among the migraineurs 30 persons (5%) had asthma and 239 persons (39%) had chronic musculoskeletal pain. Compared to non-migraineurs, migraineurs had significantly more frequent asthma (odds ratio (OR), 1.6; 95% confidence interval (CI), 1.1–2.4) and chronic musculoskeletal pain (OR, 1.7; 95% CI, 1.5–2.1).

The scores of the eight RAND-36 domains for migraineurs are shown in Fig. 16.1. Compared to non-migraineurs, migraineurs reported diminished functioning on all eight RAND-36 dimensions, which cover physical, social, and mental functioning ($p < 0.0001$). There was no difference in HRQoL among migraine subtypes. For all eight dimensions of the RAND-36, HRQoL decreased with increasing frequency of

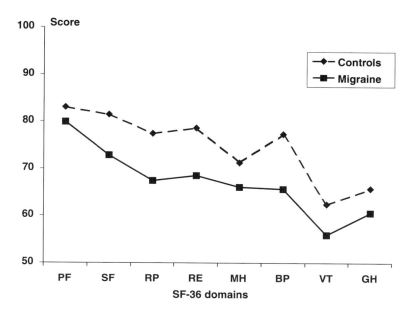

Fig. 16.1 RAND-36 scores. Migraine group ($n=620$) and control group ($n=5378$). Interpretation of scores: a lower score indicates diminished functioning or well-being. There was a significant difference between migraineurs and controls ($p<0.0001$), controlling for sex, age, socio-economic class, region of residence, and marital status, for all domains. (See Table 16.1 for an explanation of the abbreviations and a description of the domains.)

migraine attacks ($p<0.0002$). The scores of the eight RAND-36 domains for subjects with migraine, asthma, and both asthma and migraine are shown in Fig. 16.2. Compared to controls, asthma cases scored lower on three RAND-36 dimensions, including physical functioning, pain, and general health perception. Compared to asthma cases, migraineurs scored significantly lower on five of the eight RAND-36 domains, including social functioning, role limitations (emotional), mental health, pain, and vitality. There was no difference in the physical functioning domains and the general health perception domain between migraineurs and asthma cases. Compared to controls, those with both asthma and migraine had significantly lower scores on the dimensions including physical functioning, role limitations (physical), mental health, pain, vitality, and general health perception. Compared to those with migraine only, cases with both migraine and asthma had significantly lower scores on dimensions of physical functioning and general health perception. Compared to those with asthma only, cases with both migraine and asthma had significantly lower scores on the dimension of pain and general health perception.

The RAND-36 scores for migraineurs, subjects with chronic musculoskeletal pain, and subjects with both chronic musculoskeletal pain and migraine are shown in Fig. 16.3. Compared to controls, persons with chronic musculoskeletal pain scored significantly lower on all RAND-36 dimensions. Compared to migraineurs, those

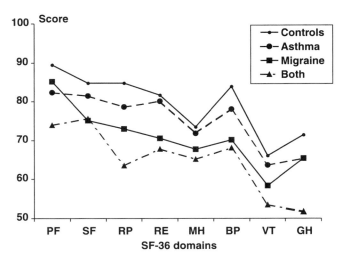

Fig.16.2 RAND-36 scores for the migraine group (n=589), asthma group (n=171), migraine+asthma group (n=30), and control group (n=5293). Fifteen persons are not included in this figure because of missing data on asthma. Interpretation of scores: a lower score indicates diminished functioning or well-being. Analysis of variance controlling for sex, age, socio-economic class, region of residence, and marital status. There was a significant difference between asthma and control groups ($p < 0.0001$ to 0.0003) for the PF, BP, and GH domains. There was a significant difference between the migraine and control groups ($p < 0.0001$) for all domains. There was a significant difference between the migraine+asthma (both) and control groups ($p < 0.0001$ to 0.0038) for the PF, RP, MH, BP, VT, and GH domains. There was a significant difference between the asthma and migraine groups ($p < 0.0006$ to 0.0030) for the SF, RE, MH, BP, and VT domains. There was a significant difference between the asthma and the migraine+asthma groups ($p < 0.0028$) for the BP and GH domains. There was a significant difference between the migraine and the migraine+asthma groups ($p < 0.0002$) for the PF and GH domains. (See Table 16.1 for an explanation of the abbreviations and a description of the domains.)

with chronic musculoskeletal pain scored significantly lower on five of the eight RAND-36 domains, including physical functioning, role limitations (physical), pain, vitality, and general health perception. Compared to controls, persons with both chronic musculoskeletal pain and migraine scored significantly lower on all RAND-36 dimensions. Compared to subjects with only migraine or chronic musculoskeletal pain, those with both migraine and chronic musculoskeletal pain had significantly lower scores for all eight RAND-36 domains.

In this population-based study we found that migraineurs, regardless of subtype, have poorer HRQoL compared to non-migraineurs. Frequency of attacks (used as a measure of disease severity) showed a clear inverse relationship indicating that HRQoL reduced with increasing migraine attack frequency.

In subanalyses we compared migraine with asthma and chronic musculoskeletal pain for HRQoL and found that migraineurs have poorer HRQoL compared to patients with asthma, but not compared to patients with chronic musculoskeletal

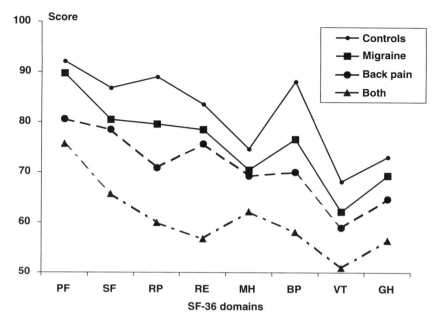

Fig. 16.3 RAND-36 scores for the migraine group (n=381), chronic musculoskeletal pain (back pain) group (n=1345), the migraine+chronic musculoskeletal pain group (n=239), and the control group (n=4033). Interpretation of scores: a lower score indicates diminished functioning or well-being. Analysis of variance controlling for sex, age, socio-economic class, region of residence, and marital status. There was a significant difference between the chronic back pain and the control groups (p<0.0001) for all RAND-36 domains. There was a significant difference between the migraine and control groups (p<0.0001 to 0.0042) for all RAND-36 domains. There was a significant difference between the chronic back pain+ migraine (both) and control groups (p<0.0001) for all RAND-36 domains. There was a significant difference between the chronic back pain and migraine groups (p<0.0001 to 0.0007) for the PF, RP, BP, VT, and GH domains. There was a significant difference between the chronic back pain and the chronic back pain+migraine (both) groups (p<0.0001) for all RAND-36 domains. There was a significant difference between the migraine and the chronic back pain+migraine (both) groups (p<0.0001) for all RAND-36 domains. (See Table 16.1 for an explanation of the abbreviations and a description of the domains.)

pain. When comparing these three disorders, we found that the impact of migraine was greater on social and mental functioning, whereas asthma and chronic musculo-skeletal pain had more impact on physical functioning. Comorbidity of migraine with asthma or chronic musculoskeletal pain results in lower social, mental, and physical functioning than one of the two conditions alone. Possibly migraineurs have a lower pain threshold. However, we cannot exclude the possibility of reporting bias resulting from more subjects with migraine self-reporting chronic musculoskeletal pain or asthma.

From this study it was concluded that migraineurs, regardless of subtype, suffer from compromised HRQoL, especially those with high frequency of attacks.

Migraineurs have a higher prevalence of asthma and chronic musculoskeletal pain, and decreased HRQoL in subjects with migraine may be partly due to these comorbid conditions.

It has been recognized that migraineurs have an increased occurrence of depression,[15,16] and depression is associated with poorer HRQoL.[12,17] In this study the (co-)occurrence of depression was not investigated and, therefore, the influence of comorbidity of depression on HRQoL in migraineurs cannot be estimated.

Migraine, quality of life, and depression

Lipton *et al.* conducted two population-based studies in the USA and UK in which 389 migraine cases (with six or more attacks per year) and 379 non-migraine controls completed the Short Form (SF)-12, and the Primary Care Evaluation of Mental Disorders (PRIME-MD), a mental health screening tool.[18] The SF-12 measures HRQoL in two domains: a mental health component score (MCS-12) and a physical health component score (PCS-12).

Depression and migraine were highly comorbid; 47% (183/389) of migraineurs had PRIME-MD defined depression compared to 17% (64/379) of the controls (adjusted prevalence ratio, 2.7; 95% CI, 2.1–3.5). Depressed subjects had lower HRQoL scores than non-depressed subjects. There were no significant differences in MCS-12 and PCS-12 scores between migraine cases and controls among depressed subjects. There were, however, significant differences in MCS-12 and PCS-12 scores between non-depressed migraine cases and controls. Both depression and migraine were significantly and independently associated with lower MCS-12 and PCS-12 scores. Depression had a larger effect than migraine on both scores. Attack frequency was a strong predictor of decreased MCS-12 and PCS-12 scores. For the MCS-12, headache-related disability (headache interfered with daily activities half the time or more) was also a strong predictor of decreased MCS-12 scores.

Lipton *et al.* concluded from this study that migraineurs have reduced HRQoL regardless of whether they are also depressed. However, HRQoL was significantly reduced in subjects with migraine and depression compared with that in those who were not depressed. Both our study and that of Lipton *et al.* found that headache frequency was an important predictor of HRQoL.

Does HRQoL differ among headache diagnoses?

To analyse the differences in HRQoL associated with different headache diagnoses Solomon *et al.* performed a clinic based study in 208 headache patients.[19] Of these 208 patients, 79 patients had migraine, 41 patients tension-type headache, 13 patients cluster headache, and 49 patients mixed headaches (chronic tension-type headache and migraine). The SF-20 was used to assess HRQoL.

Cluster headache patients had a significantly higher (worse) pain score and included a higher percentage of patients with poor health due to pain when compared to patients with migraine headache. Cluster patients had a generally well preserved physical functioning compared with that of tension-type or mixed headache patients. Cluster and tension-type headache showed more limitation in social functioning than migraine. Chronic tension-type headache was marked by a lower level of mental health compared with that associated with migraine. Solomon *et al.* concluded that distinct headache diagnoses are marked by unique patterns of impairment of HRQoL.

However, the patient sample in this study may represent the more severely afflicted headache patients who seek care at a specialized headache referral centre. Furthermore, comorbidity and confounding of depression was not investigated in this study.

HRQoL differences between patients with episodic and transformed migraine?

To investigate specifically whether there are HRQoL differences between patients with episodic migraine and those with transformed migraine Meletiche *et al.* investigated 90 patients (46 with transformed migraine, 44 with episodic migraine) using the SF-36 questionnaire.[20] Over the last 90 days prior to their first visit, patient with transformed migraine reported having a headache significantly more often compared with patients with migraine (69 days and 18 days, respectively). Compared with patients with episodic migraine, patients with transformed migraine had significantly lower mean scores on seven of the eight SF-36 domains and both the mental and physical summary scores of the SF-36.

Meletiche *et al.* concluded that patients with transformed migraine have a lower HRQoL than patients with episodic migraine and suggested that headache chronicity associated with transformed migraine has a significant influence on HRQoL. Comorbidity and confounding of depression was not investigated in this study.

HRQoL differs among headache diagnoses

Wang *et al.* evaluated HRQoL in 901 patients who visited a headache clinic by using the SF-36 and the Hospital Anxiety and Depression Scale (HADS).[21] They compared HRQoL in patients with episodic migraine (*n*=193) and chronic daily headache (CDH) (*n*=541). Of the CDH group, 310 patients were classified as transformed migraine (TM) and 231 patients as chronic tension-type headache (CTTH).

SF-36 scores were compared after controlling for the HADS, age, gender, education, and chronic illness by multiple linear regression analyses. Compared with migraine patients, the patients with TM had significantly lower scores in all scales, except for the physical functioning (PF), social functioning (SF), and role limitations–emotional (RE) scales. Patients with CTTH had SF-36 scores that were compatible with those of patients with migraine, except for bodily pain (BP; CTTH > migraine) and mental health (MH; CTTH > migraine) scales. Compared with

CTTH patients, the TM patients scored significantly lower in all SF-36 scales except for the PF and RE scales. Wang *et al.* concluded from their study that the SF-36 scores in patients with CDH depend on the percentages of the types of patients in the sample: the greater the number of TM patients, the more impaired the SF-36 scores will be.

Conclusions

Population based studies have shown that migraineurs have reduced HRQoL independent of depression. Furthermore, HRQoL is more reduced with increasing migraine attack frequency.

SF-36 scores in patients with chronic daily headache (CDH) depend on the distribution of the types of patients in the sample; the greater the number of transformed migraine (TM) cases, the more impaired the SF-36 scores will be. There are no population-based HRQoL studies with validated HRQoL questionnaires on chronic daily headache.

References

1. Lipton RB, Stewart WF. Health-related quality of life in headache research. *Headache* 1995; **35** (8): 447–8.
2. Solomon, GD, Santanello N. Impact of migraine and migraine therapy on productivity and quality of life. *Neurology* 2000; **55** (9 Suppl. 2): S29–S35.
3. Terwindt GM, Ferrari MD, Tijhuis M, Groenen SM, Picavet HS, Launer LJ. The impact of migraine on quality of life in the general population: the GEM study. *Neurology* 2000; **55** (5): 624–9.
4. Chen TC, Leviton A. Asthma and eczema in children born to women with migraine. *Arch Neurol* 1990; **47**: 1227–30.
5. Duckro PN, Schultz KT, Chibnall JT. Migraine as a sequela to chronic low back pain. *Headache* 1994; **34**: 279–81.
6. Schéle R, Ahlborg B, Ekbom K. Physical characteristics and allergic history in young men with migraine and other headaches. *Headache* 1978; **18**: 80–6.
7. Stang., Sternfeld B, Sidney S. Migraine headache in a prepaid health plan: ascertainment, demographics, physiological, and behavioral factors. *Headache* 1996; **36**: 69–76.
8. Ziegler DK, Hassanein RS, Couch JR. Characteristics of life headache histories in a nonclinic population. *Neurology* 1977; **27**: 265–9.
9. Vernon H, Steiman I, Hagino C. Cervicogenic dysfunction in muscle contraction headache and migraine: a descriptive study. *J Manipulative Physiol Ther* 1992; **15** (7): 418–29.
10. Solomon GD, Skobieranda FG, Gragg LA. Quality of life and well-being of headache patients: measurement by the Medical Outcomes Study instrument. *Headache* 1993; **33**: 351–8.
11. Stewart AL, Greenfield S, Hays RD, Wells K, Rogers WH, Berry SD, McGlynn EA, Ware JE. Functional status and well-being of patients with chronic conditions. *J Am Med Assoc* 1989; **262**: 907–13.
12. Lyons, RA, Lo SV, Littlepage BNC. Comparative health status of patients with 11 common illnesses in Wales. *J Epidemiol Commun Hlth* 1994; **48**: 388–90.

13. Beltman FW, Heesen WF, Tuinman RG, and Meyboom-de Jong B. Functionele status van patienten met chronische aandoeningen. *Tijdschr Soc Gezondheidsz* 1995; **73**: 128–34.

14. van der Zee K, Sanderman R, Heyink J. A comparison of two multidimensial measures of health status: the Nottingham Health Profile and the RAND 36-item health survey 1.0. *Qual Life Res* 1996; **5**: 165–74.

15. Breslau N, Davis GC. Migraine, physical health and psychiatric disorder: a prospective epidemiologic study in young adults. *J Psychiatr Res* 1993; **27**: 211–21.

16. Keck PE, Jr, Merikangas KR, McElroy SL, Strakowski SM. Diagnostic and treatment implications of psychiatric comorbidity with migraine [review]. *Ann Clin Psychiatry* 1994; **6**: 165–71.

17. Wells KB, Stewart A, Hays RD, Burnam MA, Rogers W, Daniels M, Berry S, Greenfield S, Ware J. The functioning and well-being of depressed patients. results from the Medical Outcomes Study. *J Am Med Assoc* 1989; **262**: 914–19.

18. Lipton RB, Hamelsky SW, Kolodner KB, Steiner TJ, Stewart WF. Migraine, quality of life, and depression: a population-based case-control study. *Neurology* 2000; **55** (5): 629–35.

19. Solomon GD, Skobieranda FG, Gragg LA. Does quality of life differ among headache diagnoses? Analysis using the Medical Outcomes Study instrument. *Headache* 1994; **34** (3): 143–7.

20. Meletiche DM, Lofland JH, Young WB. Quality-of-life differences between patients with episodic and transformed migraine. *Headache* 2001; **41** (6): 573–8.

21. Wang SJ, Fuh JL, Lu SR, Juang KD. Quality of life differs among headache diagnoses: analysis of SF-36 survey in 901 headache patients. *Pain* 2001; **89** (2–3): 285–92.

17 Assessment of the responsiveness of the Migraine-Specific Quality of Life Questionnaire (version 2.1)

Bradley C. Martin, Dev S. Pathak, W. Jackie Kwong,
Alice S. Batenhorst, and Marc Sharfman

Introduction

Migraine, a chronic headache disorder that is episodic in nature, has been known to significantly interfere with daily functioning and patient well-being. Migraineurs often have to limit their activities and make adjustments in their lifestyle due to the occurrence of migraine, or to avoid future migraine attacks. Measurement of health-related quality of life (HRQoL) is important because it allows researchers and clinicians to better describe and quantify the overall benefits of migraine treatments to the patients.

The Migraine-Specific Quality of Life questionnaire (MSQ, version 1.0) was developed in 1991 to assess the effect of migraine and treatment on patient's HRQoL in sumatriptan clinical trials.[1] Results from clinical trials and feedback from patient focus groups suggested that the instrument should be revised to reduce wording ambiguity and enhance scoring. MSQ (version 2.0) incorporated the refined items and standardized response format. Confirmatory factor analysis suggested that two items should be deleted. The deletion of two items resulted in a revised 14-item MSQ (version 2.1).[2] Although previous psychometric evaluations of the MSQ (version 2.1) had shown the instrument to be reliable and valid,[3] to be useful as an evaluative instrument, an HRQoL instrument should also be responsive and be able to detect clinically meaningful changes. We assessed the responsiveness of the MSQ (version 2.1) and the results are presented here.

Study design

Data from two non-drug, prospective, parallel-group, quasi-experimental studies were used in the assessment of responsiveness. Patients were adult migraineurs with a 1-year history of migraine as determined by the International Headache Society (IHS) criteria, and had at least one to eight moderate to severe migraine attacks per month in the last 2 months prior to study. Two groups of patients were recruited at four headache clinics in a 2:1 ratio:

(1)   new patients who had not received migraine care delivered by a headache specialist prior to the study;
(2)   stable patients who had been under the care of the study investigator prior to the study and were not expected to require any change in their migraine medications during the 12-week study period.

Both groups of patients recruited for this study were under the care of the same study investigator during the 12-week study period. The study investigators could prescribe any abortive, prophylactic, and palliative medical treatment to study patients.

Patients were asked to complete questionnaires regarding migraine characteristics, satisfaction with medication and medical care, and HRQoL at baseline, 4 weeks, and 12 weeks after enrolment. Migraine-related quality of life was assessed using the MSQ (version 2.1). The MSQ (version 2.1) is a 14-item, self-administered questionnaire with three dimensions (Table 17.1).

Table 17.1   MSQ (version 2.1) contents, an abbreviated description of the items corresponding to the three dimensions*

Dimension 1: Role function—restrictive
- Interfered with how well patient dealt with family, friends and others
- Interfered with leisure time activities such as reading or exercising
- Had difficulty in performing work or daily activities
- Kept from getting as much done at work or at home
- Limited ability to concentrate on work or daily activities
- Migraine left patient too tired to do work or daily activities
- Limited the number of days on which the patient felt energetic

Dimension 2: Role function—preventive
- Cancelled work or daily activities because of migraine
- Needed help in handling routine tasks
- Stopped work or daily activities to deal with migraine symptoms
- Inability to go to social activities such as parties, etc.

Dimension 3: Emotional function
- Felt fed up or frustrated
- Felt like a burden on others
- Afraid of letting others down

---

*Each item is rated as: none of the time; a little bit of the time; some of the time; a good bit of the time; most of the time; or all of the time.

(1) The role-restrictive dimension (7 items) examines the degree to which limitations in daily activities are due to migraine.
(2) The role-preventive dimension (4 items) examines the degree to which interruptions in daily activities are due to migraine.
(3) The emotional function dimension (3 items) examines emotional feelings that are due to migraine.

Each dimension is scored from 0 to 100, where a higher score indicates a better health status.

Assessment of responsiveness

The responsiveness of the MSQ was assessed using data from new patients at 4 weeks and 12 weeks using three methods:

(1) standardized response mean (SRM), the mean change-from-baseline MSQ score divided by the standard deviation of change-from-baseline MSQ scores;[4]
(2) Glass's effect size (GES), the mean change-from-baseline MSQ scores divided by the standard deviation of baseline MSQ scores;[5]
(3) Guyatt's responsiveness statistic (GRS), the mean change-from-baseline MSQ score for patients who reported being 'better' (responders) divided by the standard deviation of change-from-baseline MSQ scores for patients reported to have 'no change' (non-responders).[6] Operationally, patients were considered to be 'better' if they reported global change in quality of life as 'at least moderately improved' on a seven-point categorical scale (almost the same, hardly any better at all; a little better; somewhat better; moderately better; a good deal better; a great deal better; a very great deal better). Patients were considered to have 'no change' if they reported to have no change, 'hardly any better' or 'hardly any worse' in global change in quality of life on a seven-point categorical scale.

An effect size of 0.2 to 0.5 was considered as small/modest, 0.5 to 0.8 as medium/moderate, and >0.8 as large.[7]

Results

Data from 119 new patients recruited for the study were available for analysis. Mean MSQ scores at 4 weeks and 12 weeks were significantly higher than at baseline ($p < 0.001$) for all three MSQ dimensions, suggesting improvement in quality of life after seeking care at study clinics (Fig. 17.1). Mean change-from-baseline scores ranged from 10 to 16 at 4 weeks and from 15 to 18 at 12 weeks across MSQ dimensions.

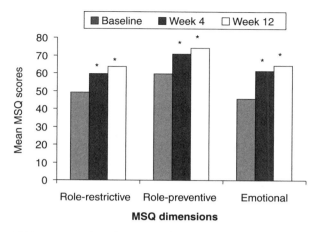

Fig. 17.1   Mean MSQ scores at baseline, 4 weeks, and 12 weeks for new subjects. *$p<0.001$ for difference with respect to baseline.

Table 17.2   Responsiveness statistics* at 4 and 12 weeks from baseline

| | Mean MSQ change of score from baseline at | | | | | |
| | 4 weeks from baseline | | | 12 weeks from baseline | | |
MSQ dimension	SRM	GES	GRS	SRM	GES	GRS
Role-restrictive	0.51	0.41	0.90	0.58	0.58	1.02
Role-preventive	0.43	0.40	0.78	0.54	0.51	0.84
Emotional function	0.53	0.55	0.96	0.60	0.65	0.89

*SRM, Mean change/standard deviation of change score; GES, mean change/standard deviation at baseline; GRS, mean change of responders/standard deviation change score of non-responders.

Results of the three types of responsiveness statistics are presented in Table 17.2. Since the standard deviation of change scores is close to the standard deviation of MSQ scores observed at baseline, it is expected that the GES estimates are similar to the SRMs. Because GRS includes only the mean change-from-baseline scores of responders (that is, those reported to be better) in the numerator, the GRS estimates are higher than the SRM and GES estimates. Overall, the responsiveness statistics ranged from 0.4 to 0.9 at 4 weeks, and ranged from 0.5 to 1.02 at 12 weeks.

Conclusions

The effect sizes of the MSQ dimension scores ranged from moderate to large, suggesting the MSQ is at least moderately responsive at 4 and 12 weeks from baseline and may be used as an evaluative tool to assess post-treatment quality of life improvements in clinical trials. Additional research is necessary to determine the minimum clinically important difference of the MSQ.

References

1. Jhingran P, Osterhaus JT, Miller DW, *et al*. Development and validation of the Migraine Specific Quality of Life Questionnaire. *Headache* 1998; **38**: 295–302.
2. Pathak D, Martin B, Kwong J, Batenhorst A. Evaluation of the Migraine-Specific Quality of Life Questionnaire (MSQ version 2.0) using confirmatory factor analysis. *Qual Life Res* 1998; **7**: 647.
3. Martin BC, Pathak DS, Sharfman MI, *et al*. Validity and reliability of the Migraine-Specific Quality of Life Questionnaire (MSQ version 2.1). *Headache* 2000; **40**: 204–15.
4. Liang MH, Fossel AH, Larson MG. Comparisons of five health status instruments for orthopedic evaluation. *Med Care* 1990; **28**: 632–42.
5. Kazis LE, Anderson JJ, Meenan RF. Effect sizes for interpreting changes in health status. *Med Care* 1989; **27**: 178–89.
6. Guyatt G, Walter S, Norman JG. Measuring change over time: assessing the usefulness of evaluative instruments. *J Chron Dis* 1987; **40**: 171–8.
7. Cohen J. *Statistical power analysis for the behavioral sciences*. New York: Academic Press, 1973.

18 Comparison of the impact of eletriptan versus sumatriptan on migraine-specific quality of life

Paula A. Funk-Orsini, Robert Miceli,
Joan Mackell, and Nicholas E.J. Wells

Introduction

Severe pain, migraine-associated symptoms, and disability frequently accompany a migraine attack, generating direct costs associated with medical care and indirect costs associated with lost productivity. Given these costs and the high prevalence of migraine worldwide, the economic burden of migraine is clearly substantial. In addition, the patient's health-related quality of life (HRQoL) is significantly reduced both during and between attacks.[1-3] Treatments that effectively relieve pain, the associated symptoms, and the functional impairment that accompanies a migraine attack should ultimately improve the patient's HRQoL.

Eletriptan is a potent, selective 5-HT$_{1B/1D}$ agonist that has previously been shown to provide rapid and effective relief of acute migraine in clinical trials.[4-8] Oral eletriptan has been shown to be clinically superior to oral sumatriptan for the treatment of migraine.[8] For both headache- and pain-free responses 2 hours postdose, oral eletriptan 40 mg and 80 mg were significantly better than oral sumatriptan 50 mg and 100 mg ($p < 0.05$).[8] Patients treated with eletriptan 40 mg also reported a greater improvement in functional status than those treated with sumatriptan 50 mg or 100 mg ($p < 0.01$).[8] Both doses of eletriptan were generally well tolerated and associated with significantly greater patient acceptability than either dose of sumatriptan ($p < 0.05$).[8]

The objective of the present study was to compare the impact of oral eletriptan 40 mg and 80 mg with that of oral sumatriptan 50 mg or 100 mg on migraine-specific QoL using data from a previously reported clinical trial.[8]

Methods

In this multicentre, double-blind, randomized, placebo-controlled, parallel-group trial, patients were randomized to one of seven treatment arms that consisted of a first and second dosing (first/second dose: eletriptan 40 mg/eletriptan 40 mg; eletriptan 40 mg/placebo; eletriptan 80 mg/eletriptan 80 mg; eletriptan 80 mg/placebo; sumatriptan 50 mg/sumatriptan 50 mg; sumatriptan 100 mg/sumatriptan 100 mg; and placebo/placebo). The second dose could be taken if a patient did not respond adequately within 2 hours or did so but experienced headache recurrence within 24 hours. For the eletriptan arms, patients received either the active treatment or placebo for their second dose; active treatment was used throughout the two sumatriptan arms.

The outcome measures were the mean scores on domains included within the 24-hour migraine-specific quality of life questionnaire (Brief 24-hour MSQoL). The Brief 24-hour MSQoL consists of 15 items across five domains: work functioning, social functioning, energy/vitality, migraine symptoms, and feelings/concerns. Each domain includes three items in which responses are recorded on a 7-point scale. A value of 1 indicates maximum impairment of HRQoL, while a value of 7 indicates no impairment. The maximum and minimum scores within each domain are 21 and 3, respectively.[9] Since the Brief 24-hour MSQoL is administered 24 h after initiating treatment for an acute migraine attack, its evaluation encompasses the patient's experience during the entire attack episode including the severity and duration of headache pain, associated symptoms, impaired functioning, efficacy and tolerability of therapy, and the need for a second dose or rescue medication.[9]

All analyses were based on 'first-attack' data and excluded patients with missing values in one or more MSQoL domains (no imputation was used). To compare treatment means between 'active–active' and 'active–placebo' treatment sequences for both doses of eletriptan, each domain of the MSQoL was analysed separately by analysis of variance (ANOVA). Since there were no significant differences between the 'active–active' and 'active–placebo' groups, patients in treatment sequences with the same first dose were pooled to increase statistical power. Treatment group differences were assessed by ANOVA followed by pair-wise treatment comparisons when the overall ANOVA was significant. The overall migraine-related QoL across all five domains for the eletriptan, sumatriptan, and placebo arms was evaluated using O'Brien's rank sum test.[10]

Results

Treatment groups were similar with respect to age, gender, and type and severity of migraine headache (Table 18.1). Patients taking either 40 mg or 80 mg of eletriptan had significantly better scores ($p < 0.05$) than placebo on all five domains of the 24-h MSQoL (Fig. 18.1 and Table 18.2). Both doses of eletriptan were significantly superior to sumatriptan 100 mg for the energy/vitality, work functioning, migraine and social functioning, and migraine symptoms domains. The MSQoL scores for eletriptan

Table 18.1 Demographic characteristics

| | | Sumatriptan | | Eletriptan | |
| | | | | | |
Characteristic	Placebo (n=79)	50 mg (n=169)	100 mg (n=152)	40 mg (n=163)	80 mg (n=154)
Gender (number (%))					
Female	70 (89)	152 (90)	133 (87)	143 (88)	133 (86)
Age (years)					
Mean ± SD*	36.8 ± 10.6	37.4 ± 10.2	38.1 ± 10.2	38.1 ± 10.1	39.5 ± 10.8
Type of migraine (number (%))					
Without aura	50 (63)	121 (71)	95 (62)	96 (59)	104 (67)
With/without aura	19 (24)	30 (18)	33 (22)	47 (29)	35 (23)
With aura	10 (13)	18 (11)	24 (16)	20 (12)	15 (10)
Baseline severity (number (%))†					
Mild	—	—	—	—	1 (1)
Moderate	46 (58)	96 (57)	88 (58)	95 (58)	92 (60)
Severe	33 (42)	73 (43)	64 (42)	68 (42)	61 (40)

*SD, Standard deviation.
†Numbers may not total 100% due to rounding.

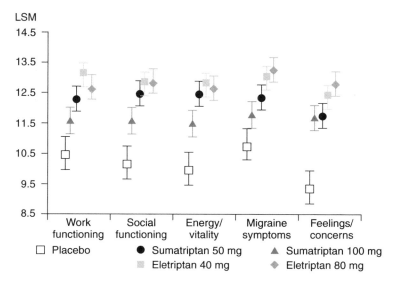

Fig. 18.1 Least square mean (LSM) scores (± SE) on the 24-hour MSQoL for patients treated with eletriptan, sumatriptan, or placebo. *$p < 0.05$ versus placebo. †$p < 0.05$ versus sumatriptan 100 mg.

Table 18.2 Least square means (± standard error (SE)) for quality of life domain by treatment group

	Work functioning	Social functioning	Energy/ vitality	Migraine symptoms	Feelings/ concerns
Placebo	10.5±0.6	10.2±0.6	10.0±0.6	10.8±0.5	9.4±0.5
Sumatriptan					
50 mg	12.3±0.4*	12.5±0.4*	12.5±0.4*	12.5±0.4*	11.8±0.4*
100 mg	11.6±0.4	11.6±0.4*	11.5±0.4*	11.8±0.4*	11.7±0.4*
Eletriptan					
40 mg	13.1±0.4*†	12.8±0.4*†	12.8±0.4*†	13.0±0.4*†	12.4±0.4*†
80 mg	12.7±0.4*†	12.9±0.4*†	12.7±0.4*†	13.3±0.4*†	12.8±0.4*†

*$p < 0.05$ versus placebo.
†$p < 0.05$ versus sumatriptan 100 mg.

(40 mg and 80 mg) were favourable across all domains in comparison to sumatriptan 50 mg, trending toward significance ($p < 0.10$) for the migraine symptoms and feelings/ concerns domains with eletriptan 80 mg. However, there were no statistically significant differences between either dose of eletriptan and sumatriptan 50 mg (Fig. 18.1 and Table 18.2).

The O'Brien's rank sum test indicated that patients receiving either dose of eletriptan experienced significantly better ($p < 0.05$) overall migraine-specific QoL than those receiving sumatriptan 100 mg. Both doses of eletriptan were also significantly better ($p < 0.0001$) than placebo in improving overall migraine-specific QoL. The improvements in QoL that eletriptan, in comparison to sumatriptan, provided are consistent with the improvements gained in relieving headache and associated symptoms previously reported with each of these drugs.[8]

Conclusions

Oral eletriptan was superior to sumatriptan 100 mg in improving overall migraine-specific QoL. Oral eletriptan was also significantly superior to placebo in improving overall migraine-specific QoL ($p < 0.0001$). The improvements in QoL that eletriptan provided compared to sumatriptan paralleled the extent of relief of headache and associated symptoms observed with each of these drugs.[8] The higher eletriptan dose can therefore be associated with increased headache response without detriment to QoL. Improvements in QoL with eletriptan were also consistent with its tolerability.

References

1. Hopkins A. The epidemiology of headache and migraine, and its meaning for neurological services. *Schweiz Med Wochenschr* 1996; **126** (4): 128–35.
2. Ferrari MD. The economic burden of migraine to society. *PharmacoEconomics* 1998; **13**: 667–76.
3. Hu HX, Markson LE, Lipton RB, *et al*. Burden of migraine in the United States: disability and economic costs. *Arch Intern Med* 1999; **159**: 813–18.
4. Solomon GD, Price KL (1997). Burden of migraine: a review of its socioeconomic impact. *PharmacoEconomics* 1997; **11** (Suppl.): 1–10.
5. Goadsby PJ, Ferrari MD, Olesen J, *et al*. (2000). Eletriptan in acute migraine: a double blind, placebo-controlled comparison to sumatriptan. *Neurology* 2000; **54**: 156–63.
6. Stark R, Dahlöf,C, Haughie S, *et al*. on behalf of the Eletriptan Steering Committee. Efficacy, safety and tolerability of oral eletriptan in the acute treatment of migraine: results of a phase III, multicentre, placebo-controlled study across three attacks. *Cephalalgia* 2002; **22** (1), 23.
7. Diener H-C, Jansen JP, Reches A, Pascual J, Pitei D, Steiner TJ. Efficacy, tolerability, and safety of oral eletriptan and ergotamine plus caffeine (Cafergot) in the acute treatment of migraine: a multicentre, randomised, double-blind, placebo-controlled comparison. *Eur Neurol* 2002; **47** (2): 99–107.
8. Pryse-Phillips W on behalf of the Eletriptan Steering Committee. Comparison of oral eletriptan (40–80mg) and oral sumatriptan (50–100mg) for the treatment of acute migraine: a randomised, placebo-controlled trial in sumatriptan-naïve patients [abstract]. *Cephalalgia* 1999; **19** (4): 355–6.
9. Santanello N, Polis A, Hartmaier S, *et al*. Improvement in migraine-specific quality of life in a clinical trial of rizatriptan. *Cephalagia* 1997; **17**: 867–72.
10. Tandon P. Applications of global statistics in analyzing quality of life data. *Stat Med* 1990; **9**: 19–27.

19 Impact of cluster headache on health-related quality of life

D. D'Amico, A. Rigamonti, A. Solari, M. Leone,
S. Usai, L. Grazzi, and G. Bussone

Introduction

Over the last decade several studies have demonstrated that patients with primary headaches report markedly impaired quality of life and ability to function. Standardized instruments to assess health-related quality of life (HRQoL), such as the Medical Outcomes Study 'short forms' SF-36 and SF-20, have been used by several authors.[1–6] However, most studies have focused on migraine and more recently on chronic headache forms; little work has been done on cluster headache.[1,3] Cluster headache (CH) is characterized by excruciatingly painful unilateral headaches associated with ocular/nasal autonomic phenomena, occurring one or several times per day. Two main clinical forms are recognized: episodic CH, when periods lasting days/months with daily attacks (cluster phase) are separated by periods lasting months/years without headache (remission phase); and chronic CH, in which remission periods are absent or last less than 14 days.[7]

The purpose of the study was to administer the SF-36 to a sample of CH patients in order to investigate the impact of this severe primary headache form on different quality of life domains and patients' sense of well-being.

Materials and methods

Fifty-six consecutive patients with an International Headache Society (IHS) diagnosis of CH[7] were recruited. Thirty-four patients had episodic CH, and 22 had chronic CH. There were 40 men and 16 women; the mean age was 45 years (range 21–72) and the mean illness duration was 12.6 years (range 2 months–41 years). All patients completed the validated Italian version of the SF-36.[8] The Student t-test with

Bonferroni correction was used to compare scores for each of the SF-36 components in patients with those of the Italian normative population. The two-sample Wilcoxon rank-sum test was used to compare the SF-36 scores of episodic versus chronic CH patients.

Results

CH patients' mean scores for each of the SF-36 scales were worse than those in the Italian general population, significantly so ($p < 0.0001$) for most components (bodily pain, role functioning—physical, general health, social functioning, role functioning–emotional, and mental health), The difference was not significant for vitality ($p = 1.59$) and physical functioning ($p = 2.28$) (Table 19.1). No significant differences were found when SF-36 scores in episodic and chronic CH patients were compared.

Conclusion

Our results show that patients with cluster headache have markedly impaired quality of life (QoL). As expected, pain had a major influence on QoL. Patients also had poor scores on the scales indicating the extent to which physical health (role functioning–physical) and emotional problems (role functioning–emotional) interfere with work and social activities (social functioning), and also in scales that tap personal evaluation of health (general health, mental health).

These findings are partially concordant with those reported by Solomon et al.[1] in 1994 after administration of the SF-20 to 13 CH patients. Like us, these workers found that pain markedly influenced QoL, and that there were evident limitations in social functioning; However, health perception was preserved. The patients in our study therefore reported that CH had a more pervasive impact on QoL than

Table 19.1   SF-36 scores in 56 cluster headache (CH) patients compared to Italian normative data (Student *t*-test with Bonferroni correction)

SF-36 components	Scores (mean ± standard deviation)		p-value
	CH patients	Italian normative data	
Physical functioning	82.68±19.63	84.46±23.18	2.28
Role functioning–physical	37.5±37.45	78.21±35.93	<0.0001
Bodily pain	53.75±10.88	73.67±27.65	<0.0001
General health	52.2±22.30	65.22±22.18	<0.0001
Vitality	59.55±11.88	61.89±20.69	1.59
Social functioning	44.87±22.71	77.43±23.34	<0.0001
Role functioning–emotional	38.09±37.83	76.16±37.25	<0.0001
Mental health	52.86±19.94	66.59±20.89	<0.0001

those in Solomon *et al.*'s study. This difference may be due to different instruments used (SF-36 versus SF-20) and also differences in patient characteristics. Our patients had high morbidity: chronic or episodic CH and long illness duration (mean 12.6 years), while the patients reported in the US study were not so clearly characterized; in particular, it was not clear if all subjects were surveyed in the cluster phase, or if they had episodic or chronic CH.

Further studies on larger samples are needed to better evaluate the extent of the impairment of HRQoL in CH. Ongoing research to compare SF scores of episodic CH patients during the active with those in the remission phase, and to compare CH with migraine will lead to a better understanding of QoL impairment in CH.

References

1. Solomon GD, Skobieranda FG, Gragg LA. Does quality of life differ among headache diagnoses? Analysis using the Medical Outcomes Study instrument. *Headache* 1994; **34**: 143–7.
2. Osterhaus JT, Townsend RJ, Gandeck B, Ware JE. Measuring the functional status and well-being of patients with migraine headache. *Headache* 1994; **34**: 337–43.
3. Monzon MJ, Lainez MJA. Quality of life in migraine and chronic daily headache patients. *Cephalalgia* 1998; **18**: 638–43.
4. Wang SJ, Fuh JL, Lu SR, Juang KD. Quality of life differs among headache diagnoses: analysis of SF-36 survey in 901 headache patients. *Pain* 2001; **89**: 285–92.
5. D'Amico D, Grazzi L, Usai S. Quality of life and disability in transformed migraine with drug overuse. *Cephalalgia* 2001; **21**: 484.
6. Meletiche DM, Lofland JH, Young WB. Quality-of-life differences between patients with episodic and transformed migraine. *Headache* 2001; **41**: 573–8.
7. Headache Classification Committee of the International Headache Society. Classification and diagnostic criteria for headache disorders, cranial neuralgias and facial pain. *Cephalalgia* 1988; **8** (Suppl. 7): 1–96.
8. Apolone G, Mosconi P. The Italian SF-36 health survey: translation, validation and norming. *J Clin Epidemiol* 1998; **51** (11): 1025–36.

20 Improvement in migraine-specific quality of life with eletriptan (Relpax™) as compared to Cafergot®

Paula A. Funk-Orsini, Robert Miceli, Joan Mackell, and Nicholas E.J. Wells

Introduction

Migraine is a highly prevalent and chronic disorder, characterized by a combination of neurological, gastrointestinal, and autonomic symptoms that can markedly impair the sufferer's ability to function normally. In Europe, the total annual direct and indirect costs of migraine, including medication, productivity losses, and the use of emergency services, were recently estimated at 10 billion euros and, in the USA, as up to US \$30 billion.[1,2] In addition, migraine has a negative impact on the patient's health-related quality of life (HRQoL), both during and between attacks.[3,4] Thus, relieving headache pain and migraine-associated symptoms with effective treatment should also improve HRQoL by shortening the duration of the attack and reducing functional impairment.

Eletriptan is a potent, selective $5\text{-HT}_{1B/1D}$ agonist that has been shown to provide rapid and effective relief of acute migraine in clinical trials.[5–8] Oral eletriptan has been demonstrated as clinically superior to Cafergot®.[7] Both headache- and pain-free responses at 2 hours post-dose were reported by significantly more patients ($p < 0.0001$) treated with eletriptan 40 mg and 80 mg than those treated with Cafergot (two tablets of 1 mg ergotamine tartrate with 100 mg of caffeine).[7] Additionally, eletriptan 40 mg and 80 mg were significantly more effective than Cafergot in reducing functional impairment ($p < 0.0001$) and the associated symptoms of migraine (nausea, photophobia, and phonophobia) ($p < 0.005$) at 2 hours postdose. Both doses of eletriptan were also generally well tolerated, with the majority of adverse events being mild to moderate and transient in nature.[7]

The objective of this study was to compare the effects of oral eletriptan 40 mg and 80 mg with those of oral Cafergot (two tablets of 1 mg ergotamine tartrate with 100 mg caffeine) on migraine-specific QoL, using data from a previously reported clinical trial.[7]

Methods

In this multicentre, double-blind, randomized, placebo-controlled, parallel-group trial, patients were randomized to one of seven treatment arms that consisted of a first and second dosing (first/second dose: eletriptan 40 mg/eletriptan 40 mg; eletriptan 40 mg/placebo; eletriptan 80 mg/eletriptan 80 mg; eletriptan 80 mg/placebo; Cafergot/Cafergot; placebo/eletriptan 40 mg; and placebo/eletriptan 80 mg). The second dose could be taken if a patient did not respond adequately within 2 hours or experienced headache recurrence within 24 hours. For the eletriptan arms, patients received either the active treatment or placebo for their second dose; active treatment was used throughout the Cafergot arm. Due to the lack of a true placebo group and the 24-hour time frame measured by the 24-hour Migraine-specific Quality of Life Questionnaire (MSQoL), the two placebo sequences were excluded from analyses.

Outcome measures were the mean scores on domains included in the 24-h MSQoL. The MSQoL consists of 15 items across five domains: work functioning, social functioning, energy/vitality, migraine symptoms, and feelings/concerns. Each domain includes three items in which responses are recorded on a 7-point scale. A value of 1 indicates maximum impairment of QoL, while a value of 7 indicates no impairment. The maximum and minimum scores within each domain are 21 and 3, respectively.[9] Since the 24 hour MSQoL is administered 24 hours after initiating treatment for an acute migraine attack, its evaluation encompasses the patient's experience during the entire attack episode including the severity and duration of headache pain, migraine-associated symptoms, impaired functioning, efficacy and tolerability of therapy, and the need for a second dose or rescue medication.[9]

All analyses were based on 'first-attack' data and excluded patients with missing values in one or more MSQoL domains (no imputation was used). Each domain of the MSQoL was analysed separately with analysis of variance (ANOVA) to compare treatment means between 'active–active' and 'active–placebo' treatment sequences for both doses of eletriptan. Since there were no significant differences between the 'active–active' and 'active–placebo' groups, patients in treatment sequences with the same first dose were pooled to increase statistical power. Treatment group differences were assessed by ANOVA followed by pair-wise treatment comparisons when the overall ANOVA was significant. O'Brien's rank sum test was used to evaluate the overall migraine-related QoL across all five domains for the eletriptan and Cafergot.[10]

Results

Treatment groups were similar with respect to age, gender, and type and severity of migraine headache (Table 20.1).

Compared with patients who received Cafergot, patients who took eletriptan 80 mg had significantly better ($p<0.001$) scores for energy/vitality, migraine symptoms, and feelings/concerns (Fig. 20.1 and Table 20.2). Patients treated with eletriptan 80 mg also had significantly better ($p<0.05$) scores for work functioning and social functioning (Fig. 20.1 and Table 20.2).

Patients who took eletriptan 40 mg had significantly better scores than those who took Cafergot on social functioning ($p<0.05$), energy/vitality ($p<0.05$), and

Table 20.1   Demographic characteristics

Characteristic	Cafergot ($n=185$)	Eletriptan, 40 mg ($n=194$)	Eletriptan, 80 mg ($n=196$)
Gender (number (%))			
Female	158 (85)	166 (86)	175 (89)
Age (years)			
Mean ± SD*	39.7 ± 10.7	39.5 ± 10.7	40.2 ± 10.8
Type of migraine (number (%))			
Without aura	96 (52)	126 (65)	122 (62)
With/without aura	57 (31)	44 (23)	55 (28)
With aura	32 (17)	24 (12)	19 (10)
Baseline severity (number (%))†			
Mild	1 (1)	1 (1)	1 (1)
Moderate	97 (52)	103 (53)	103 (53)
Severe	87 (47)	90 (46)	92 (47)

*SD, Standard deviation.
†Numbers may not total 100% due to rounding.

Table 20.2   Least square means (±standard error) for MSQoL domain by treatment group

	Functioning		Energy/ vitality	Migraine symptoms	Feelings/ concerns
	Work	Social			
Cafergot	10.6 ± 0.4	10.5 ± 0.4	10.5 ± 0.4	11.6 ± 0.4	10.8 ± 0.4
Eletriptan					
40 mg	11.4 ± 0.4	11.5* ± 0.4	11.5* ± 0.4	13.2† ± 0.4	11.7 ± 0.4
80 mg	11.8* ± 0.4	11.8* ± 0.4	12.2† ± 0.4	13.4† ± 0.4	12.4† ± 0.4

*$p<0.05$ for difference with Cafergot.
†$p<0.001$ for difference with Cafergot.

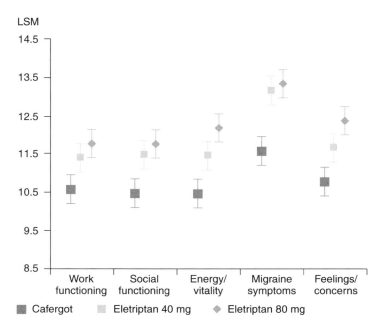

Fig. 20.1   Least square mean (LSM) scores (±standard error) on the 24-h MSQoL for patients treated with eletriptan or Cafergot. *$p < 0.05$ for difference with Cafergot. †$p < 0.001$ for difference with Cafergot.

migraine symptoms ($p < 0.001$), and trended toward significance for work function-ing and feelings/concerns scores ($p < 0.10$) (Fig. 20.1 and Table 20.2). The O'Brien's rank sum test indicated that patients receiving both eletriptan 80 mg ($p < 0.001$) and eletriptan 40 mg ($p < 0.01$) experienced significantly superior overall migraine-specific QoL to that of those taking Cafergot.

Conclusions

Oral eletriptan was clinically superior to Cafergot in improving migraine-specific QoL as indicated by scores from the 24 hour MSQoL. The findings of this study reflect the improved clinical benefits and overall tolerability of eletriptan compared to Cafergot.

References

1. Hopkins A. The epidemiology of headache and migraine, and its meaning for neurological services. *Schweiz Med Wochenschr* 1996; **126** (4): 128–35.
2. Ferrari MD. The economic burden of migraine to society. *PharmacoEconomics* 1998; **13**: 667–76.

3. Hu HX, Markson LE, Lipton RB, *et al.* Burden of migraine in the United States: disability and economic costs. *Arch Intern Med* 1999; **159**: 813–18.
4. Solomon GD, Price KL. Burden of migraine: a review of its socioeconomic impact. *PharmacoEconomics* 1997; **11** (Suppl.): 1–10.
5. Goadsby PJ, Ferrari MD, Olesen J, *et al.* Eletriptan in acute migraine: a double blind, placebo-controlled comparison to sumatriptan. *Neurology* 2000; **54**: 156–63.
6. Stark R, Dahlöf C, Haughie S, *et al.* on behalf of the Eletriptan Steering Committee. Efficacy, safety and tolerability of oral eletriptan in the acute treatment of migraine: results of a phase III, multicentre, placebo-controlled study across three attacks. *Cephalalgia* 2002; **22** (1): 23.
7. Diener H-C, Jansen JP, Reches A, Pascual J, Pitei D, Steiner TJ. Efficacy, tolerability, and safety of oral eletriptan and ergotamine plus caffeine (Cafergot) in the acute treatment of migraine: a multicentre, randomised, double-blind, placebo-controlled comparison. *Eur Neurol* 2002; **47** (2): 99–107.
8. Pryse-Phillips W on behalf of the Eletriptan Steering Committee. Comparison of oral eletriptan (40–80mg) and oral sumatriptan (50–100mg) for the treatment of acute migraine: a randomised, placebo-controlled trial in sumatriptan-naïve patients [abstract]. *Cephalalgia* 1999; **19** (4): 355–6.
9. Santanello N, Polis A, Hartmaier S, *et al.* Improvement in migraine-specific quality of life in a clinical trial of rizatriptan. *Cephalalgia* 1997; **17**: 867–72.
10. Tandon P. Applications of global statistics in analyzing quality of life data. *Stat Med* 1990; **9**: 19–27.

21 Improvements in health-related quality of life with long-term use of sumatriptan therapy for migraine

T.A. Burke, W. Jackie Kwong, and Alice S. Batenhorst

Background

Migraine is associated with significant impairments in health-related quality of life (HRQoL), reflecting the considerable mental, physical, and social burden of this condition. HRQoL assessment is an important endpoint of migraine therapy because it measures the patient's perception of his or her own health and provides information regarding impairments between attacks, such as the inability to anticipate migraine-induced interruptions in daily activities.[1] HRQoL assessments supplement traditional treatment endpoints (such as relief of pain or other symptoms) in providing a more comprehensive assessment of treatment benefits.

HRQoL may be measured using generic or disease-specific instruments. Disease-specific instruments are developed to measure unique limitations or restrictions associated with a given disease. The Migraine-Specific Quality of Life Questionnaire (MSQ) is a disease-specific instrument developed to study the effects of migraine on HRQoL.[2,3] Generic instruments measure limitations in functional status and well-being and they may be used across a variety of conditions. An example of a widely used generic instrument is the Medical Outcomes Study short form 36 (SF-36) health survey.[4] Compared to disease-specific instruments, generic instruments are generally less sensitive at detecting treatment effects. Therefore, generic and disease-specific instruments are frequently used together to provide a comprehensive assessment of HRQoL.

Sumatriptan has been associated with statistically significant quality of life improvements using generic and disease-specific quality of life instruments.[5–8] However, these studies have studied the quality of life benefits of sumatriptan treatment for only up to 12 months. The objective of this study was to examine changes in HRQoL with long-term (up to 42 months) use of sumatriptan therapy for migraine and to characterize the quality of life changes from clinical and statistical significance perspectives.

Methods

Study design

Three consecutive, prospective, open-label, multicentre clinical trials were conducted to examine the efficacy and safety of sumatriptan treatment. Patients who were 18 years or older, with at least a 6-month history of migraine, as diagnosed by the study investigator, and gave informed consent were eligible for the study. Patients with ischaemic heart disease, unstable angina, Raynaud's syndrome, Prinzmetal's angina, or blood pressure over 160/95 were excluded. Patients completing the first trial were given the option of participating in a second trial consisting of both sumatriptan-naïve patients and patients previously exposed to sumatriptan. Patients completing the second trial were given the option of participating in a third trial.

Quality of life assessments were not performed in the first trial. In the second and third trials, patients completed the SF-36 and the MSQ (version 1.0) at 6-month intervals. During the second trial, patients could treat an unlimited number of migraines in the clinic for up to 24 months using subcutaneous sumatriptan (6 mg). Patients were eligible to receive either one tablet of oral sumatriptan (100 mg) or alternative rescue medications. During the third trial, patients could treat an unrestricted number of acute migraine attacks 'at home' using subcutaneous sumatriptan (6 mg) over a period of 24 months. The second trial accounted for HRQoL assessments from baseline through 18 months. The third trial accounted for HRQoL assessments for months 24 through 42. Analyses were performed on data obtained on patients who completed the second trial and enrolled in the third trial.

Quality of life measurements

The SF-36 consists of 36 items that measure general HRQoL in eight multi-item dimensions: social functioning (SF); general health perceptions (GH); mental health (MH); vitality (VT); bodily pain (BP); physical functioning (PF); role–physical (RP); and role–emotional (RE).

The MSQ (version 1.0) is a 16-item instrument that measures quality of life related to migraine in the following three dimensions:

- role function-restrictive (7 items): examines the degree to which limitations in performance of daily activities are due to migraine;
- role function-preventive (5 items): examines the degree to which interruptions in performance of daily activities are due to migraine;

◆ emotional function (4 items): examines feelings of frustration and helplessness due to migraine.

For both the SF-36 and MSQ dimensions are scored from 0 to 100, where a higher score indicates a better health status. A five-point change on any particular dimension of the SF-36 is considered to be clinically significant.[4] The clinical significance of changes in MSQ dimension scores has yet to be examined.

Statistical analyses

Separate repeated-measures analyses of variance (ANOVA) with time as the repeated factor were performed for each of the SF-36 and MSQ dimensions as an overall test of significance. Pair-wise comparisons between baseline and subsequent time periods were performed contingent on the significance of the repeated-measures ANOVA. An intent-to-treat analysis was performed using last observation carried forward (LOCF) to impute missing SF-36 and MSQ dimension scores. A p-value of less than 0.05 was considered statistically significant.

Results

The intent-to-treat analysis population included 126 patients. The average age of patients at baseline was 45 years and the majority were females (92%) and Caucasian (98%). A total of 90 patients completed the follow-up trial and 36 (29%) patients withdrew before completion. Patients withdrew for a variety of reasons including: failure to treat a migraine ($n=15$), and adverse events ($n=5$). Seventy-four patients (59%) were previously exposed to sumatriptan at the time of the baseline quality of life assessment. Previous exposure to sumatriptan probably affected baseline quality of life scores for these patients.

Sumatriptan was associated with clinically and statistically significant improvements across several aspects of general and disease-related HRQoL. Five SF-36 dimensions demonstrated statistically significant improvements over time (Table 21.1

Table 21.1 SF-36 dimensions demonstrating clinical (c) and statistically significant (s) improvements over time

Dimension	Months from baseline						
	6	12	18	24	30	36	42
Social functioning		c, s	c, s	c, s	c, s	c, s	c, s
General health		s	s	s			
Mental health			s	s	s	s	s
Vitality			c, s	c, s	c, s	c	c, s
Bodily pain	c, s	c, s	c, s	c, s	c, s	c, s	c, s

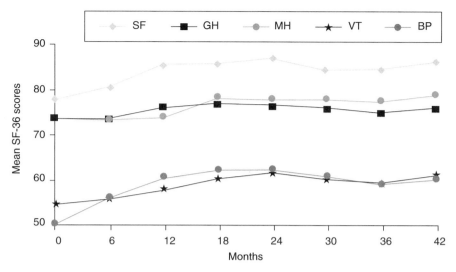

Fig. 21.1 Mean SF-36 scores over time. SF, Social functioning; GH, general health; MH, mental health; VT, vitality; BP, bodily pain.

Table 21.2 MSQ dimenstions demonstrating statistically significant (s) improvements over time

Dimension	Months from baseline						
	6	12	18	24	30	36	42
Role-restrictive	s	s	s	s	s	s	s
Role-preventive		s	s	s	s	s	s
Emotional function	s	s	s	s	s	s	s

and Fig. 21.1), namely, SF, GH, MH, VT, and BP. Clinically significant improvements (equal to or great than a 5-point change) were observed for three dimensions, SF, VT, and BP. Each of the three MSQ dimensions demonstrated statistically significant improvements over time (Table 21.2 and Fig. 21.2).

For both SF-36 and MSQ, the most notable improvements in mean HRQoL scores occurred during the first 6 to 12 months of study participation. These improvements were generally sustained over the 42-month study period, suggesting that long-term use of sumatriptan provides a sustained improvement in HRQoL.

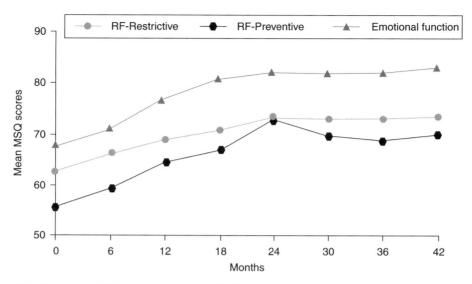

Fig. 21.2   Mean MSQ scores over time. RF, Role function.

Conclusion

The results of this study demonstrate that the long-term benefits in HRQoL after using sumatriptan therapy are both statistically and clinically significant. Both generic and disease-specific quality of life instruments detected the improvements. By including patients previously exposed to sumatriptan, baseline HRQoL estimates may be elevated. Thus, the results presented here may represent a conservative estimate of quality of life improvements associated with sumatriptan. Further research employing a randomized study design is warranted.

References

1. Dahlöf CGH, Dimeas E. Migraine patients experience poorer subjective well-being/quality of life even between attacks. *Cephalagia* 1995; **15**: 31–6.
2. Jhingran P, Osterhaus JT, Miller DW, *et al.* Development and validation of the Migraine Specific Quality of Life Questionnaire. *Headache* 1998; **38**: 295–302.
3. Martin BC, Pathak DS, Sharfman MI, *et al.* Validity and reliability of the Migraine-Specific Quality of Life Questionnaire (MSQ version 2.1). *Headache* 2000; **40**: 204–15.
4. Ware JE, Snow K, Kosinski M, Gandek B. *SF-36 health survey: manual and interpretation guide*. Boston: Nimrod Press, 1993.
5. Dahlöf C, Bouchard J, Cortelli P, *et al.* A multinational investigation of the impact of subcutaneous sumatriptan: health-related quality of life. *PharmacoEconomics* 1997; **11** (Suppl. 1): 24–34.

6. Cohen JA, Beall D, Beck A, *et al*. Sumatriptan treatment for migraine in a health maintenance organization: economic, humanistic and clinical outcomes. *Clin Therapeut* 1999; **21**: 190–204.
7. Adelman JU, Sharfman M, Johnson R, *et al*. Impact of oral sumatriptan on workplace productivity, health-related quality of life, healthcare use, and patient satisfaction with medication in nurses with migraine. *Am J Managed Care* 1996; **2**: 1407–16.
8. Gross MLP, Dowson AJ, Deavy L, Duthie T. Impact of oral sumatriptan 50 mg on work productivity and quality of life in migraineurs. *Br J Med Econ* 1996; **10**: 231–46.

22 Psychometric evaluation of a computerized program to assess migraine-specific quality of life in clinical practice

Lisa K. Mannix, W. Jackie Kwong, Elizabeth P. Skinner,
and Todd A. Dimsdale

Introduction

The Migraine-Specific Quality of Life Questionnaire (MSQ version 2.1) is included in the Medical Outcomes Trust library of outcomes instruments (http://www.outcomes-trust.org). Although the paper-and-pencil format of the MSQ has been available for several years, the use of MSQ has been limited to clinical trials, mostly because additional data entry and separate scoring programming are required.

Since the publication of the MSQ in 1998,[1] there has been growing interest among physicians in using the MSQ to evaluate health-related quality of life (HRQoL) relating specifically to migraine. Accordingly, the MSQ was included in the GlaxoSmithKline Migraine Matrix Program, a disease management offering for health plans to use in developing quality improvement initiatives for migraine.

To facilitate the administration and scoring of the MSQ in physician practice groups, managed care organizations, and other groups interested in assessing quality of life for migraineurs, the MSQ Analyzer, a computerized format with automatic scoring capabilities, was developed. The MSQ Analyzer allows patients to complete the MSQ by directly entering their responses into a computer. Data that are captured by the paper-and-pencil format also can be entered into the program via a batch entry mode. MSQ data entered into the program are scored automatically and results are presented in a graphical format.

Although the psychometric properties of MSQ version 2.1 were previously assessed,[2] the reliability and validity of a computerized format of the questionnaire is yet to be determined. Pilot testing of the software in a real-life practice setting is also necessary to ensure the applicability of the software in a clinical practice environment.

Methods

Study design

This study was conducted in two phases. In phase I, two site personnel were recruited at the study centre to receive training on how to use the MSQ Analyzer and they provided feedback regarding the administration functions. Modifications to the MSQ Analyzer and user's manual were made based on the comments received. The revised MSQ Analyzer was used in phase II of this study. In phase II, 48 patients with migraine were recruited at the study site to provide data for the assessment of the reliability and validity of the MSQ via the computerized MSQ Analyzer at the screening visit (visit 1) and 1 week after the screening visit (visit 2). In addition to completing the MSQ via the Analyzer, patients also completed the following questions: migraine characteristics (visits 1 and 2); ease of use of the MSQ Analyzer (visit 1); and overall satisfaction with migraine care (visit 1).

Patients who participated in the study were adult migraineurs with at least a 1-year history of migraine with or without aura using the International Headache Society (IHS) criteria 1.1, had no change in pharmacotherapy during the 1-week study period, were willing and able to give informed consent prior to entry in the study, and returned to the study clinic to complete follow-up visit 1 week after study entry.

Reliability and validity assessment

The reliability of data collected by the MSQ Analyzer in terms of internal consistency was assessed by Cronbach's alpha using MSQ data from visit 1. One-week test–retest reliability was evaluated using Pearson correlation coefficients between MSQ scores at visit 1 and visit 2. A reliability estimate greater or equal to 0.50 was considered acceptable.[3]

The clinical validity of the data collected by MSQ Analyzer was examined by Pearson correlation coefficients of MSQ scores with self-reported migraine frequency in the past 4 weeks, average pain intensity, frequency, duration of migraines, time since last migraine attack, and ability to function during migraine attack using data from visit 1. Because a higher MSQ score indicates better health status, it was hypothesized that MSQ scores would decrease with migraine severity and increase with time since the last migraine attack.

Results

Data from 48 patients were available for analysis (Table 22.1). About 96% were females and 96% were White; the mean age was 44.0 years (SD, 7.92). Over 79% of patients were very satisfied with their migraine care at baseline. On a five-point rating scale, over 90% of patients rated the MSQ Analyzer as easy to use.

The internal consistency reliability and test–retest reliability estimates of the MSQ exceeded the acceptable criteria of 0.50 (Table 22.2). Correlation coefficients of MSQ scores with migraine symptoms were in the expected direction (Table 22.3). Self-reported average ability to function during migraine was significantly correlated with MSQ scores ($p < 0.05$).

Table 22.1 Patient characteristics

Characteristic	Visit 1	Visit 2
Number of patients	48	47
Number reporting migraine*	48	32
Frequency of attacks in last 4 weeks	2.8	1.7
Mean duration of attacks in hours (SD)	25.0 (34.74)	14.4 (17.46)
Mean average pain rating[†] (SD)	2.3 (0.61)	2.1 (0.67)
Average ability to function (number (%))		
Normal	8 (16.7)	4 (12.5)
Mildly impaired	17 (35.4)	15 (46.9)
Moderately impaired	17 (35.4)	10 (31.3)
Severely impaired	6 (12.5)	3 (9.4)
Presence of symptoms (number (%))		
Nausea	37 (77.1)	19 (59.4)
Vomiting	6 (12.5)	3 (9.4)
Sensitivity to light	43 (89.6)	27 (84.3)
Sensitivity to sound	40 (83.3)	25 (78.1)
Mean number of days since last attack (SD)	8.63 (7.29)	2.57 (2.51)

*Patients were asked if they experienced migraines in the past 4 weeks at visit 1, and if they experienced migraines since visit 1 at visit 2.

Table 22.2 Mean MSQ scores and reliability estimates

SQ dimension	Mean score (SD)	Cronbach's alpha	Test–retest reliability
Role restrictive	62.61 (17.99)	0.93*	0.53*
Role preventive	76.63 (19.92)	0.86*	0.72*
Emotional function	67.82 (25.62)	0.86*	0.78*

*Exceeded acceptable criteria of 0.50.

Table 22.3   Pearson correlation matrix between MSQ scores and migraine symptoms

	MSQ domains		
Symptoms	Role-restrictive	Role-preventive	Emotional function
Migraine frequency	−0.273*	−0.174	−0.101
Average pain intensity	−0.214	−0.224	−0.139
Time since last attack	0.219	0.262	0.208
Average duration of migraine	−0.119	−0.205	−0.132
Ability to function	−0.463*	−0.473*	−0.396*

*$p < 0.05$.

Conclusion

The study suggested that the computerized MSQ Analyzer demonstrates reliability and validity in assessing migraine-related quality of life. It is a useful tool in facilitating collection of outcomes data in clinical settings where support on data entry and analysis may not be readily available.

References

1. Jhingran P, Osterhaus JT, Miller DW, *et al*. Development and validation of the Migraine Specific Quality of Life Questionnaire. *Headache* 1998; **38**: 295–302.
2. Martin BC, Pathak DS, Sharfman MI, *et al*. Validity and reliability of the Migraine Specific Quality of Life Questionnaire (MSQ version 2.1). *Headache* 2000; **40**: 204–15.
3. Helmstadter GC. *Principles of psychological measurement*. New York: Appleton-Century-Crofts, 1964.

23 Quality of life and disability in transformed migraine with drug overuse

D. D'Amico, L. Grazzi, S. Usai, A. Solari, M. Leone,
A. Rigamonti, and G. Bussone

Introduction

Transformed migraine is a distinct form of chronic daily headache that develops from episodic migraine or is characterized by the presence of typical migrainous features in some attacks. This condition is often associated with overuse of symptomatic medications.[1] Little is known about the functional impact of chronic headaches in general and transformed migraine in particular on patients' lives, particularly when associated with regular intake of symptomatic medications.

The aim of this study was to investigate functional status in a sample of patients with transformed migraine and drug overuse, using well-reported tools: the Migraine Disability Assessment Score (MIDAS) questionnaire and the Medical Outcomes Study short form 36 (SF-36). MIDAS is a brief and reliable headache-specific tool,[2] which captures headache-related disability in different domains by means of five questions. The MIDAS score can then be used to assign a disability grade ranging from grade I (little or no disability) to grade IV (severe disability). The SF-36 is widely used to assess health-related quality of life (HRQoL).[3] It is a generic HRQoL questionnaire that indicates the influence of any given disorder on patients' functioning in different roles, and on their perception of their health status.

Materials and methods

One hundred forty-five consecutive patients with transformed migraine and drug overuse were studied. Diagnoses were according to the criteria of Silberstein *et al.*[1] There were 121 women and 24 men of mean age 45.5 years (range 19–72) and mean

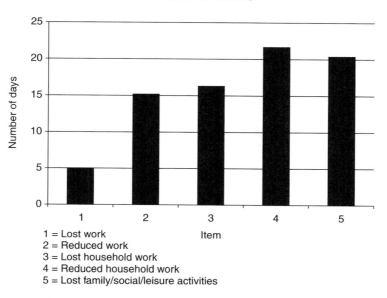

DISABILITY IN DIFFERENT DOMAINS
MIDAS ITEMS

1 = Lost work
2 = Reduced work
3 = Lost household work
4 = Reduced household work
5 = Lost family/social/leisure activities

Fig. 23.1 Disability in different activity domains in 145 patients with transformed migraine and drug overuse: scores on MIDAS questionnaire items.

illness duration 26.86 years (range 2–55 years). The mean number of symptomatic drug consumptions/month was 53 (range 20–200). All patients completed the MIDAS questionnaire and 65 also completed the SF-36. The validated Italian versions of both questionnaires were used.[4, 5]

Results

The mean MIDAS score (corresponding to the number of days over the preceding 3 months on which patients were totally or severely impaired in everyday duties) was quite high (78.83; SD 64.63). Disability was evident in all activity domains (work and non-work activities) as shown in Fig. 23.1. Fourteen patients (9.7%) had grade I disability; 5 (3.4%) had grade II, disability; 11 (7.6%) had grade III disability, and 115 (79.3%) had grade IV disability. Thus, most patients with transformed migraine had a moderate/severe disability (MIDAS grades III + IV in 86.9% patients).

Patients' SF-36 scores were significantly lower ($p < 0.001$, Student's t-test with Bonferroni correction) than those of the normative Italian population (see Table 23.1) and this difference was also clinically significant (difference > 5 points).

Table 23.1 SF-36 scores in 65 patients with transformed migraine and drug overuse in comparison to Italian normative data (Student's *t*-test with Bonferroni correction)

SF-36 scales	Transformed migraine (mean (SD))	Italian normative data (mean (SD))	*p*-value
Physical functioning	72.40 (20.09)	84.46 (23.18)	0.0001
Role functioning–physical	19.44 (29.93)	78.21 (35.93)	0.0001
Bodily pain	53.23 (9.03)	73.67 (27.65)	0.0001
General health	36.63 (16.78)	65.22 (22.18)	0.0001
Vitality	57.93 (12.56)	61.89 (20.69)	NS*
Social functioning	41.40 (23.97)	77.43 (23.34)	0.0001
Role functioning–emotional	36.92 (38.69)	76.16 (37.25)	0.0001
Mental health	47.80 (17.76)	66.59 (20.89)	0.0001

*NS, Not significant.

Conclusions

Few studies have assessed impact of chronic daily headache forms on HRQoL or disability,[6-8] and only one specifically focused on transformed migraine.[9] Our findings are consistent with the results of the latter study, in that transformed migraine has a significant influence on quality of life. Our patients were characterized by a markedly lower QoL than normal and had severe limitations in their ability to function in work and non-work activities, and in all roles (involving physical, social, and emotional components).

These findings shed light on the personal and social burden of transformed migraine and suggest the need for effective treatment interventions in these patients but also the importance of management programmes for migraine patients that can, on the one hand, avoid increases in headache frequency and, on the other, discourage drug overuse so as to prevent the development of transformed migraine, which is a chronic, difficult to treat, and severely disabling condition.

References

1. Silberstein SD, Lipton RB, Sliwinski M. Classification of daily and near-daily headaches: field trial of revised IHS criteria. *Neurology* 1996; **47**: 871–87.
2. Stewart WF, Lipton RB, Kolodner K, Liberman J, Sawyer J. Reliability of the migraine disability assessment score in a population sample of headache sufferers. *Cephalalgia* 1999; **19**: 107–14.
3. Stewart AL, Hays RD, Ware JE. The MOS short-form. A general health survey. Reliability and validity in a patient population. *Med Care* 1988; **26**: 724–35.
4. D'Amico D, Mosconi P, Genco S, *et al.* The Migraine Disability Assessment (MIDAS) questionnaire: translation and reliability of Italian version. *Cephalalgia* 2001; **21**: 947–52.

5. Apolone G, Mosconi P. The Italian SF-36 health survey: translation, validation and norming. *J Clin Epidemiol* 1998; **51** (11): 1025–36.
6. Monzon MJ, Lainez MJA. Quality of life in migraine and chronic daily headache patients. *Cephalalgia* 1998; **18**: 638–43.
7. Villarreal SS, Mathew NTT, Shahlai N, Kalaisam J. Disability in chronic daily headache: factors affecting MIDAS scores. *Headache* 1999; **39** (5): 384.
8. Guitera V, Munoz P, Castello J, Pascual J. Impact of chronic daily headache in the quality of life: a study in the general population. *Cephalalgia* 1999; **19**: 412–13.
9. Meletiche DM, Lofland JH, Young WB. Quality-of-life differences between patients with episodic and transformed migraine. *Headache* 2001; **41**: 573–8.

24
Quality of life and migraine: a multicentre Spanish study

M.J.A. Láinez, R. Leira, J. Pascual, E. Díez Tejedor,
F. Morales, F. Titus, and R. Alberca

Introduction

The unpredictable and episodic nature of migraine, together with its debilitating symptomatology, has a profound effect on the lives of many sufferers and can cause a significant impairment in the quality of life of many patients. In Spain, migraine is the most common reason for visits to general out-patient clinics in neurology departments.[1] We knew the prevalence and socio-economic impact of migraine in our country,[2,3] which are very similar to those in other Western countries, but we didn't know the impact of the disease in the life of our patients. In 1998 we decided to perform the multicentre study reported here, using healthy volunteers and diabetic patients as control groups, to determine the impact of migraine on the quality of life of Spanish patients suffering from migraine and to establish the relation between migraine characteristics and different items affecting the quality of life.

Material and methods

The survey was undertaken in seven Spanish hospitals from different geographical areas, all of which have migraine units. Consecutive patients with a diagnosis of migraine sent to these units for a first consultation for evaluation were included. The criteria for including the migraineurs were: diagnosis of migraine with or without aura according to International Headache Society (IHS) criteria; migraine with at least 1 year of evolution; age between 18 and 65 years; and agreement to fill in the questionnaires. Patients with more than 6 days of tension-type headache per month and patients affected by chronic daily headache or by chronic disorders were excluded.

The migraineurs were compared with a group of diabetics and a group of healthy people matched by sex and age. The healthy group were people subjectively healthy and without a history of chronic diseases. The diabetic group were patients with a diagnosis of diabetes mellitus and without a history of migraine or other chronic diseases.

All the patients and controls were interviewed by a senior neurologist and asked about general health, headache characteristics, and previous use of treatment. The neurologist had the patients answer the Hamilton test for depression. All the interviewed people completed the Spanish version of the Medical Outcomes Study short form 36 (SF-36) questionnaire[4] and, in addition, the migraine group completed the Migraine-Specific Quality of Life Questionnaire (MSQoL).[5]

The results were compared using one-factor analysis of variance (ANOVA) and Fisher and chi square tests.

Results

A total of 518 people were included: 305 patients with migraine; 105 diabetics; and 105 healthy people.

Both groups of patients (migraineurs and diabetics) had a statistically significant lower scores in all of the items of the SF-36. Diabetics had a lower score only in the general health parameter. Migraineurs showed statistically lower scores compared with the diabetic group in the items 'role functioning–physical', 'bodily pain', and 'social functioning' (Fig. 24.1).

In the migraine group there were not any differences per type of migraine, sex, or age group. Neither were there differences in function related to duration or frequency (by month) of migraine crisis. There were small differences in relation to the social status and level in the physical items and general health.

With the MSQoL there were also no differences in function between different types of migraine, sex, or age groups. However, the score in the MSQoL had a good relationship to the frequency and duration of migraine attacks (Fig. 24.2), but not to the intensity.

Hamilton's test allowed us to see significant differences between healthy people and both groups of patients with higher scores among the diabetics and migraineurs (Table 24.1). The number of migraineurs scoring more than 17 points in Hamilton's test was small (8.1%). In any case, the score in Hamilton's test correlated with a significant difference in all items of SF-36 and also in the MSQoL (Table 24.2).

Conclusions

The SF-36 is able to discriminate between migraineurs and the general population in terms of quality of life and can be useful in the general evaluation of therapeutic programmes. It also makes it possible to establish differences with other chronic diseases such as diabetes mellitus. The items more affected by migraine are: bodily pain, role functioning–physical, and social functioning. Our results are very similar, even in the scores, to those of other clinical[6] and general population studies.[7,8]

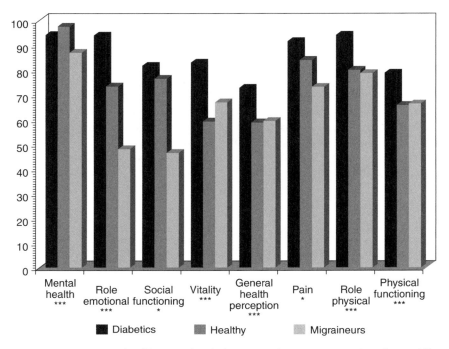

Fig. 24.1 SF-36 scores in healthy people, diabetics, and migraineurs. *Significant differences between migraineurs and healthy controls: $p < 0.01$. ***Significant differences between migraineurs and diabetics: $p < 0.01$.

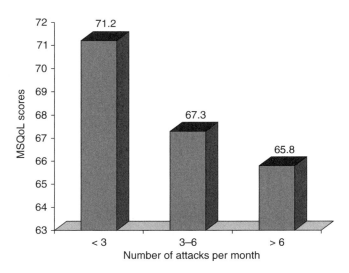

Fig. 24.2 MSQoL scores (0–100) versus number of migraine attacks per month. ANOVA: $p = 0.0276$.

Table 24.1   Scores in Hamilton's test in the three groups: healthy people, diabetics, and migraineurs. The score in Hamilton's test was significantly higher in both groups of patients*

	Group			Total
	Healthy	Diabetes	Migraine	
N	105	108	303	516
Mean	3.5	7.1	7.1	6.4
Standard deviation (SD)	3.4	7.0	5.9	5.9
Minimum	0.0	0.0	0.0	0.0
Maximum	19.0	32.0	30.0	32.0

*Healthy group versus migraineurs and diabetics: $p = 0.0001$.

Table 24.2   Hamilton's test scores in the migraine group compared with scores in MSQoL. The patients who had a score > 17 in Hamilton's test scored significantly lower in the MSQoL*

	Score on Hamilton's test			Total
	0–8	9–16	>17	
N	193	85	25	303
Mean	71.4	66.4	26.3	68.8
Standard deviation (SD)	12.7	15.0	13.1	14.1
Minimum	37.5	35.0	30.0	30.0
Maximum	98.8	97.5	87.5	98.8

*Hamilton's test score 0–8 versus > 17: $p = 0.0001$.

The SF 36 doesn't permit, in our experience, the establishment of differences in relation to the severity of migraine. For this purpose, the MSQoL probably is better, because patients score significantly less in this test when the frequency and duration of their crisis are higher. It could be a good instrument for evaluating acute or preventive treatments

It would be interesting to continue studying the relation between social and educational status and score in the SF-36 to confirm whether or not the social status can determine differences in some of the items of the questionnaire.

When using quality of life scales it is necessary to perform a test such as Hamilton's test to know the emotional status of our patients. A high score in Hamilton's test leads to a score reduction in all items of the quality of life tests. For this reason, in the quality of life studies in migraineurs, it could be important to include tests that measure the patient's level of depression.

References

1. Gracia Naya M, Usón-Martín NM, Grupo de Estudio de Neurólogos Aragoneses. Estudio transversal multicéntrico de las consultas externas de la Seguridad Social en Aragón. Resultados globales. *Rev Neurol* 1997; **25**: 194–9.

2. Láinez JM, Titus F, Cobaleda S, *et al.* Socioeconomic impact of migraine [abstract]. *Funct Neurol* 1996; **11**: 133.

3. Láinez JM. Impacto socieconómico del dolor de cabeza. *Continua Neurológica* 1999; **2**: 7–16.

4. Alonso J, Regidor E, Barrio G, *et al.* Valores poblacionales de referencia de la versión española del Cuestionario de Salud SF-36. *Med Clin (Barc)* 1998; **111**: 410–16.

5. McKenna SP, Doward LC, Davey KM. The development and psychometric properties of the MSQOL. A migraine-specific quality-of-life instrument. *Clin Drug Invest* 1998; **15**: 413–23.

6. Osterhaus JT, Trownsend RJ, Gandeck B, Ware JE. Measuring functional status and well-being of patients with migraine headache. *Headache* 1994; **34**: 337–43.

7. Terwindt GM, Ferrari MD, Tijhuis M, *et al.* The impact of migraine on quality of life in the general population. The GEM study. *Neurology* 2000; **55**: 624–9.

8. Lipton RB, Hamelsky SW, Kolodner KB, *et al.* Migraine, quality of life and depression. A population-based case-control study. *Neurology* 2000; **55**: 629–35.

9. Mathew N, Shetfell F, Silberstein S, *et al.* Evaluation of the improvement in migraine-specific quality of life test: impact of zolmitriptan [abstract]. *Headache* 1997; **37**: 323.

25 Patient-centred measures: health-related quality of life: discussion summary

Hartmut Göbel

The first main point of the discussion concerned the methods for measuring health-related quality of life (HRQoL). The question of whether there was an ideal method was discussed. It became clear that the different measuring instruments have to be selected depending on the requirements and the project objectives. A number of different principal objectives can be distinguished, in particular: reducing the number of headache days; reducing the need to take painkillers or anti-migraine products; improving the general quality of life in both physical and psychological terms; reducing the use of health-care facilities; and increasing satisfaction with the results of the health services. Different measuring instruments are necessary for registering these dimensions, whether it is a matter of analysing short- or long-term effects. For example, the MSQ (Migraine-Specific Quality of Life Questionnaire) has 14 items covering three different dimensions: role-restrictive, role-preventive, and emotional function. It was pointed out that this measuring instrument can be used to measure improvements in HRQoL over a period of 4 to 12 weeks. Other measuring instruments, such as the 24-hour Migraine Specific Quality of Life Questionnaire (24-hour MSQoL), are suitable for recording short-term effects in the context of attack therapy. It was suggested that it should be possible to use the measuring methods both in clinical studies and in the practical field.

The second part of the discussion was devoted to a detailed consideration of the effect of various headache syndromes on HRQoL. The different primary and secondary headache syndromes can evidently bring about very specific changes in the dimensions of quality of life. It was pointed out that measuring this effect was also of relevance for practical therapy planning. This makes it possible to focus the therapeutic efforts specifically on the different restrictions. It was pointed out that cluster headache, for instance, could—in addition to the pain—influence role behaviour and social function, but that in practical therapy it was largely only the pain attacks that received attention. Since cluster headache may involve both active periods and remission phases, there should in future be targeted analysis of the HRQoL situation in these phases. Moreover, drug-induced continuous headache displayed distinct effects on all scales in both the Migraine Disability Assessment (MIDAS) and the Medical Outcomes Study short form 36 (SF-36) tests. The emphasis here was on serious impairment of role and work function. This, in particular, is evidence of the serious impairment of the patients affected, and of the need for intensive therapeutic efforts. Attention was also drawn to the importance of measuring clinical dimensions such as depression. Many headache patients who have suffered pain for a long time exhibit marked depressive impairment that moulds the HRQoL. It was also pointed out that, compared with diabetic patients and healthy individuals, migraine had much greater negative effects on HRQoL. This too underlined the need for intensive therapeutic efforts in the treatment of migraine.

Finally, the discussion considered what positive effects on HRQoL could be achieved by treating migraine and other headache syndromes. Numerous studies confirm the positive short-term and also long-term effects of acute therapy. Triptans, for example, can bring about an improvement in HRQoL in a highly targeted and effective manner. It is evidently possible, however, to show differences between the different triptans in individual dimensions. This indicates that the triptans differ not only in their pharmacological properties, but also in their effects on complex physical and psychological dimensions of the quality of life. This appears to be due to both the efficacy and the tolerance of the different active ingredients. It is interesting to note that such an improvement has not been demonstrated for the ergot alkaloids used in the past, and new studies show that the improvements due to treatment with ergot alkaloids are essentially in the placebo region. It is a surprising fact that, to date, there are hardly any data on long-term treatment with prophylactic medication that confirms a positive effect on HRQoL as a result of preventive-medication-based therapeutic methods.

Section

III

Family burden, comorbidities, and health-care utilization

26 Family impact of migraine

Robert Smith and Lora A. Hasse

Introduction

The family is a key functioning social unit that can exert a powerful influence on the health and well-being of its members.[1] Health problems, particularly those involving a major family care-giver, such as a spouse or parent, may seriously threaten and destabilize the whole family.[2] There is an extensive literature on the impact of chronic pain on the family. Much of this work deals with back-pain and work-related injuries; little deals directly with the disabling effect of headache.[3] What data there are strongly suggest that migraine's impact on the family is a widespread problem.

Lipton and his colleagues have shown that the greater prevalence of migraine in women increases during the years of reproduction and peaks before the average age of menopause.[4] The same group has shown that, over a 3-month period, 92% of migraine sufferers reported some level of disability and 53% reported severe disability or the need for bed rest.[5] On these occasions when a major care-giver is partially or totally disabled, families are unlikely to function normally. Between attacks migraine's negative effects on the family appear to continue. Kopp *et al.*[6] have shown that, compared with backache families and pain-free families, migraine families show 'less openness in expressing feelings', are 'less able to tolerate criticism', and 'are more readily annoyed'. Basolo-Kunzer, Diamond, and colleagues[7] have shown that married couples where one spouse has severe migraine, compared with non-migraine couples, have 'more frequent disagreements, and less affection for each other'. There are also reduced family cohesion and problems with sexual relations. Rueveni[8] has reported that headache sufferers 'experience a sense of guilt and isolation' and 'other family members experience confusion, anger and frustration at their failed efforts to help during attacks' and they wonder 'if the headaches are sometimes faked or used as a tool to control others'. In families with a chronic pain problem, patient compliance with treatment has been shown to be greater in more supportive families.[9] Parental response to paediatric headache ranges widely from positive to negative.[10] Physician failure to recognize the importance of family in chronic pain cases has been reported.

We report on a nationwide study in the USA on the impact of migraine on the family.

Methods

Sampling

Four thousand households in the USA were telephoned by trained interviewers using a structured questionnaire. The households were chosen by random digit selection to represent a national sample. The interviewer asked to speak to the male or female head of household and explained to him or her that a national survey was being undertaken concerning health-related issues and that nothing was being sold. If at home, the respondent was asked if he, she, spouse, or partner had suffered a severe headache or migraine in the past year. If not available, the name of the sufferer was obtained and a call-back was arranged. If the respondent failed to qualify, the spouse or partner sufferer was questioned and, if not available, a call-back was arranged. If neither head of household, spouse, nor partner were present or if answers were 'don't know', the interview was terminated.

The first priority was to complete one migraine-sufferer interview per household. The second priority was to call back to speak to the non-sufferer/spouse or partner. This was only done upon completing the sufferer interview first. There was a maximum of two completed interviews per household (one sufferer and one non-sufferer spouse or partner). Only sufferers whose symptoms conformed with the International Headache Society (IHS) criteria for migraine with or without aura were included in the study.

Diagnostic interview

Sufferers were asked if their headaches had ever been diagnosed by a physician. Validation of migraine was based on replies to a series of questions on headache symptoms structured on IHS criteria for migraine with and without aura. These questions were as follows.

(1) During the headache was the pain focused on one side of the head?
(2) Was the pain throbbing or pulsating?
(3) Was the pain aggravated by physical exercise such as walking upstairs or lifting boxes?
(4) Was the pain moderate or severe which affected ability to work or engage in general activities or required bed rest or seclusion in a dark quiet area?

The interview was terminated if three or more of the above questions were answered with 'no' or 'don't know'.

(5) During a headache did you feel nauseated or have a feeling of a 'weak' or queasy stomach, or did you vomit?
(6) During a headache, were you sensitive to bright lights or loud noises?

The interview was terminated if both 5 and 6 were answered 'no' or 'don't know'.

(7) Before the start of the headache, did you see shimmering lights, circles, blind spots, or other shapes or colours in your field of vision ('before your eyes')?
(8) Before the start of the headache did you feel numbness of the eye, tongue, fingers, or legs?
(9) Did you have speech difficulty?

The interview continued irrespective of the answers given to questions 7–9.

Family impact interview

A series of questions followed directed at the sufferer's perception of:

(1) the impact their migraine had on the family as a whole;
(2) the amount of family time and time doing household chores lost each month due to migraine;
(3) the feelings of the family towards their migraine;
(4) delays or postponement or cancellation of domestic and social activities due to migraine;
(5) the effect of the patient's migraine on his or her children;
(6) the effect of the patient's migraine on the spousal or partnership relation.

Results

The physicians' migraine-diagnosis rate (Table 26.1) is higher than that reported by others.[5] It is possible that our screening method of selecting migraine sufferers ('severe headache or migraine in the past year') identified more severe migraine sufferers and so resulted in more migraine diagnoses being made by physicians.

   In response to question 1 of the family impact interview, 61% of sufferers reported that their migraine attacks had a significant impact on their families (Table 26.2). In response to question 3 of the family impact interview, positive descriptors of family response to migraine were more frequently selected by sufferers than negative descriptors (Table 26.3).

Table 26.1 Population base

	Number (%)
Households	4000
Migraine sufferers (total)	350 (8.9)
Females	269 (5.7)
Males	81 (2.0)
Physician-diagnosed*	220 (5.5)
Not physician-diagnosed*	130 (3.3)
Non-sufferer spouse or partner	77 (1.9)

*Diagnosed as having symptoms conforming to IHS criteria.

Table 26.2 Impact level on migraine sufferers (N=350)

Impact of migraine	Number (%) of sufferers reporting
Extremely significant	27 (8)
Very significant	47 (13)
Somewhat significant	139 (40)
Not very significant	90 (26)
Not significant at all	43 (12)
Don't know	4 (1)

Table 26.3 Feelings of family of migraine sufferers (N=350)

Feeling of family	Number (%) of sufferers reporting
Understanding	225 (64)
Sympathetic	164 (47)
Resigned/accepting	157 (45)
Frustrated	83 (24)
Resentful	42 (12)
Indifferent	16 (5)

Table 26.4 Domestic activities delayed or postponed as reported by migraine sufferers (N=350)*

Activity delayed or postponed	Number (%) of sufferers reporting
Housecleaning, yard work	283 (81)
Laundry, shopping	277 (79)
Activities with spouse	265 (76)
Activities with children	243 (69)
Driving/car pooling activities	216 (62)
All domestic activities (stayed in bed)	63 (18)

*Estimated time lost with family or on chores each month, 50 hours.

In response to question 2 of the family impact interview, it was reported that household duties were most commonly delayed or postponed (79–81%). Activities with spouse (76%) and children (69%) were also frequently affected (Table 26.4). In response to question 4 of the family impact interview it was found that cancellation or postponement of social activities, although significant, was at a lower level of interference than that that occurred with household duties (Table 26.5).

Table 26.5   Social activities cancelled or postponed as reported by migraine sufferers (N=350)

Social activity cancelled or postponed	Number (%) of sufferers reporting
Entertainment of family, friends, colleagues	136 (39)
Birthday, anniversary celebrations	107 (31)
Week-end pleasure trips	76 (22)
Holiday celebrations	74 (21)
Other social activities outside home	47 (14)

Table 26.6   Impact of parent's migraine (N=350) on their children under age 12

Impact	Number (%) of sufferers reporting
Parent cancels plans for playing, helping with homework	79 (61)
Parent cancels outings	73 (56)
Others take care of children	55 (42)
Parent arranges for baby-sitter	24 (14)
Children keep quiet	85 (66)
Children keep their distance	47 (36)
Children become confused	32 (25)
Children become hostile	23 (17)
Children become afraid	15 (12)
Children try to be helpful	9 (7)
Children rub parent's head, neck	4 (3)

In response to question 5 of the family impact interview it was reported that, for children under 12 years of age (Table 26.6), parental care was abandoned in 61% of cases, 56% of outings were cancelled, and alternative child-care arrangements were made on 42% of occasions. As expected, children aged 12 to 17 were more understanding (87%), more helpful (42%), and less hostile (12%) (Table 26.7).

Table 26.7   Impact of parent's migraine (N=350) on their children aged 12 to 17

Impact	Number (%) of sufferers reporting
Children stop playing music, other loud activities	76 (87)
Children stop asking questions, asking for homework help	53 (61)
Children cancel plans to have friends visit	37 (42)
Children go to friends' homes	30 (34)
Children want to stay home from school	18 (21)
Children prepare meals	10 (12)
Children become hostile	10 (12)
Children do household chores	6 (6)

Table 26.8 Impact of migraine on relationship with spouse as reported by migraine sufferers (N=350)

Impact	Number (%) of sufferers reporting
Affects frequency or quality of sexual relations	86 (24)
Resulted in need for personal counselling with therapist	21 (6)
Resulted in divorce or end of relationship	18 (5)
Resulted in separation from spouse	16 (5)

In response to question 6 of the family impact interview, one in four migraine sufferers reported that their headaches affected their sexual relations. Divorce or ending of relationships was reported in 5% of cases (Table 26.8).

Conclusion

Migraine may interfere with many aspects of family life. The family response to the sufferer in most cases appears supportive. Most families are understanding and ready to help the sufferer to cope. The physician should always recognize the possible negative effects of migraine on the family, which may have headache-aggravating effects on the patient.

In cases of severe disabling migraine and other chronic severe headaches, particularly when there is poor response to treatment, family dysfunction should be considered as a possible contributing cause. The readiness or not of the spouse to accompany the patient at an office visit, when requested by the physician, may be a useful indicator of the level of support the patient is receiving at home.

Little is known about the benefits of taking family response into account in the overall care of the migraine patient. Rectifying family dysfunctional problems may be beyond the scope of the busy practitioner and introducing additional health professionals for family counselling and therapy, if available, would generate additional costs. The indications and methods of intervention to be used remain unclear. Further study in this area is required.

Acknowledgements

Funding was provided by GlaxoSmithKline.

References

1. Litman TJ. The family as a basic unit in health and medical care: a social–behavioral overview. *Soc Sci Med* 1974; **8**: 495–519.
2. Flor H, Turk DC, Rudy TE. Pain and families, II. Assessment and treatment. *Pain* 1987; **30**: 29–45.

3. Turk DC, Flor H, Rudy TE. Pain and families I. Etiology, maintenance, and psychosocial impact. *Pain* 1987; **30**: 3–27.
4. Stewart WF, Lipton RB, Celentano DD, Reed ML. Prevalence of migraine headache in the United States. Relationship to age, income, race and other sociodemographic factors. *J Am Med Assoc* 1992; **267**: 64–9.
5. Lipton RB, Stewart WF, Diamond S, Diamond ML, Reed M. Migraine diagnosis and treatment: results from the American Migraine Study II. *Headache* 2001; **41**: 646–57.
6. Kopp M, Richter R, Rainer J, Kopp-Wilfling P, Rumpold G, Walter MH. Differences in family functioning between patients with chronic headache and patients with chronic headache and patients with chronic low back pain. *Pain* 1995; **63**: 219–24.
7. Basolo-Kunzer M, Diamond S, Maliszewski M, Weyermann L, Reed J. Chronic headache patients' marital and family adjustment. *Issues Ment Hlth Nursing* 1991; **12**: 133–48.
8. Rueveni U. Brief consultation with headache sufferers. *Am J Fam Ther* 1992; **20**: 168–78.
9. Painter JR, Seres JL, Newman RI. Assessing benefits of the pain center: why some patients regress. *Pain* 1980; **8**: 101–13.
10. Wall BA, Holden EW, Gladstein J. Parent responses to pediatric headache. *Headache* 1997; **37**: 65–70.

27 Migraine comorbidity with stroke, epilepsy, and major depression

Naomi Breslau

Introduction

The development of explicit diagnostic criteria for neurological and psychiatric disorders in the 1980s provided an essential prerequisite for the scientific investigation of the associations between migraine and psychiatric disorders or other neurological disorders. Despite controversies regarding the validity of diagnostic categories, the use of standard definitions has facilitated communication among researchers and clinicians. Case-control studies of consecutive admissions of stroke patients, recruited from hospitals serving defined geographical areas, have yielded information on migraine as a risk factor for stroke and on the comorbidity of migraine with epilepsy. The risk for stroke in persons with a history of migraine was also examined in large data sets from general population studies in the USA. The comorbidity of migraine with psychiatric disorders has been also examined in samples of the general population. The driving question in studies on the migraine–stroke association concerns the pathogenic role of migraine in the subsequent occurrence of stroke events. By contrast, the research questions in studies on the association of migraine with epilepsy and with psychiatric disorders concern lifetime comorbidity and, in regard to psychiatric disorders, also the temporal order between the onset of migraine and the onset of the comorbid disorders.

This review summarizes results from recent studies on the association of migraine with stroke, epilepsy, and major depression. The studies selected for this summary have used the 1988 International Headache Society (IHS) criteria for migraine (or an approximation of these criteria) and applied the standard explicit definition for the second disorder, that is, that of the International Classification of Diseases (ICD) 9th edition for stroke, that of the International League Against Epilepsy for epilepsy, and the definitions of the DSM-III (3rd edition of the *Diagnostic and statistical manual of mental disorders*, or later DSM editions) for psychiatric disorders.

Migraine and the risk of stroke

Apart from the very rare occurrence of migraine-induced stroke and the possible migraine-like manifestation of stroke, there is evidence suggesting an association between history of migraine and the subsequent occurrence of stroke. In the past decade, several case-control studies compared the prevalence of migraine in patients hospitalized for stroke with the prevalence of migraine in sex- and age-matched hospitalized controls. Additionally, analyses of data from two longitudinal studies of the general population reported on the association between history of migraine and the subsequent occurrence of stroke during a follow-up period. Table 27.1 presents a summary of these studies.

Two case-control studies that included both sexes[1,2] reported an increased risk of stroke associated with history of migraine in women but not in men. Both studies suggested that the increased risk applied to young women, that is, those <45 years of age, but not to young men or older men and women. Furthermore, Carolei et al.[2] reported a higher odds ratio (OR) for stroke associated with migraine in women <35 years of age than in their total sample of women 15–44 years of age. However, despite the higher ORs in younger women (<45 in Tzourio et al.[1] and <35 in Carolei et al.[2]), the confidence intervals (CI) of these estimates were wide and the question of the specificity of the increased risk to young women could not be reliably demonstrated. This is due to the very low incidence of stroke in young women (10 per 100 000 per year).[1]

Three case-control studies of women <45 years of age[3–5] confirmed the finding of an increased risk for stroke in younger women with a history of migraine. Additionally, two of the studies identified smoking and current use of oral contraceptives as effect-modifiers, increasing the risk for stroke in women with migraine. High blood

Table 27.1   Migraine as a risk factor for stroke

Reference number	Age (years)	Odds ratio (95% CI)	
		Males	Females
1	18–80	1.1 (0.5–2.2)	1.6 (0.7–3.5)
1	<45	0.7 (NS)*	4.3 (1.2–16.3)
2	15–44	1.2 (0.4–3.2)	1.9 (1.1–3.3)
2	<35	—	3.7 (1.5–9.0)
3	<45	—	3.5 (1.8–6.4)
4	15–44	—	2.8 (p<0.01)
5	20–44	—	1.8 (1.1–2.8)
6	40–84	1.8 (1.1–3.2)†	
7	25–74	1.5‡	1.5

*NS, Not significant.
†Relative risk and 95% CI.
‡Hazards ratio.

pressure was identified in one of the studies as an effect-modifier as well.[5] On the basis of these five case-control studies, the estimated risk of stroke associated with history of migraine in women <45 years of age ranges from 1.8 to 4.3.

Of the two studies that used large-scale longitudinal data sets, one included only men[6] and the other included both sexes.[7] Buring *et al.*[6] reported results from a longitudinal study of 22 071 male physicians 40–84 years of age. The authors reported that men with history of migraine were at a nearly twofold-increased risk for the incidence of stroke during a 5-year follow-up period, compared to men with no history of migraine. Merikangas *et al.*[7] reported results from analysis of the US National Health and Nutrition Examination Study (NHANES) longitudinal data of 12 220 persons of both sexes, 25–74 years of age. The estimated relative risk for stroke during a 10-year follow-up period in persons with migraine was 1.5. Sex did not modify the effect of migraine on stroke. The association of migraine with stroke did not vary significantly between men and women. This study found that the risk of stroke associated with pre-existing migraine decreased as the age at the stroke events increased. For example, it was 2.8 ($p<0.05$) at age 40, 1.7 ($p<0.05$) at age 60, and 1.4 (not significant) at age 70. These results suggest that migraine plays a greater role in early stroke, when the incidence of stroke is low, than in later stroke.

In sum, the case-control studies of patients with stroke and longitudinal studies of samples of the general population have reported an increased risk for stroke in persons with a history of migraine. The case-control studies reported no increased risk in men, whereas the studies of samples of the general population found a statistically significant increased risk in men. The inconsistency in the results from case-control studies and epidemiological studies with respect to the pathogenic role of migraine in stroke among men calls for further research. Most studies reported evidence that supports an increased risk only for ischaemic stroke.[5] Some studies suggested that the risk for stroke is stronger in migraine with aura than in migraine without aura.

Migraine comorbidity with epilepsy

Ottman and Lipton[8] examined the association between migraine and epilepsy, using data on 1948 adult patients with epilepsy and 1411 of their parents and siblings from the Epilepsy Family Study of Columbia University. The sex-adjusted hazards ratio for migraine in probands with epilepsy was 2.4 (95% CI 2.0–2.9) and in relatives with epilepsy, 2.4 (95% CI 1.6–3.8), using relatives without epilepsy as reference. When probands were stratified by seizure type, age of onset, and aetiology, the risk of migraine was significantly increased in all subgroups, with little variation across subgroups. The highest relative risk, 4.1 (95% CI 2.9–5.7), was observed in epilepsy attributable to head trauma, a category that included a very small subset of all probands with epilepsy (8% of all probands). The relative risk associated with idiopathic seizure, the largest subgroup of probands with epilepsy (80% of all probands), was 2.3 (95% CI 1.9–2.7). These results are consistent with results from previous studies.[9]

In a separate analysis, Ottman and Lipton[10] examined the possibility that the comorbidity of migraine with epilepsy results from a shared genetic susceptibility to both disorders. Testing several proxy measures for genetic forms of epilepsy, the authors failed to find support for a shared genetic susceptibility for the migraine–epilepsy association. The authors concluded that the comorbidity between migraine and epilepsy cannot be accounted for by genetic mechanisms and that both disorders might be caused by abnormal neuronal excitability that results from genetic and environmental factors.

Migraine comorbidity with psychiatric disorders

General population studies have reported positive lifetime associations between migraine and psychiatric disorders.[11-17] Associations between migraine and affective and anxiety disorders have been consistently reported across studies, whereas reports of associations with alcohol and drug use disorders have been inconsistent. Table 27.2 presents estimates of lifetime associations between migraine and specific psychiatric disorders from two recent population-based studies. The first study is a report by Swartz et al.[18] based on data from a 12–14 year follow-up study of the 1981 Baltimore ECA study. Unadjusted and sex- and age-adjusted ORs were reported for the lifetime associations between migraine and major depression, specific anxiety disorders, and alcohol and/or drug abuse defined according to DSM-III. Of all the comorbid disorders examined in that

Table 27.2 Lifetime association of migraine with specific psychiatric disorders in the Baltimore ECA Study and the Detroit Area Study of Headache

	Baltimore ECA Study*		Detroit Area Study†	
Disorder	OR (95% CI)‡	AOR (95% CI)§	OR (95% CI)‡	AOR (95% CI)§
Major depression	3.1 (2.0–4.8)	2.2 (1.4–3.5)	3.6 (2.7–4.8)	3.6 (2.7–4.7)
Panic disorder	5.1 (2.6–9.8)	3.4 (1.7–6.7)	5.0 (3.5–7.5)	4.9 (3.3–7.4)
Agoraphobia	2.5 (1.8–3.5)	1.9 (1.3–2.7)	2.4 (1.6–3.8)	2.4 (1.6–3.7)
Social phobia	1.4 (1.1–2.0)	1.3 (0.9–1.8)	2.2 (1.5–3.2)	2.1 (1.5–3.1)
Simple specific phobia	1.7 (1.3–2.2)	1.4 (1.02–1.8)	2.2 (1.7–2.9)	2.2 (1.6–2.9)
Any phobia	1.8 (1.4–2.4)	1.4 (1.1–1.9)	2.3 (1.8–3.0)	2.2 (1.7–2.9)
Alcohol/drug abuse	0.8 (0.6–1.2)	1.0 (0.7–1.6)	—	—
Alcohol abuse disorder	—	—	1.3 (1.0–1.6)	1.4 (1.1–1.8)
Drug abuse disorder	—	—	1.5 (1.1–2.1)	1.7 (1.2–2.4)

*Swartz et al.'s (2000) Baltimore ECA study (ref. 18) presents DSM-III disorders.
†The Detroit Area Study (ref. 19) presents DSM-IV disorders.
‡OR, Unadjusted odds ratios.
§AOR, Sex- and age-adjusted odds ratios.

study, the highest association was found for panic disorder for which the OR was 5.1 (95% CI 2.6–9.8). The sex- and age-adjusted OR was lower, but remained the highest of all the similarly adjusted estimates (3.4, 95% CI 1.7–6.7). The association between migraine and major depression ranked second in magnitude. The combined category of alcohol and/or drug abuse was reported to be unrelated to migraine.[18]

Table 27.2 also presents estimates from the Detroit Area Study of Headache, conducted in 1997 in southeast Michigan.[19] This study was designed to identify representative samples of persons 25–55 years of age with (1) migraine, (2) other severe headaches, and (3) controls with no history of headache in order to estimate the prevalence of psychiatric disorders in each group. The study was conducted in two phases. In the first phase, a large-scale random-digit dialling telephone interview was used to identify the three population groups. Migraine was defined by the 1998 IHS criteria. Severe headache was defined as headache not meeting migraine criteria, with no history of nausea, vomiting, photophobia, or phonophobia; with a duration similar to the duration specified in the IHS definition of migraine; and with a severity level corresponding to that of migraine. In the second phase, face-to-face interviews were conducted with subsets of persons identified in the telephone survey, that is, those with migraine, those with other severe headaches, and controls, in order to assess psychiatric disorders according to DSM-IV. A structured diagnostic interview for DSM-IV psychiatric disorders—the WHO CIDI 2.1—was used. (Detailed information on the sample, measurement, and data were presented previously.[19])

The lifetime associations between migraine and specific psychiatric disorders in the Detroit Area Study of Headache follow a similar pattern to the pattern reported from the Baltimore ECA follow-up study (Table 27.2). The psychiatric disorder with the highest lifetime association with migraine was panic disorder, for which the sex- and age-adjusted OR was 4.9 (95% CI 3.3–7.4). The second in magnitude was major depression. In contrast with the Baltimore ECA results, in the Detroit Area Study of Headache the association between migraine and drug abuse disorder was significant; the adjusted OR was 1.7 (95% CI 1.2–2.4). However, the association between migraine and alcohol abuse disorder was not significant. Of all the anxiety disorders, agoraphobia had the highest lifetime association with migraine in both studies.

These two recent studies replicate previous reports on the lifetime associations between migraine headaches and psychiatric disorders, especially major depression and anxiety disorders.[11–17] However, the previous reports were based on samples of young adults, whereas these recent studies included a wider age range, subjects >30 years of age in the Baltimore ECA follow-up study and 25–55 years of age in the Detroit Area Study of Headache. The extent to which the observed lifetime associations among persons older than 30 years of age reflect comorbid disorders with onset before age 30 years cannot be inferred from the estimates of lifetime associations. For this purpose, information is needed on the incidence of migraine in adults with pre-existing psychiatric disorders and on the incidence of psychiatric disorders in adults with pre-existing migraine.

Migraine and major depression: investigating temporal order

Of all the psychiatric disorders reported to be associated with migraine, major depression has received the greatest attention. The association between migraine headache and major depression might have several explanations. The association might be noncausal, reflecting shared genetic or environmental factors. Alternatively, migraine might cause major depression or might be caused by it. A finding that each disorder increases the risk of the first onset of the other would support the hypothesis of shared aetiology. In contrast, the hypothesis that major depression in persons with migraine reflects a psychological response to recurrent pain would predict an influence only from migraine to major depression but not from major depression to migraine.

Both retrospective and prospective epidemiological data have been used to examine potential causal pathways between migraine and major depression. Based on retrospective data of a sample of 1007 young adults,[15] we reported estimates from Cox proportional hazards models for censored survival data of the relative risk for major depression associated with prior migraine and the relative risk for migraine associated with prior major depression. Using migraine as a time-dependent covariate, the hazards ratio for subsequent first onset of major depression was 3.3 (95% CI 2.1–5.2). The sex- and education-adjusted hazards ratio was 2.9 (95% CI 1.9–4.7). Analysis that examined the reverse direction, that is, from major depression to the subsequent first onset of migraine, yielded a similar estimate. The hazard ratio was 4.1 (95% CI 2.3–7.4) and the sex- and education-adjusted hazards ratio was 3.8 (95% CI 2.1–6.7).[15]

Analysis of retrospective data from the 1997 Detroit Area Study of Headache, which included persons aged 25 to 55 years, replicated the results of our previous study.[19] Using the same survival analytical approach, the sex-adjusted hazards ratio for the subsequent first onset of major depression associated with prior migraine was 2.4 (95% CI 1.8–3.0). The sex-adjusted hazards ratio for the subsequent first onset of migraine associated with prior major depression was 2.8 (95% CI 2.2–3.5). Additional analyses of these retrospective data indicated that the associations applied to both migraine with aura and migraine without aura, with only small differences in the estimates.[19]

Results from *prospective* data from the Study of Young Adults confirmed the results from the retrospective data. The prospective data covered 3.5 years in young adulthood, specifically in persons who were 21–30 years of age at baseline. The adjusted estimate of the risk for the first onset of major depression in persons with prior migraine was 4.1 (95% CI 2.2–7.4) and for the first onset of migraine in persons with prior major depression, 3.3 (95% CI 1.6–6.6).[19] The estimates from the prospective data were not significantly different from the estimates based on the retrospective data (p > 0.20). Recent analysis of prospective data from a 2-year follow-up assessment of the Detroit Area Study of Headache replicated these results.

These data indicate that the previously observed cross-sectional association between migraine and major depression might result from bi-directional influences, with each disorder increasing the risk for the first onset of the other. The explanation that major depression in persons with migraine represents a psychological response to recurrent severe pain would have been more plausible had there been evidence of an influence only from migraine to major depression. The findings of bi-directional influences are consistent with the explanation that both disorders share common aetiologies, although a more complex causal explanation cannot be ruled out.

Is the bi-directional association with major depression specific to migraine?

Apart from migraine, major depression has been linked to other pain conditions. Reciprocal psychological effects of pain and depressive symptoms have been postulated: pain precipitates worry and pessimism, while distress impairs the ability to cope with pain.[20–23] Headaches and other pain conditions also have been viewed as somatic symptoms of depression.[24,25] These findings on the relationship of depression with pain call into question the specificity of the migraine–major depression association. Are other severe headaches also associated with major depression? Are there bi-directional influences in relation to other headaches of similar severity?

This question was addressed in the Detroit Area Study of Headache.[19] Lifetime prevalence of major depression in persons with migraine was 40.7%, in persons with other headaches of comparable severity 35.8%, and in controls with no history of severe headaches 16.0%. The sex-adjusted ORs that measure the association of major depression with migraine and with other severe headache, relative to persons with no history of severe headaches, were similar in magnitude, 3.5 (95% CI 2.6–4.6) and 3.2 (95% CI 2.1–4.7), respectively. Results from survival analysis models with time-dependent covariates did not support a bi-directional relationship between other severe headaches and major depression. The hazards ratio for the first onset of major depression in persons with severe headaches other than migraine was 3.6 (95% CI 2.4–5.3). However, the hazards ratio for the first onset of severe headaches in persons with major depression was not significant, 1.6 (95% CI 0.9–2.8). In sum, in contrast to the evidence of a bi-directional relationship between migraine and major depression, there was evidence of an influence from other severe headaches to depression, but not for an influence in the reverse direction, that is, from major depression to severe headache.

Conclusions

Recent evidence suggests that migraine might constitute a risk factor for subsequent stroke. A lifetime association between migraine and epilepsy has been reported, but the temporal order between the two disorders has not been examined. New evidence on the association between migraine and major depression suggests a bi-directional association, with each disorder increasing the risk for the subsequent first onset of the other. The evidence suggests that this association might not apply to other headaches of similar severity. The specificity of the bi-directional association between migraine and major depression provides further support for the hypothesis that both disorders share a common aetiology.

References

1. Tzourio C, Iglesias S, Hubert J-B, *et al*. Migraine and risk of ischaemic stroke: a case-control study. *Br Med J* 1993; **307**: 289–92.
2. Carolei A, Marini C, De Matteis G, and the Italian National Research Council Study Group on Stroke in the Young. History of migraine and risk of cerebral ischaemia in young adults. *Lancet* 1996; **347**: 1503–6.
3. Tzourio C, Tehindrazanarivelo A, Iglesias S. Case-control study of migraine and risk of ischaemic stroke in young women. *Br Med J* 1995; **310**: 830–3.
4. Lidegaard O. Oral contraceptives, pregnancy and the risk of cerebral thromboelism: the influence of diabetes, hypertension, migraine and previous thrombotic disease. *Br J Obstetr Gynaecol* 1995; **102**: 153–9.
5. Chang CL, Donaghy M, Poulter N, and World Health Organisation Collaborative Study of Cardiovascular Disease and Steroid Hormone Contraception. Migraine and stroke in young women: case-control study. *Br Med J* 1999; **318**: 13–18.
6. Buring JE, Hebert P, Romero J, *et al*. Migraine and subsequent risk of stroke in the Physicians' Health Study. *Arch Neurol* 1995; **52**: 129–34.
7. Merikangas KR, Fenton BT, Cheng SH, Stolar MJ, Risch N. Association between migraine and stroke in a large-scale epidemiologic study of the United States. *Arch Neurol* 1997; **54**: 362–8.
8. Ottman R, Lipton RB. Comorbidity of migraine and epilepsy. *Neurology* 1994; **44**: 2105–10.
9. Andermann E, Andermann F. Migraine–epilepsy relationships: epidemiological and genetic aspects. In *Migraine and epilepsy* (ed. Andermann FA, Lugaresi E). Boston: Butterworths, 1987: 281–91.
10. Ottman R, Lipton RB. Is the comorbidity of epilepsy and migraine due to a shared genetic susceptibility? *Neurology* 1996; **47**: 918–24.
11. Merikangas KR, Risch NJ, Merikangas JR, Weissman MM, Kidd KK. Migraine and depression: association and familial transmission. *J Psychiatr Res* 1988; **22**: 119–29.
12. Merikangas KR, Angst J, Isler H. Migraine and psychopathology: results of the Zurich Cohort Study of young adults. *Arch Gen Psychiatry* 1990; **47**: 849–53.
13. Breslau N, Davis GC, Andreski P. Migraine, psychiatric disorders and suicide attempts: an epidemiologic study in young adults. *Psychiatr Res* 1991; **37**: 11–23.
14. Breslau N, Davis GC. Migraine, physical health and psychiatric disorder: a prospective epidemiologic study of young adults. *J Psychiatr Res* 1993; **27**: 211–21.
15. Breslau N, Davis GC, Schultz LR, Peterson EL. Migraine and major depression: a longitudinal study. *Headache* 1994; **34**: 387–93.
16. Merikangas KK, Merikangas JR, Angst J. Headache syndromes and psychiatric disorders: association and familial transmission. *J Psychiatr Res* 1993; **27**: 197–210.
17. Breslau N, Merikangas K, Bowden CL (1994). Comorbidity of migraine and major affective disorders. *Neurology* 1994; **44** (Suppl. 7): S17–S22.
18. Swartz KL, Pratt LA, Armenian HK, Lee LC, Eaton WW. Mental disorders and the incidence of migraine headaches in a community sample. *Arch Gen Psychiatry* 2000; **57**: 945–50.
19. Breslau N, Schultz LR, Stewart WF, Lipton RB, Lucia VC, Welch KMA. Headache and major depression: is the association specific to migraine? *Neurology* 2000; **54**: 308–13.

20. Von Korff M, Le Resche L, Dworkin SF. First onset of common pain symptoms: a prospective study of depression as a risk factor. *Pain* 1993; **55**: 251–8.
21. Dworkin SF, Von Korff M, Le Resche L. Multiple pains and psychiatric disturbance: an epidemiologic investigation. *Arch Gen Psychiatry* 1990; **47**: 239–44.
22. Fields H. Depression and pain: a neurobiological model. *Neuropsychiatry Neuropsychol Behav Neurol* 1991; **4**: 83–92.
23. Von Korff M, Simon G. The relationship between pain and depression. *Br J Psychiatry* 1996; **30** (Suppl.): 101–8.
24. Katon W, Kleinman A, Rosen G. Depression and somatization: a review. Part 1. *Am J Med* 1982; **72**: 127–35.
25. Katon W, Kleinman A, Rosen G. Depression and somatization: a review. Part II. *Am J Med* 1982; **72**: 241–7.

28 Health-care utilization for headache

Birthe Krogh Rasmussen

Headache disorders constitute a public health problem of enormous proportions with an impact on both the individual sufferer and on society. The public health significance of headaches is often overlooked, probably because of their episodic nature and lack of mortality, but headache disorders are often incapacitating with considerable impact on social activities and work, and may lead to a significant consumption of drugs. Epidemiological knowledge is required to quantitate the significance of these disorders. The effects on individuals can be assessed by examining prevalence, distribution, attack frequency and duration, and headache-related disability. On the basis of data on the size and nature of the headache problem, you could estimate the need for health care to alleviate these disorders. However, there is compelling evidence that, worldwide, these disorders are both underdiagnosed and undertreated. One reason is that health-care resources are insufficient for all needs both in terms of availability and effectiveness. But another reason is that the general information in society about these disorders and their possible treatments is insufficient with the result that many sufferers never contact their general practitioner. In this chapter, health-care utilization for headache is described on the basis of the results of population-based studies using the criteria of the International Headache Society (IHS).[1]

Consultation rates: sex- and age-distribution

In a Danish epidemiological study of headache disorders nearly all persons with migraine stated that the pain impaired or abolished working capacity as well as social activities. This was also described by 60% of persons with tension-type headache.[2] Nevertheless, according to several studies, nearly half of the persons with migraine and more than four-fifths of persons with tension-type headache had never contacted their general practitioner because of the headache.[3–11]

Among subjects with migraine, 56% had, at some time, consulted their general practitioner because of migraine (Fig. 28.1). The corresponding figure among subjects with tension-type headache was 16%. One or more specialists had been consulted by 16% of migraine sufferers and by 4% of subjects with tension-type headache.[4,5,8]

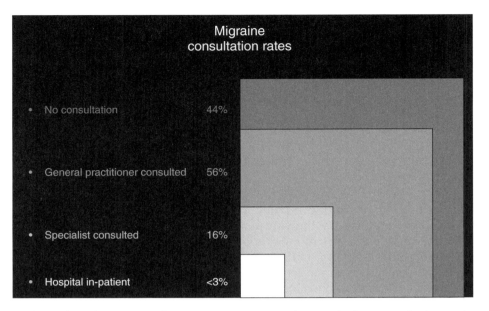

Fig. 28.1 Consultation rates due to migraine among subjects who have ever had migraine.

In both migraineurs and in subjects with tension-type headache, the consultation of a general practitioner is positively correlated to the frequency of attacks.[4–6,12,13]

The reported consultation rates in Western countries may be somewhat different from those in other areas due to varying cultural and social backgrounds and to variations in the availability of general practitioners.[14,15] The consultation rates are found to be higher among women than among men in most studies.[4,6,7,11,13,16–19] Consultation rates among men and women have only been reported to be equal in one study.[20] The consultation rates of chiropractors and physiotherapists ranged from 5% to 8%,[4] which is somewhat higher than rates reported in a study in the USA,[16] but the latter study included only young adults, and regional variations in the health service systems as well as different traditions may influence the parameters.

Lipton and associates found that, in women, consulting behaviour was associated with pain intensity, the number of migraine symptoms, attack frequency and duration, and disability.[5] Table 28.1 lists factors reported in the literature to be associated with consulting behaviour among headache sufferers. Predictors of higher consultation rates include female gender and advancing age.[7,21–23] With advancing age, duration of illness increases creating a longer window for diagnosis. Type of headache, including severity and disability and number of headache types, influences the consultation rates. Higher consultation rates in subjects with coexisting migraine and tension-type headache[4,21] and in headache sufferers with comorbidities are in concordance with Berkson's view[24] that subjects with more than one disease are more likely to seek medical care than subjects with only one disease.

Table 28.1 Factors associated with consulting behaviour among primary headache sufferers

Gender
Age
Length of the disease
Type of headache
Number of headache types
Comorbidity
Belief in the effectiveness of medical care
Pain intensity
Attack frequency
Attack duration
Disability
Number of migraine symptoms

Admission rates

Hospitalization rates for treatment of primary headache disorders are low. In a Danish population-based study only 2% of the population had been admitted to hospital because of headache[4] and in a US study hospitalization rates for migraine are reported as about 7% of migraineurs.[19] Supplementary laboratory investigations (electroencephalography (EEG), computerized tomography (CT) scan, etc.) and emergency department visits due to headache are rare (< 3%).[4,5]

Medication

Our present knowledge of medication habits in headache sufferers is poor and mainly based on headache-prone populations. In a Danish study of an unselected population, about half of migraineurs and one-seventh of persons with tension-type headache managed without medication in the current year. About one-quarter of migraineurs and one-third of subjects with tension-type headache used one or more forms of medicine for 1–3 times a month. Among those who used medicine, over-the-counter (OTC) drugs were the most frequently used.[4] The most commonly used analgesics were acetylsalicylic acid preparations and paracetamol, that is, the same as those reported in other studies.[16,17,23,25–29] Specific antimigraine drugs are less frequently used. Prescription medication is only used by about one-third of migraine sufferers and in afew with tension-type headache.[4,6,25–28] Prophylactics are used by 6–7% of migraineurs.[4,21]

Utilization of medical services

The headaches strike individuals early in life and usually continue to affect them through the majority of their productive years, not infrequently continuing even after retirement. A large proportion of headache sufferers are never diagnosed or regularly treated.[4,5] The relatively low consultation rate and low consumption of medicine could be interpreted to mean that medical care is unnecessary for a large proportion of the sufferers. However, the majority of headache sufferers stated that their daily activities were inhibited due to the headaches. Therefore, it is plausible that many headache sufferers are unaware that effective treatment exists and therefore do not consult a physician. In a population-based US sample of headache sufferers, it is reported that, among subjects absent from work during the week preceding the interview, only 31% of females and 18% of males had consulted a physician during the previous 12 months.[6] Thus, measures of medical care expenditure due to the disorders do not reflect the true burden of the diseases. Estimates of socio-economic loss should include direct costs associated with medical care as well as indirect costs associated with lost workplace productivity.

The reasons previously reported for not seeking medical attention were low frequency of headaches, insufficient severity of headaches, and the availability of OTC medications (Table 28.2).[25] Reasons cited for not returning for further medical attention encompass the availability of OTC medications as effective or more effective and with fewer side-effects than prescribed medications, as well as dissatisfaction with the primary care physician not taking the problem seriously, that is, poor patient–physician communication (Table 28.2).[25,27,30] In France, 65% of migraineurs thought that migraine could never been cured, and 43% believed that nothing could be done for migraine.[26]

The episodic nature of the headache disorders may be another reason for not consulting physicians. Between acute attacks, the sufferer is perfectly well, at least as far as the headache features are concerned. This may delay contact with health care. On the other hand, between attacks, fear of the occurrence of the next attack may provoke anxiety and avoidance behaviour. Because of worry about the next attack, there is a tendency amongst migraine sufferers to use symptomatic therapy, not for the attack they actually have but for the attack they fear they are about to have. Frequently, this may lead to recurrent misuse of medication and a subsequent chronic and more disabling headache.

Table 28.2 Factors associated with non-consulting behaviour among primary headache sufferers

Availability of OTC drugs
Therapeutic inadequacies
No belief/information about possible effective treatments
Low frequency
Low pain intensity

Conclusion

The burden associated with headaches has previously been underestimated. Primary headache disorders are highly prevalent and frequently disabling disorders. Considerable benefits can be gained by strategies leading to reductions in the amount of work absence caused by headache. The impact of the headache disorders on the sufferer's quality of life may, however, be the most substantial burden. In addition to the disability related to attacks, many headache sufferers live with a fear of the next attack and restrict their lifestyles, which may disrupt their ability to meet social obligations. Thus, the individual and societal burden of headache is substantial. Nonetheless, a large proportion of headache sufferers are never diagnosed or regularly treated. Combined with the fact that primary headache disorders cause about 20% of all absenteeism due to sickness, this dictates a call for an improved health-care service especially concerning strategies leading to adequate primary prevention, diagnosis, and treatment.

References

1. Headache Classification Committee of the International Headache Society. Classification and diagnostic criteria for headache disorders, cranial neuralgias and facial pain. *Cephalalgia* 1988; **8** (Suppl. 7): 1–96.
2. Rasmussen BK, Jensen R, Olesen J. A population-based analysis of the diagnostic criteria of the International Headache Society. *Cephalalgia* 1991; **11**: 129–34.
3. O'Brien B, Goeree R, Streiner D. Prevalence of migraine headache in Canada: a population-based survey. *Int J Epidemiol* 1994; **23**: 1020–6.
4. Rasmussen BK, Jensen R, Olesen J. Impact of headache on sickness absence and utilisation of medical services. A Danish population study. *J Epidemiol Commun Hlth* 1992; **46**: 443–6.
5. Lipton RB, Stewart WF, Simon D. Medical consultation for migraine: results from the American Migraine Study. *Headache* 1998; **38**: 87–96.
6. Stewart WF, Celentano DD, Linet MS. Disability, physician consultation, and use of prescription medications in a population-based study of headache. *Biomed Pharmacother* 1989; **43**: 711–18.
7. Lipton RB, Stewart WF, Celentano DD, Reed ML. Undiagnosed migraine headaches. a comparison of symptom-based and reported physician diagnosis. *Arch Intern Med* 1992; **152**: 1273–8.
8. Rasmussen, Birthe Krogh. Epidemiology of headache. Thesis. *Cephalalgia* 1995; **15**: 48–68.
9. Ekbom K, Ahlborg B, Schèle R. Prevalence of migraine and cluster headache in Swedish men of 18. *Headache* 1978; **18**: 9–19.
10. Waters WE, O'Connor PJ. Epidemiology of headache and migraine in women. *J Neurol Neurosurg Psychiatry* 1971; **34**: 148–53.
11. Newland CA, Illis LS, Robinson PK, Batchelor BG, Waters WE. A survey of headache in an English City. *Res Clin Stud Headache* 1978; **5**: 1–20.
12. Fitzpatrick R, Hopkins A. Referrals to neurologists for headaches not due to structural disease. *J Neurol Neurosurg Psychiatry* 1981; **44**: 1061–7.
13. Post D, Gubbels JW. Headache: An epidemiological survey in a Dutch rural general practice. *Headache* 1986; **26**: 122–5.
14. Sakai F, Igarashi H. Epidemiology of migraine in Japan: a nationwide survey. *Cephalalgia* 1997; **17**: 15–22.

15. Roh JK, Kim JS, Ahn YO. Epidemiologic and clinical characteristics of migraine and tension-type headache in Korea. *Headache* 1998; **38**: 356–65.

16. Linet MS, Stewart WF, Celentano DD, Ziegler D, Sprecher M. An epidemiologic study of headache among adolescents and young adults. *J Am Med Assoc* 1989; **261**: 2211–16.

17. Hollnagel H, Nørrelund N. Headache among 40 year-olds in Glostrup. *Ugeskr Laeger* 1980; **142**: 3071–7.

18. Waters WE. *Headache* (ed. Bourke GJ), Series in Clinical Epidemiology. London and Sydney: Croom Helm, 1986.

19. Stang PE, Osterhaus JT. Impact of migraine in the United States: data from the National Health Interview Survey. *Headache* 1993; **33**: 29–35.

20. Nikiforow R. Headache medication habits in Northern Finland. *Headache* 1980; **20**: 274–8.

21. Linet MS, Celentano DD, Stewart WF. Headache characteristics associated with physician consultation: a population-based survey. *Am J Prevent Med* 1991; **7**: 40–6.

22. Stewart WF, Lipton R. Migraine headache: epidemiology and health care utilization. *Cephalalgia* 1993; **13** (Suppl. 12): 41–6.

23. Stang PE, Osterhaus JT, Celentano DD. Migraine: patterns of health care use. *Neurology* 1994; **44** (Suppl. 4): S47–S55.

24. Berkson J. Limitations of the application of fourfold table analysis to hospital data. *Biometrics Bull* 1946; **2**: 47–53.

25. Edmeads J, Findlay H, Tugwell P, Pryse-Philips W, Nelson RF, Murray TJ. Impact of migraine and tension-type headache on life-style, consulting behaviour, and medication use: a Canadian population survey. *Can J Neurol Sci* 1993; **20**: 131–7.

26. Michel P, Pariente P, Duru G, Dreyfuss J-P, Chabriat H, Henry P. Mig Access: a population-based, nationwide, comparative survey of access to care in migraine in France. *Cephalalgia* 1996; **16**: 50–5.

27. Lipton RB, Diamond S, Reed M, Diamond ML, Stewart WF. Migraine diagnosis and treatment: results from the American Migraine Study II. *Headache* 2001; **41**: 638–45.

28. Celentano DD, Stewart WF, Lipton RB, Reed ML. Medication use and disability among migraineurs: a national probability sample survey. *Headache* 1992; **32**: 223–8.

29. Clarke CE, MacMillan L, Sondhi S, Wells NEJ. Economic and social impact of migraine. *Quart J Med* 1996; **89**: 77–84.

30. Holmes WF, MacGregor EA, Sawyer JP, Lipton RB. Information about migraine disability influences physicians' perceptions of illness severity and treatment needs. *Headache* 2001; **41**: 343–50.

29 Functional improvement in migraine patients treated with oral eletriptan versus sumatriptan: a pooled analysis

Volker Limmroth and Jayasena Hettiarachchi

Background

Migraine is a highly prevalent and chronic disorder, characterized by a combination of neurological, gastrointestinal, and autonomic symptoms that can markedly impair the sufferer's ability to function normally. Thus, migraine is associated with a high degree of disability.[1,2] Eletriptan is a potent, selective $5\text{-HT}_{1B/1D}$ agonist that has previously been shown to provide rapid and effective relief of acute migraine in clinical trials.[3–6] Additionally, oral eletriptan has been shown to be significantly better than sumatriptan at relieving migraine.[6] Eletriptan has also been associated with significantly greater patient acceptability than sumatriptan.[6]

In a previous meta-analysis of three pooled sumatriptan–eletriptan comparator trials, oral eletriptan was found to be superior to oral sumatriptan for relief of headache and migraine-associated symptoms.[7,8] The objective of the present study was to establish whether the superior efficacy and tolerability of oral eletriptan over oral sumatriptan in relieving headache and migraine-associated symptoms translate into a greater improvement in patient functional status with eletriptan.

Methods

A total of 2102 patients were included in this pooled analysis of three randomized, double-blind, placebo-controlled clinical trials of similar design. These patients treated up to three migraine attacks with either eletriptan 20 mg, 40 mg, or 80 mg; sumatriptan 50 mg or 100 mg; or placebo.

Functional response was measured prospectively, and was defined as an improvement from bed rest or doing nothing or very little, to returning to normal function or being able to do something. A post-hoc analysis was conducted to examine the functional response of patients with nausea and phonophobia/photophobia at baseline.

Results

Patient demographic data were comparable between treatment groups (Table 29.1).

Patients taking eletriptan at 40 mg (62%) and 80 mg (65%) achieved superior functional response at 2 h compared with patients taking sumatriptan at 50 mg (51%, $p < 0.01$) or 100 mg (49%, $p < 0.005$), or placebo (35%, $p < 0.0001$). Functional response with eletriptan 20 mg was significantly better than placebo at 2 h (53%, $p < 0.005$) (Fig. 29.1). Eletriptan rapidly improved the functional status of patients, as eletriptan at 80 mg (37%) achieved significantly greater functional improvement over sumatriptan at 50 mg and 100 mg (26%, 24%, $p < 0.005$) and placebo (21%, $p < 0.0001$) as early as 1 h postdose (Fig. 29.1). Eletriptan 40 mg (31%) was also statistically superior to placebo (21%, $p < 0.005$) at 1 h (Fig. 29.1).

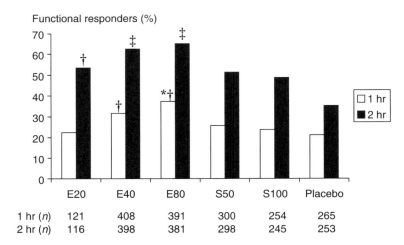

Fig. 29.1 Percentage of functional responders in migraine patients treated with eletriptan, sumatriptan, or placebo. E20, E40, and E80 are eletriptan 20 mg, 40 mg, and 80 mg, respectively; S50 and S100 are sumatriptan 50 mg and 100 mg, respectively. *$p < 0.005$ versus S50, S100. †$p < 0.005$ versus placebo. ‡$p < 0.01$ versus S50; $p < 0.005$ versus S100; $p < 0.0001$ versus placebo. Sumatriptan versus placebo was not tested.

Table 29.1 Patient demographics

Patient characteristics	Eletriptan			Sumatriptan		Placebo (n=319)
	20 mg (n=144)	40 mg (n=494)	80 mg (n=485)	50 mg (n=362)	100 mg (n=298)	
Age (years ± SD)	40.1±11.34	37.9±10.45	37.9±10.62	36.0±9.93	39.0±10.11	38.5±10.32
Female, number (%)	118 (82)	418 (85)	415 (86)	300 (83)	256 (86)	266 (83)
Male, n (%)	26 (18)	76 (15)	70 (14)	62 (17)	42 (14)	53 (17)
Migraine type, number (%)						
With aura	18 (13)	66 (13)	55 (11)	41 (11)	39 (13)	38 (12)
Without aura	99 (69)	342 (69)	357 (74)	284 (78)	201 (67)	233 (73)
With/without aura	27 (19)	86 (17)	72 (15)	37 (10)	58 (19)	48 (15)
Baseline nausea, number (%)						
Present	93 (65)	273 (56)	281 (58)	188 (52)	204 (69)	185 (58)
Absent	51 (35)	215 (44)	202 (42)	171 (48)	93 (31)	133 (42)
Baseline phonophobia/photophobia, number (%)						
Present	117 (81)	423 (86)	405 (84)	311 (87)	256 (86)	269 (84)
Absent	27 (19)	67 (14)	77 (16)	48 (13)	41 (14)	50 (16)
Baseline functional impairment, number (%)						
Absent	2 (1)	5 (1)	8 (2)	7 (2)	6 (2)	6 (2)
Mild	12 (8)	63 (13)	68 (14)	46 (13)	27 (9)	38 (12)
Moderate	90 (63)	292 (60)	294 (61)	221 (61)	174 (59)	199 (62)
Severe	40 (28)	130 (27)	112 (23)	86 (24)	89 (30)	76 (24)

In patients with nausea at baseline, eletriptan at both 40 mg (59%) and 80 mg (62%) was superior to placebo (32%, $p<0.0001$) and sumatriptan at 50 mg and 100 mg (47% and 46%, respectively, $p<0.05$) at 2 h. Eletriptan 20 mg was also statistically superior to placebo at 2 h (54%, $p<0.005$) (Fig. 29.2). At 1 h, eletriptan at 80 mg (34%) was significantly superior to sumatriptan at 50 mg (19%, $p<0.005$) and 100 mg (22%, $p<0.05$) in patients with nausea at baseline (Fig. 29.2). When compared to placebo, eletriptan at both 40 mg (28%) and 80 mg (34%) was significantly better at improving functional status in patients with nausea 1 h postdose (16%, $p<0.005$) (Fig. 29.2).

Eletriptan at 40 mg and 80 mg provided functional improvement at 2 h in patients with phonophobia/photophobia at baseline (62% and 64%, respectively) that was significantly superior to that of placebo (36%, $p<0.0001$) and sumatriptan at 50 mg (49%, $p<0.005$) and 100 mg (46%, $p<0.0005$). Eletriptan 20 mg was also significantly superior to placebo at 2 h (51%, $p<0.05$) (Fig. 29.3). At 1 h, both doses of eletriptan (40 mg, 31%; 80 mg, 35%) provided statistically significant functional improvement over sumatriptan at 100 mg (20%, $p<0.01$) in patients with baseline phonophobia/photophobia. Eletriptan 80 mg was also significantly better than sumatriptan 50 mg at 1 h (24%, $p<0.005$), while eletriptan 40 mg tended toward a significant difference ($p=0.0522$) (Fig. 29.3). Both 40 mg (31%) and 80 mg (35%) doses of eletriptan were significantly better at improving functional status in patients with phonophobia/photophobia at baseline 1 h postdose compared to placebo (19%, $p<0.001$) (Fig. 29.3).

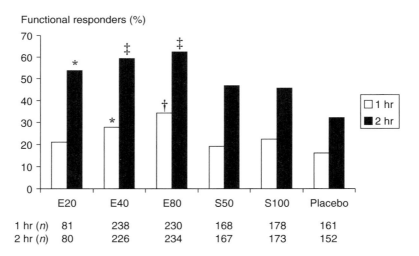

Fig. 29.2 Percentage of functional responders in migraine patients with nausea at baseline treated with eletriptan, sumatriptan, or placebo. E20, E40, and E80 are eletriptan 20 mg, 40 mg, and 80 mg, respectively; S50 and S100 are sumatriptan 50 mg and 100 mg, respectively. *$p<0.005$ versus placebo. †$p<0.0001$ versus placebo; $p\leq0.005$ versus S50; $p<0.05$ versus S100. ‡$p<0.05$ versus S50 and S100; $p<0.0001$ versus placebo. Sumatriptan versus placebo was not tested.

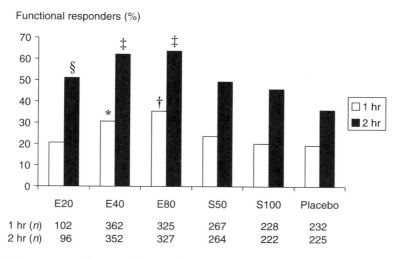

Fig. 29.3 Percentage of functional responders in migraine patients with phonophobia/photophobia at baseline treated with eletriptan, sumatriptan, or placebo. E20, E40, and E80 are eletriptan 20 mg, 40 mg, and 80 mg, respectively; S50 and S100 are sumatriptan 50 mg and 100 mg, respectively. $*p=0.001$ versus placebo. $^\dagger p<0.0001$ versus placebo; $p<0.005$ versus S50; $p=0.0005$ versus S100. $^\ddagger p<0.01$ versus S50; $p<0.0005$ versus S100; $p<0.0001$ versus placebo. $^\S p<0.005$ versus placebo. Sumatriptan versus placebo was not tested.

Conclusions

Overall, eletriptan was found to confer high functional improvement in this patient population. Eletriptan at 40 mg and 80 mg doses elicited a significantly better and faster functional response than sumatriptan or placebo. Similar percentages of patients with and without nausea or phonophobia/photophobia had an improved functional response with eletriptan, indicating that the presence of nausea or phonophobia/photophobia did not impair eletriptan's ability to achieve a superior functional response over sumatriptan.

References

1. Lipton RB, Stewart WF, Diamond S, *et al.* Prevalence and burden of migraine in the United States: data from the American Migraine Study II. *Headache* 2001; **41** (7): 646–57.
2. Solomon GD, Price KL. Burden of migraine: a review of its socioeconomic impact. *Pharmacoeconomics* 1997; **11** (Suppl.): 1–10.
3. Goadsby PJ, Ferrari MD, Olesen J, *et al.* Eletriptan in acute migraine: a double blind, placebo-controlled comparison to sumatriptan. *Neurology* 2000; **54**: 156–63.
4. Stark R, Dahlöf C, Haughie S, Hettiarachchi J, on behalf of the Eletriptan Steering Committee. Efficacy, safety and tolerability of oral eletriptan in the acute treatment of

migraine: results of a phase III, multicentre, placebo-controlled study across three attacks. *Cephalalgia* 2002; **22** (1): 23.

5. Diener H-C, Jansen JP, Reches A, Pascual J, Pitei D, Steiner TJ. Efficacy, tolerability, and safety of oral eletriptan and ergotamine plus caffeine (Cafergot) in the acute treatment of migraine: a multicentre, randomised, double-blind, placebo-controlled comparison. *Eur Neurol* 2002; **47** (2): 99–107.

6. Pryse-Phillips W on behalf of the Eletriptan Steering Committee. Comparison of oral eletriptan (40–80mg) and oral sumatriptan (50–100mg) for the treatment of acute migraine: a randomised, placebo-controlled trial in sumatriptan-naïve patients [abstract]. *Cephalalgia* 1999; **19** (4): 355–6.

7. Hettiarachchi J. Comparison of the efficacy of oral eletriptan (20 mg, 40 mg, 80 mg) and sumatriptan (50 mg, 100 mg) for the treatment of acute migraine: pooled analysis of randomized clinical trials [abstract]. *Eur J Neurol* 2000; **7** (Suppl. 3): 118.

8. Hettiarachchi J, Taylor K. Comparison of oral eletriptan and sumatriptan for the improvement of functional disability and the relief of migraine-associated symptoms: a pooled analysis of three randomized clinical studies [abstract]. *Neurology* 2001; **56** (Suppl. 3): A312.

30 Health-care utilization for in-patient headache therapy

Hartmut Göbel, Peter Buschmann, and Axel Heinze

Introduction

A number of fundamental changes can currently be observed in the health-care system. The main driving forces behind these changes are rising costs and the desire to get these costs better under control while at the same time improving health care for the insured population. It is only in recent years that the need for systematically organized headache care has become evident. One main reason for this new thinking is that the usual form of headache care—'on the side' and 'among other things'—is inefficient from the patients' point of view. The results are inadequate pain alleviation, short- and long-term side-effects of inadequate self-medication, frequent changes of doctors, incapacity to work, and social disadvantages. From the medical and academic points of view, the lack of specially organized treatment means that systematic training, experience, and scientific knowledge are being wasted. From an economic point of view the situation gives rise to horrendous follow-on costs for health insurance funds, employers, and patients. For this reason we undertook, in cooperation with the Allgemeine Ortskrankenkasse (AOK) Schleswig-Holstein, the biggest statutory health insurance fund in the federal state Schleswig-Holstein, a first exact quantitative analysis of the costs involved in in-patient care of chronic headache and pain patients. Unfortunately, it is not possible to make a diagnosis-specific breakdown of the direct costs of out-patient health care of the insured population in Germany, because there is no coding and computer storage of the individual diagnoses in the out-patient sector. At present, this is only possible in the in-patient sector. To make it possible to evaluate the costs for the insured community of the AOK in Schleswig-Holstein, the exact expenditure on chronic pain problems in the federal state of Schleswig-Holstein was therefore determined with the aid of the coded International Classification of Diseases, 9th edition (ICD-9) diagnoses. To date, there are no comparable analyses available.

Methods

The exact numbers of patients treated because of chronic headaches in the federal state of Schleswig-Holstein were determined with the aid of the coded ICD-9 diagnoses in the year 1995. These data could be directly collected in the database of the health insurance fund AOK consisting of a total of about 1.3 million insured persons. The costs per case treated and the duration of treatment were analysed and the total costs for the group of AOK members in Schleswig-Holstein were calculated.[1,2]

Results

The selection of diagnoses of chronic pain conditions on the basis of the ICD-9 coding revealed that, of a total of about 1.3 million insured persons, 16 614 patients with an initial diagnosis of chronic pain conditions received in-patient treatment. Thus, in about 1.5% of the general population a chronic pain disorder required hospitalization. The average time spent in hospital was 14 days. This analysis only takes account of patients admitted to acute hospitals, not to rehabilitation centres. The average costs per case were 6911 DM. Thus for the treatment of chronic headache and other neurological pain syndromes in Schleswig-Holstein, the total cost in 1995 for the insured community of the AOK in Schleswig-Holstein alone came to 108 million DM (Table 30.1).

Thanks to the exact ICD coding it was possible to make a diagnosis-specific analysis of costs. Some 5788 insured persons were treated in hospital for chronic headache conditions. This means that every year about one person in 200 in the population requires headache therapy on an in-patient basis. The average length of stay was around 12 days. The average costs per case were 5856 DM. As a result of chronic headache syndromes a total of 23.2 million DM was spent on hospital treatment for members of the insured community (Table 30.1).

The codes revealed a diagnosis of 'analgesic abuse' for 818 patients. These patients spent an average of 16 days in an acute hospital. The average costs per case were 5897 DM amounting to a total of 4.8 million DM for the treatment of chronic drug-induced headache. It should be remembered here that these are only the costs of

Table 30.1 Financial impact of in-patient treatment of chronic pain disorders in 1995 (AOK Schleswig-Holstein: 1.3 million members)

	All chronic pain disorders	Chronic headache disorders	Drug-induced headache
Number of patients	16 614	5788	818
Average time spent in hospital (days)	14.3	11.9	16.4
Average costs per case (DM)	6911	5856	5897
Total cost for AOK in 1995 (DM)	108 million	23.2 million	4.8 million

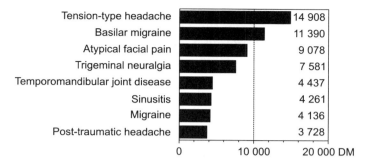

Fig. 30.1   Hit list. Average costs per case for in-patient treatment of chronic headache disorders in 1995 (insured community of AOK Schleswig-Holstein) ($n=470$) or episodic tension-type headache ($n=321$).

acute measures for treating analgesic abuse not including any consequential costs (Table 30.1).

A completely unexpected picture emerges if a hit-list of the costs of pain syndromes is drawn up (Fig. 30.1). Chronic tension-type headache, which one might think of as a minor problem, heads the list of causes of in-patient treatment costs. The average costs per case for this diagnosis were nearly 15 000 DM. The next most expensive headache diagnosis, at 11 390 DM, is basilar migraine. Even atypical facial pain is very expensive, with in-patient treatment costs of 9078 DM. A relatively inexpensive item, by contrast, is 'migraine without aura' with an average cost of about 4000 DM per case.

Discussion

These figures show that particularly those pain syndromes that are especially long-lasting and relate to the nervous system can only be treated at high cost in terms of time and money. Especially for these conditions it is obviously necessary to provide specific treatment measures and to concentrate efforts on the pain syndromes themselves. Extrapolated for the entire population of 80 million Germans, this means that a total of about 3.2 billion DM a year has to be spent on in-patient treatment of headache and neurological pain syndromes. A total of 500 000 people per year in Germany have such strong pains that they have to undergo in-patient treatment. Also extrapolated for the total population of Germany, 171 496 patients a year have to receive in-patient treatment for headache. This results in expenditure of 1 billion DM. In Germany a total of 26 785 patients a year have to be treated in hospital for analgesic abuse. This costs the society 142 million DM. To this end there is a need for facilities that provide not only efficient withdrawal therapy, but also specific follow-up treatment of the underlying pain syndrome. Also extrapolated for the total population of Germany, 29 601 patients a year have to receive in-patient treatment for neuralgia syndromes. For this purpose the nation has to spend 184 million DM.

This analysis of costs, which was made for the first time on the basis of exact empirical data, reveals extremely surprising results. Non-specific conditions that cannot be attributed to a precise causal factor, such as primary headaches, are the principal causes of costs among chronic pain syndromes. For these chronic pain syndromes, however, it is only in isolated cases that the standard health-care system provides specialized strategies and specific organizational forms. In the interests of cost reduction and effective treatment it is therefore necessary to offer and evaluate specialized treatment strategies for these syndrome groups, which are particularly widespread.

References

1. Göbel H, Buschmann P, Heinze A, Heinze-Kuhn K. Epidemiologie und sozioökonomische Konsequenzen von Migräne und Kopfschmerzerkrankungen. *Versicherungsmedizin* 2000; **52** (1): 19–23.
2. Göbel H, Buschmann P, Heinze A, Heinze-Kuhn K. Nutzen spezialiserter Schmerzbehandlung. *Versicherungsmedizin* 2000; **52** (2): 57–65.

31
Self-described 'sinus headache' and headache-related impact

Curtis P. Schreiber and Roger K. Cady

Introduction

Headache with symptoms involving the frontal or maxillary regions is a common complaint among headache sufferers in the USA. Because of the location of these symptoms, many of these patients are diagnosed as having 'sinus headache'. Involvement of these locations may occur early in the headache process, which accounts for the apparent 'cause and effect' relationship perceived by those with these headaches. In many cases, the patients themselves make the diagnosis. The belief in a sinus origin for these individuals may be reinforced by the massive direct-to-consumer advertising campaigns made for non-prescription sinus treatments. 'Sinus headache' remains a common clinical diagnosis.

In the guidelines for diagnosis of headache disorders established by the International Headache Society (IHS) in 1988,[1] the only category in which 'sinus headache' is identified is in association with acute sinusitis. The criterion (IHS 11.5.1) explicitly defines the headache as having onset occurring simultaneously with sinusitis and disappearing after treatment of acute sinusitis. Other components of this diagnostic criteria include evidence of purulent discharge in the nasal passage and evidence of pathological finding on at least one test (X-ray, computerized tomography (CT), magnetic resonance imaging (MRI), or transillumination of the sinuses). The IHS criteria go on to state (IHS 11.5.2) that chronic sinusitis is not validated as a cause of headache or facial pain. In 1997, the recommendations of a task force of the American Academy of Otorhinolaryngology—Head and Neck Surgery (AAO-HNS) regarding factors associated with the diagnosis of rhinosinusitis were published.[2] In the proposed AAO-HNS diagnostic scheme rhinosinusitis is diagnosed by having 2 of 6 major factors or a combination of 1 major factor with 2 of 7 minor factors. Headache is among the 7 minor factors associated with rhinosinusitis.

'Sinus headache' is considered by most headache specialists and general neurologists in the USA to be a rare condition. This may be due in part to referral patterns for sinus-related diseases. However, in primary care, it is a commonly made diagnosis. In the American Migraine Study II,[3] it was found that 39.6% of individuals with recurrent headaches complained of 'sinus headaches' and that 42% of undiagnosed migraine sufferers had been diagnosed as having 'sinus headache'. Despite the lack of diagnostic criteria for recurrent 'sinus headache' without signs of infection, it is commonly diagnosed.

Methods and results

In order to further investigate 'sinus headache', we have enrolled three separate clinical studies. In these studies, the Headache Impact Test (HIT-6) was used to determine headache-related disability. All three studies enrolled subjects with patient self-defined 'sinus headaches' and with at least a 1-year history of this type of headache. Subjects were required to have had at least one 'sinus headache' per month over the preceding 3 months. Specifically excluded were individuals with symptoms of infectious sinusitis within the past year as defined by headaches with fever and purulent nasal discharge, or radiographic evidence of sinus involvement. A history of headache occurring more than 15 days a month was also exclusionary for enrolment in all three studies.

Study 1 was conducted with a group of subjects with self-defined 'sinus headache'. Exclusionary criteria included prior diagnosis of migraine by a clinician or use of triptan-class medication. At study enrolment, subjects provided detailed information regarding symptoms associated with their sinus headaches. These symptoms were used to determine a headache diagnosis according to IHS diagnostic criteria. All subjects completed the HIT-6 at the time of their enrolment. Forty-seven subjects were enrolled in this study. By applying IHS criteria to the symptoms, it was found these individuals fulfilled criteria for the following IHS diagnoses (Fig. 31.1): 68% (32/47) migraine without aura (IHS 1.1); 2% (1/47) migraine with aura (IHS 1.2); 28% (13/47) migrainous headache (IHS 1.7); and 2% (1/47) episodic tension-type headache (IHS 2.1).

The HIT-6 scores were recorded at enrolment (Table 31.1). For all subjects in study 1, the HIT-6 scores indicated the following levels of headache-related impact: 70% (33/47) very severe impact; 19% (9/47) substantial impact; 9% (4/47) some impact; and 2% (1/47) little or no impact. The impact was similar for both the group which fulfilled criteria for migraine without aura (IHS 1.1) and that which fulfilled the criteria for migrainous headache (IHS 1.7).

Study 2 enrolled 11 individuals with self-described 'sinus headache' features that met IHS diagnostic criteria for migraine-type headaches (IHS 1.1, 1.2, or 1.7). Subjects with a previous physician's diagnosis of migraine or previous exposure to triptans were excluded. The subjects were queried about the symptoms they experienced with their self-described 'sinus headaches'. At enrolment subjects completed the HIT-6. Of this group, based on the symptoms described with 'sinus headaches',

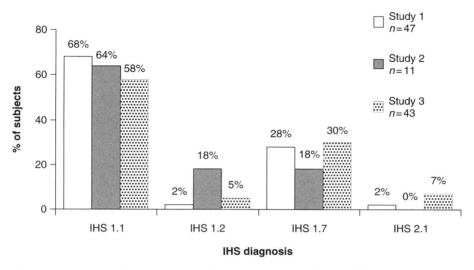

Fig. 31.1   Percentage of subjects in the three studies fitting different IHS diagnostic criteria.

it was found these individuals fulfilled criteria for the following IHS diagnoses (Fig. 31.1): 64% (7/11) migraine without aura (IHS 1.1); 18% (2/11) migraine with aura (IHS 1.2); and 18% (2/11) migrainous headache (IHS 1.7).

The HIT-6 scores for all subjects recorded at entry to study 2 (Table 31.1) indicated very severe impact in 55% (6/11), substantial impact in 36% (4/11), and some impact in 9% (1/11). In this smaller sample, the impact on those subjects who met criteria for migrainous headache (IHS 1.7) was very similar to that on those who met criteria for migraine without or with aura (IHS 1.1, 1.2).

Study 3 enrolled 43 subjects with self-described 'sinus headache' in addition to clinician-diagnosed migraine headaches. They were required to be able to distinguish between their migraine and 'sinus headache' attacks. A history of prior triptan use was allowed for their migraine attacks but not for their 'sinus headache' attacks. At study enrolment, subjects provided detailed information regarding symptoms associated with their 'sinus' and migraine headaches. These symptoms were used to classify the 'sinus headache' attacks according to IHS diagnostic criteria. By applying IHS criteria to the symptoms of the 'sinus headache' attacks, it was found these attacks fulfilled criteria for the following IHS diagnoses (Fig. 31.1): 58% (25/43) migraine without aura (IHS 1.1); 5% (2/43) migraine with aura (IHS 1.2); 30% (13/43) migrainous headache (IHS 1.7); and 7% (3/43) episodic tension-type headache (IHS 2.1).

The HIT-6 scores were recorded at enrolment (Table 31.1). For all subjects in study 3, the HIT-6 scores indicated the following levels of headache-related impact: 86% (37/43) very severe impact and 14% (6/43) substantial impact. Impact was similar for the groups who fulfilled criteria for migraine without or with aura (IHS 1.1, 1.2) and migrainous headache (IHS 1.7).

Table 31.1 Impact table. Results from the HIT-6 test in the three studies reported here

HIT-6 impact range	Percentage of subjects (number in impact range/number satisfying IHS criterion)		
	Study 1 (n=47)	Study 2 (n=11)	Study 3 (n=43)
Subjects satisfying IHS 1.1			
Very severe impact	72 (23/32)	57 (4/7)	88 (22/25)
Substantial impact	22 (7/32)	43 (3/7)	12 (3/25)
Some impact	6 (2/32)	—	—
Little or none	—	—	—
Subjects satisfying IHS 1.2			
Very severe impact	100 (1/1)	50 (1/2)	100 (2/2)
Substantial impact	—	50 (1/2)	—
Some impact	—	—	—
Little or none	—	—	—
Subjects satisfying IHS 1.7			
Very severe impact	69 (9/13)	50 (1/2)	92 (12/13)
Substantial impact	15 (2/13)	50 (1/2)	8 (1/13)
Some impact	8 (1/13)	—	—
Little or none	8 (1/13)	—	—
Subjects satisfying IHS 2.1			
Very severe impact	—	—	33 (1/3)
Substantial impact	—	—	66 (2/3)
Some impact	100 (1/1)	—	—
Little or none	—	—	—
All subjects			
Very severe impact	70 (33/47)	55 (6/11)	86 (37/43)
Substantial impact	19 (9/47)	36 (4/11)	14 (6/43)
Some impact	9 (4/47)	9 (1/11)	—
Little or none	2 (1/47)	—	—

Conclusion

In summary, recurrent 'sinus headache' without evidence of sinus infection is a diagnosis commonly made by patients and clinicians alike in the USA. On the basis of the results presented here, there is strong evidence that a significant majority of individuals with self-described 'sinus headache' actually have headaches that fulfil IHS criteria for migraine-type headaches (IHS 1.1, 1.2, and 1.7). In the physician and lay community alike, there is a generally accepted feeling that 'sinus headaches' are less likely to be disabling to the sufferer than are migraine headaches. The results shown here indicate that, for many sufferers, self-described 'sinus headache' can have significant impact on their ability to perform routine daily activities. Also, after applying IHS diagnostic criteria to the symptoms of the attacks, we found that individuals with attacks that fulfil the migrainous criteria (IHS 1.7) experienced headache-related impact equal to that of those that fulfilled criteria for migraine without or with aura (IHS 1.1, 1.2).

The results of these three studies indicate that 'sinus headache', for many individuals, represents a distinct clinical presentation of the migraine process. Recognition of this presentation of migraine may expand the treatment options available to those who suffer with 'sinus headache'.

References

1. Headache Classification Committee of the International Headache Society. Classification and diagnostic criteria for headache disorders, cranial neuralgias and facial pain. *Cephalalgia* 1988; **8** (Suppl. 7): 1–96.
2. Lanza DC, Kennedy DW. Adult rhinosinusitis defined. *Otolaryngol Head NeckSurg* 1997; **117** (Pt. 2): S1–S7.
3. Lipton RB, Stewart WF, Diamond S, Diamond M, Reed M. Prevalence and burden of migraine in the United States. Data from the American Migraine Study II. *Headache* 2001; **41**: 646–57.

32 Reducing the personal burden of migraine: a patient's perspective

Anne Bülow-Olsen

Introduction

The burden of migraine on a patient is twofold: (1) *personal* (pains and discomfort) and (2) problems and misunderstandings arising from *society* (family, friends, work, etc.). Migraine is a debilitating disease that is exacerbated by lack of information. The personal burden could be reduced if information were available about: (1) how to avoid migraine and (2) how to treat migraine. The burden imposed by society relates to a lack of understanding of our disease by other people. *Information* to patients and society is the best way to alleviate these burdens!

The personal burden

A patient has two strategies that can be used against migraine attacks: (1) to reduce the number and severity of attacks as much as possible; (2) to get the best possible treatment for the remaining attacks.

Reducing the number of attacks

The triggers of many migraine attacks are known and identifiable, but far too little information about them is disseminated to patients and general practitioners. If the patient and his or her doctor take the trouble to record details in a diary and to analyse the data carefully, it is possible to identify many triggers. Far too often this does not happen. Patients are not informed about the importance of a detailed diary, and the doctors have only a short time for consultation, so only blatantly obvious patterns are identified. The patients' burdens could be alleviated if more time and effort could be devoted to *information about triggers*—how to identify them, how to avoid them, and how to exclude erroneously identified triggers.

Specific medication

Even if triggers are identified, patients may not be able to avoid migraine attacks entirely. Today's medication relieves symptoms, but does not counteract the problem that caused the attack to develop in the first place. If taken to excess, medication causes even more attacks. Triptans influence the arteries not only in the brain, but also in the heart, and can cause serious and unpleasant side-effects.

Patients would find it much more satisfying to have treatment that is specific for each type of migraine, for example, hormonal migraine (control of the rate of change of oestrogen concentration) or food migraine (supplying the enzymes that the body lacks). If patients and doctors had more *information* about the importance of triggers, the pressure on the producers of medicine would increase, and we would—hopefully—soon get more specific medication with fewer side-effects.

Lack of reliable information

Most migraine patients have a general understanding that attacks are triggered by 'something'. However, most information in popular pamphlets and on the internet is provided by the medical companies that sell the medication for migraine. This information is provided with the aim of selling medicine. Patients feel frustrated when reading the popularized information because the amount of information from the industry is overwhelming and is disguised as 'objective'. Nonetheless, it still leaves patients in limbo with respect to much sought after concrete information about the causes and triggers of migraine, and what the individual herself may do to have fewer attacks.

Most medical information is first published as a scientific paper in a reputable international journal. There was a period when acknowledgements were not included in many papers, so readers could not see who had sponsored—and perhaps influenced—the data and conclusions. Publications without indication of sponsors have been observed to contain inconsistencies, data that seem to be based on biased samples, and conclusions that are not supported by the data. The conclusions drawn are, however, often cited, and penetrate to the media and pamphlets for the general public.

The lack of distinction between reliable information and promotional material drives patients to try alternative treatments. As there is no particular difference to the patient in reliability between the information from the medical companies and the information provided by alternative healers and the like, many migraine patients try all available alternative treatments. Better information, provided by sources not involved in selling services or medicine to the patients, might reduce the waste of time and effort on treatments that have no documented effect.

The burden imposed by society

Migraine is a disease with a bad image. Patients are classified (wrongly) as unable to tolerate stress, as overly zealous people who should live a quiet life with regular sleeping habits and fixed meal times, and as generally unreliable because their disease can strike at any inconvenient time. Patients meet these preconceptions throughout society—from doctors, from colleagues and bosses, and from friends and partners. Many migraine patients even believe that they are delicate and cannot participate in fast-paced modern life. The only viable strategy to overcome these preconceptions is through *honest and reliable information*.

Some patients have been able to 'get a grip' on their disease. Honest information about how well they perform in society could increase the acceptance of other migraine patients at work and at home. Patients believe that employers sack migraine patients preferentially because migraine patients on average have more sick days than others. So migraine patients keep their disease secret. Better information about the ability of patients to cope with their attacks might alleviate this preconception.

Marriages may break up because the migraine patient's partner gets frustrated and annoyed by the sufferer's inability to cope with or avoid migraine. More information to relatives and spouses about triggers and about what they themselves can do to alleviate the attacks might provide the frustrated partners with the necessary background to accept and cope with the disease.

Conclusion

The primary way to lessen the burden of migraine on the patient is to *make information readily available* to doctors, patients, and society at large. Information about how to improve life quality of migraine patients already exists, but is not distributed. More information, perhaps through research funded by sources outside the medical industry, is still needed to provide information that is not related to the marketing of medicine.

33
The burden of migraine in a sample of doctors of an Italian general hospital in Rome

T. Catarci, F. Baldinetti, and F. Granella

....

Migraine represents an important burden for patients and society,[1] but is still largely underdiagnosed[2] and undertreated[3] worldwide. In order to better understand the possible causes of this situation, we decided to perform an epidemiological study on doctors with migraine. We investigated the impact of migraine on their work and social activities, with the assumption that a low impact of migraine on their life could lead doctors to have an unrealistic perception of the migraine burden in the community and possibly explain their lack of interest in this disabling pathological condition.

Methods

A simple screening questionnaire for migraine, previously validated in the Danish general population,[4] was distributed to all 561 physicians of a general hospital in Rome, Italy. This questionnaire was deemed to be the most appropriate because it was easy and quick to use and validated in a 'well-educated' population, and thus suitable for using with doctors. Two hundred-fifteen physicians responded to the screening questionnaire (27% females, 73% males). Among these, 116 potential migraineurs were identified, 87 of whom could be interviewed (75%) directly (68%) or by phone (32%). A headache specialist (FG), who made diagnoses following International Headache Society (IHS) criteria, conducted the interview. The burden of migraine during the last 12 months was investigated through the following items: lost workdays due to migraine; workdays with migraine; mean residual efficiency when working with migraine; domestic and social activities lost because of migraine.

We calculated workdays lost from reduced effectiveness at work (LWD) and lost workday equivalents (LWDE), as a composite of work-related disability, combining information on missed days and LWD due to migraine, as described by Stewart et al.[5]

Results

Sixty-three of the 87 potential migraineurs (72%) had the migraine diagnosis confirmed (migraine without aura 63%, migraine with aura 17%, migrainous disorder 20%). Forty-eight (76%) physicians (54% males, 46% females, mean age 45.3±6.8 years) had experienced at least one attack during the previous 12 months (active migraineurs). Of these, 44% worked in the Internal Medicine Department, 35% were surgeons or anaesthetists; and 21% worked in radiology and pathology services.

The mean frequency of attacks was 2 days per month and the mean duration of attacks was 5.5±6.5 hours. Sixty-five per cent of physicians reported severe attacks; only 19% of them, however, experienced severe attacks in at least 50% of the cases.

Only three doctors (6%) had missed 1–2 workdays during the previous year because of migraine. Forty physicians (83%), however, had worked at least once (mean: 1.8±3.0 days per month) during a migraine attack in the last year, with a mean residual efficiency of 65%. Absenteeism was 0.08±0.35 days per year. LWD during the last year was 5.7±8.9 days; LWDE was 5.8±9.0 days (females, 7.1±9.3 days; males, 4.7±8.6 days) (Table 33.1 and Fig. 33.1).

The physicians lost 8.2±14.4 days of domestic activities (females, 10.4±16.7 days; males, 6.2±12.2 days) and 2.3±7.5 days of social activities (females, 1.9±3.7 days; males, 2.6±9.8 days) in the previous year (Table 33.2 and Fig. 33.2). In particular, 27 doctors (56%) reported a loss of 14 days per year of domestic activities and 15 (31%) reported a loss of 7 days per year of leisure activities.

Discussion

The burden of migraine in our sample of hospital doctors is similar to that found in the general population. In some European studies, estimates of LWDE ranged from 1.8 to 7.1 days per year in men and 0.9 to 10.5 days per year in women,[6] compared to 4.7 and 7.1 days per year, respectively, in men and women, in our survey. Similarly, the days of missed household activities in our sample (8.2 days per year) are not too far from those (13.2 days per year) reported in a recent UK study in the general population.[7]

However, some relevant differences from the general population emerge, the most striking being the extremely low absenteeism found among our doctors

Table 33.1 Burden of illness in doctors with active migraine in the previous year

Number of days	Percentage of		
	Females (n=22)	Males (n=26)	Total (n=48)
Workdays missed			
0	96	92	94
1–2	4	8	6
Workdays lost from reduced effectiveness at work (LWD)			
0	14	19	17
1–2	32	50	41
3–5	14	4	8
6–10	18	15	17
>10	22	12	17
Lost workday equivalents (LWDE)			
0	14	19	17
1–2	32	42	35
3–5	14	12	14
6–10	18	15	17
>10	22	12	17
Days of missed domestic activities			
0	41	46	44
1–2	18	15	17
3–5	9	15	13
6–10	0	12	6
>10	32	12	20
Days of missed social activities			
0	64	73	69
1–2	14	12	12
3–5	9	12	11
6–10	4	0	2
>10	9	3	6

(0.08 days per year). This finding is in agreement with the observation of Blau[8] who reported a work loss of 0.44 days per year in a sample of 50 doctors in the UK. This is possibly due to the physicians' strong commitment to carry out their work anyway. In addition, social activities were also remarkably less impaired among our physicians (2.3 days lost per year) than in the general UK population (7.2 days per year).[7] Such differences were not the result of doctors using a better or faster acute treatment than the general population (data not shown).

We can therefore speculate that, whereas the migraine disability is not (and could not be) different in physicians compared with the general population, the coping

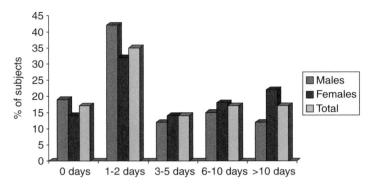

Fig. 33.1 Lost workday equivalents (LWDE) in the last year by gender in physicians with active migraine (*n*=48).

Table 33.2 Burden of illness in doctors with active migraine: differences between males and females

Variable	Females (mean ± SD)	Males (mean ± SD)
LWDE	7.1±9.3	4.7±8.6
Days of missed domestic activities	10.4±16.7	6.2±12.2
Days of missed social activities	1.9±3.7	2.6±9.8

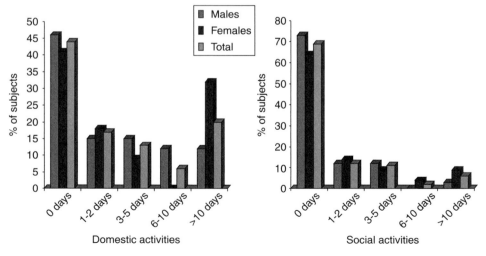

Fig. 33.2 Days of domestic and social activities lost in the last year by gender in physicians with active migraine (*n*=48).

with migraine is deeply different in physicians with respect to lay people. In some ways, doctors seem to minimize the impact of migraine on their lives. It is possible that such behaviour induces an underestimation of the real impact of migraine on individuals and may even affect migraine treatment. A recent American study has demonstrated that many physicians interested in headache do not collect information about disability. Yet, when available, a history of disability powerfully influences physicians' perception of the severity of the illness and appropriate treatment urgency.[9] The reasons why physicians are less affected in their work and social life than lay people are purely speculative and could be linked to a different approach to the concept of illness due to their professional training.

References

1. Holmes WF, MacGregor EA, Dodick D. Migraine-related disability. Impact and implications for sufferers' lives and clinical issues. *Neurology* 2001; **56** (Suppl. 1): 13–19.
2. Lipton RB, Stewart WF, Celentano DD, Reed ML. Undiagnosed migraine headaches. A comparison of symptom-based and reported physician diagnosis. *Arch Intern Med* 1992; **152**: 1273–8.
3. Lipton RB, Amatniek JC, Ferrari MD, Gross M. Migraine. Identifying and removing barriers to care. *Neurology* 1994; **44** (Suppl. 4): 63–8.
4. Gervil M, Ulrich V, Olesen J, Russell MB. Screening for migraine in the general population: validation of a simple questionnaire. *Cephalalgia* 1998; **18**: 342–8.
5. Stewart WF, Lipton RB, Simon D. Work-related disability: results from the American Migraine Study. *Cephalalgia* 1996; **16**: 231–8.
6. Ferrari MD. The economic burden of migraine to society. *PharmacoEconomics* 1998; **13**: 667–76.
7. Stewart WF, Lipton RB, Sawyer J. An international study to assess the reliability of the Migraine Disability Assessment (MIDAS) score. *Neurology* 1999; **53**: 988–94.
8. Blau JN. Migraine in doctors: work loss and consumption of medication. *Lancet* 1994; **344**: 1623–4.
9. Holmes WF, MacGregor EA, Sawyer JP, Lipton RB. Information about migraine disability influences physicians' perceptions of illness severity and treatment needs. *Headache* 2001; **41**: 343–50.

34
The Framig 2000 (II) survey: therapeutical data

C. Lucas, M. Lantéri-Minet, and C. Chaffaut

Framig 2000 was an epidemiological survey on migraine performed on the general population in France in 2000, 1 year after Framig 99[1,3] and 10 years after the first epidemiological survey of migraine in France.[2] Framig 2000 (II) focused on therapeutical data during the migraine attack, calculating Migraine Disability Assessment (MIDAS) scores and a mean headache intensity score (range 1–10) based on 10 attacks.

Methods

A phone survey was carried out by Ipsos, a statistical institute, from 12 to 28 December 2000 on 4689 subjects aged 18 to 65 years, who were representative of the French general population. Migraine was diagnosed using an algorithm based on International Headache Society (IHS) criteria, and a 'decision-tree' questionnaire was administered to subjects. We studied subjects with 'active' migraine (at least one attack in the last 3 months) with reference to acute treatment (treatment taken during the attack), improvement or absence of improvement with the treatment, and recurrence of the attacks.

Results

A total of 312 migraineurs took part in the survey. Twenty-two per cent scored grade III or IV on the MIDAS scale. Forty-eight per cent of migraineurs with MIDAS scores of grade I or II had severe attacks. An acute treatment was systematically taken by 97% of migraineurs with a mean delay of 6.4 hours after the beginning of the attack. The acute treatment was non-specific in 90% of migraineurs (Fig. 34.1). Seventy-one per cent of patients had taken at least three units of acute treatment for the same attack (Fig. 34.2) with an absence of improvement in 50% of these

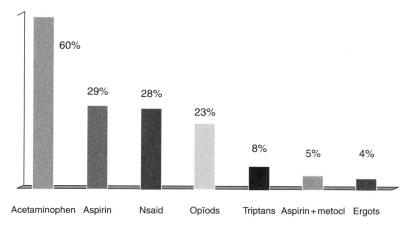

Fig. 34.1   Data on the treatment of migraine (*n*=312). NSAID, Nonsteroidal anti-inflammatory drug; Asp, aspirin; metoclo, metoclopramide.

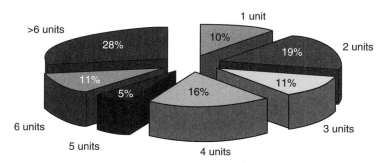

Fig. 34.2   Number of units of acute treatment taken during the same migraine attack (*n*=306).

Table 34.1   Evolution of attacks distributed according to MIDAS scores. Mean performed on 10 attacks

	Percentage of subjects having MIDAS grade			
	I (*n*=15)	II (*n*=59)	III (*n*=33)	IV (*n*=28)
Absence of improvement	15	34	33	35
Partial improvement without relief	36	30	37	35
Partial improvement with relief	28	21	22	18
Headache-free	21	15	8	12

(Table 34.1). One-quarter of patients experienced a recurrence of the attack. Patients who used triptans (7.6%) considered that their treatment had a faster onset and was more efficacious than non-specific treatment. Triptans were taken as the second or third option during the same attack in one-third of patients.

Comments

Framig 2000 (II) showed that non-specific treatments are overused with a frequent absence of improvement and with recurrence in one-quarter of patients in the French general population. The therapeutic strategy should probably be based on the severity of the disease as given by the MIDAS grade and also on the intensity of each attack.

References

1. Lantéri-Minet M, Lucas C, Leroy L. Framig 99-I. Caractéristiques des patients migraineux. *Lett Neurologue* 2000; **4** (Suppl. 5): 8–10.
2. Henry P, Duru G, Chazot G, *et al. La migraine en France*: *étude épidémiologique, impact socio-économique et qualité de vie*. Paris: John Libbey Eurotext, 1993.
3. Lucas C, Lantéri-Minet M, Leroy L. Framig 99-III. Comportements thérapeutiques des migraineux. *Lett Neurologue* 2000; **4** (Suppl. 5): 14–16.

35
The Framig 2000 (III) survey: health-care use

C. Lucas, M. Lantéri-Minet, and C. Chaffaut

Framig 2000 was an epidemiological survey on migraine performed on the general population in France in 2000, 1 year after Framig 99[1,3] and 10 years after the first epidemiological survey of migraine in France.[2] Framig 2000 (III) focused on the relationship between patients and practitioners.

Methods

A phone survey was carried out by Ipsos, a statistical institute, from 12 to 28 December 2000 on 4689 subjects aged 18 to 65 years who were representative of the French general population. Migraine was diagnosed using an algorithm based on International Headache Society (IHS) criteria, and a 'decision-tree' questionnaire was administered to subjects. We studied subjects with 'active' migraine (at least one attack in the last 3 months). We evaluated the relationship between the patients and their practitioners and the patients' use of the health-care system.

Results

A total of 312 migraineurs took part in the survey. Twenty-two per cent scored grade III or IV on the MIDAS scale.[3-5] Forty-eight per cent of migraineurs with MIDAS scores of grade I or II had severe attacks. The large majority of migraineurs (82%) did not consult practitioners specifically for migraine, and 23% had never seen a general practitioner for migraine. Neurologists were only rarely consulted (7%). 'Shopping for a doctor' was uncommon (an average of 2.1 general practioners consulted in 10 years). Of the patients who had never seen a general practioner for migraine, 56% thought that consultation would not be useful, 55% thought that migraine is not a real disease, and 45% thought that there is no real treatment for migraine. Of the patients who had consulted a general practitioner for migraine, 58% thought that there was no change in their condition. We also considered the therapeutical management of the migraine attack in terms of the relationship

Table 35.1 Migraineurs and general practitioners (GPs): choice of acute treatment for migraine attack

	Percentage of migraineurs	
	Never seen by GP for migraine	Not followed-up by a GP for migraine
Last consultation	—	44
Advice from family/friend	41	22
Advice from pharmacist	25	15

between general practitioners and patients (Table 35.1). Many patients were found to have followed the advice of family, friends, or pharmacists in treating their migraine.

Comments

Framig 2000 (III) confirmed that French migraineurs do not make sufficient use of the health-care system for their disease and showed the deficit of information on migraine in France.

References

1. Lantéri-Minet M, Lucas C, Leroy L. Framig 99-I. Caractéristiques des patients migraineux. *Lett Neurologue* 2000; **4** (Suppl. 5): 8–10.
2. Henry P, Duru G, Chazot G, *et al*. La migraine en France: étude épidémiologique, impact socio-économique et qualité de vie. Paris: John Libbey Eurotext, 1993.
3. Lucas C, Lantéri-Minet M, Leroy L. Framig 99-III. Comportements thérapeutiques des migraineux. *Lett Neurologue* 2000; **4** (Suppl. 5): 14–16.
4. Steward WF, Lipton RB, Whyte J, *et al*. An international study to asses the reliability of the Migraine Disability Assessment (MIDAS) score. *Neurology* 1999; **53**: 988–94.
5. McGregor EA, Lantéri-Minet M, Lucas C. The clinical utility of the Migraine Disability Assessment (MIDAS) questionnaire. Abstract at the Fifth Congress of the European Federation of Neurological Societies, Copenhagen, October 2000.

36
Family burden, comorbidities, and health-care utilization: discussion summary

Richard B. Lipton

Robert Smith pointed out that, from the perspective of family medicine, migraine influences not just individuals but the family system and, in turn, the family system influences the health of its members. He presented survey data indicating that most but far from all migraine sufferers often feel that their families are supportive (64%) and sympathetic (47%) to their condition. In addition, because migraine is a familial disorder, many households have more than one migraine sufferer. The behaviour of each family member may influence other household members. The need for additional research on patterns of health-care behaviour and disability for migraine was discussed. It was pointed out that, when migraine sufferers and their spouses were directly interviewed, the migraine sufferer reported that their illness had a higher degree of family impact than reported by the unaffected spouse. It is not clear if the migraine sufferers overestimate the burden of their illness on others or if their spouses underestimate the burden. This was identified as an area for future research.

Naomi Breslau reviewed the relationship of migraine to depression, anxiety, stroke, and epilepsy. Her recent study showed that, although migraine influences the risk of depression, it does not influence the clinical course of depression. The discussion highlighted the need for a high index of suspicion of migraine in persons with anxiety disorders and depression. The need to suspect comorbid illnesses in migraine sufferers was also emphasized.

Lantéri-Minet presented data from the Framig study showing that 73% of migraine sufferers say yes to the question, 'You are a migraine sufferer. Did you know this?' There was a concern that some people may be embarrassed to confess their ignorance and may therefore report that they know they had migraine, even if their diagnosis was in doubt. These authors showed that migraine awareness was greatest in those with higher occupational status, longer duration of disease (episodic attacks over more years), and greater disruption of daily life.

Catarci *et al.* showed that the prevalence of migraine in Italian doctors was surprisingly high while the rate of absenteeism during migraine was low. The authors noted that efficiency was reduced while at work ('presenteeism'). It was pointed out that, across a range of conditions, the level of absenteeism versus presenteeism may be determined in part by the demand–control conditions of the job. Individuals with highly demanding jobs over which they have little control tend to stay at home when they are ill to escape from otherwise unmanageable demands. Individuals with high control over their jobs, including physicians, may come to work despite illness and attempt to regulate the pace and demands of work.

Section IV

Economics of headache

37 General principles of disease-costing

Bengt Jönsson

Basic principles

The basic principle in costing is that resources should be valued according to their 'opportunity cost' (that is, the cost in terms of opportunities lost). This means that we should consider the best alternative use for the resources and consider the cost in relationship to that. Since this opportunity cost cannot be directly observed, we are in practice limited to the observation of 'accounting costs'. A common mistake is to equate costs with charges. What is charged for a certain good or service can be both more or less than the cost of providing it.

It is also important to include all relevant cost consequences of a disease, regardless of when and where they occur.[1] Very often the costing is considered from a limited perspective, which may lead to suboptimization if significant cost consequences are ignored.

Identification, quantification, and valuation

The process of costing starts with the identification of all relevant resources. The next step is to find a quantitative measure for each resource item. For some resources it may be difficult to find an adequate measure or data. But it is always useful to have a list of what are judged to be the relevant resources, even if they cannot be measured. When the result is presented and interpreted, it is important to consider what was left out.

The final and most difficult step is the valuation. Usually, it is this step that we think of when we talk about costing. But it is important to separate the quantification of resource use from the costing.

Perspective

The societal perspective includes all costs. It may very well be that a specific decision-maker will only take part of the costs into account, because the other part does not concern him or her. However, from an analytical point of view, it is important to include everything. It is then always possible to look at the costs from different perspectives. Such an analysis can very often explain certain types of behaviour and help to identify suboptimizations.

Marginal and average cost

Marginal cost is defined as the cost of producing one more unit of production, for example, an extra bed/day in hospital or an extra visit from a physician. Marginal cost will differ from average cost when there are fixed costs, for example, overheads that are, within limits, independent of the level of production. What is a fixed or a variable cost usually depends on the time perspective. In the long run, most resources will have an opportunity cost, even if, in the short run, it is difficult to imagine any other use of resources than the present one.

Opportunity cost versus monetary flow

An example of monetary flow without an opportunity cost is a transfer payment. In health care transfer payments are commonly found in terms of compensation for lost income due to illness. These transfer payments represent no cost for society, since there are two parties to the transaction, one who gives and one who receives. Thus, for society as a whole, there is no cost. The cost is the loss of production or other real resources spent due to the disease. Also, the real costs used in the transfer process represent a social cost. Insurance cannot be provided without real cost and sometimes the 'loading factor', that is, the difference between premiums paid and benefits received, can be substantial.

The provision of 'informal care' is an example of a resource that is not paid for but can still have an opportunity cost. The time given up by the carer could have been used for other production or for consumption.

In well-functioning markets, the monetary flow and the opportunity costs coincide. When markets are imperfect, the prices must be corrected to better reflect opportunity cost.

Different types of costs

A distinction is often made between direct, indirect, and intangible costs.[2]

Direct costs can occur within or outside the health-care sector. Direct health-care costs include hospitalizations, physician visits, diagnostic and therapeutic interventions, and drugs. Direct costs outside the health-care sector can be costs for specific accommodation and transportation. In many countries, nursing homes are counted as social services rather than health services. For diseases like dementia and multiple sclerosis a major part of the direct costs are outside the health-care sector. They are used to compensate for the disability that follows with the progression of the disease.

Indirect costs relate to both morbidity and mortality. Morbidity costs can be estimated from data on absenteeism or early retirement. But loss of production while at work, for example, due to migraine or depression, should also be included when relevant. A major problem with these costs is to arrive at reliable and valid estimates of the value of the resource loss, which is not directly observable or accounted for.

Calculations of mortality costs are complicated by the fact that mortality is associated with the loss of not only a producer but also a consumer. While the prevailing method is to calculate these costs without the deduction of consumption, there are theoretical arguments for calculating the net loss as consumption minus production.[3] A consequence of this is that mortality cost becomes negative for older persons. Depending on the age distribution of mortality, the total mortality cost may also be positive or negative.

The controversy surrounding the calculation of mortality costs makes it important to separate them in the calculation. An alternative may also be to present this cost as number of (quality-adjusted) life years lost, without any monetary valuation.

Separation of price and quantity

It is an important principle to separate price and quantity in the calculation and presentation of costs. There is uncertainty in estimates of both quantities and prices and it is important to separate these. A sensitivity analysis can be undertaken with different prices. When quantities are reported separately, it is also easy to undertake an analysis, for example, with unit costs for another country.

Market prices and opportunity costs

For prices to reflect opportunity cost, there needs to be no significant market imperfection.[4] When market imperfections are present, the market price has to be adjusted to better reflect opportunity cost. For a monopolist, the market price is higher than opportunity cost. The same is true of the price of labour, the salaries in a situation with unemployment. An example where the marker price is too low, is when negative external circumstances are present.

In a well functioning labour market, the salaries reflect the opportunity cost. An alternative method for calculating the value of production lost due to illness is the 'friction method'.[5,6] The friction method assumes that there is always someone available after some time to take over a job if illness strikes the person who has the job in the first instance. The problems with this method are not only the questionable empirical foundation and difficulties in estimation, but it also introduces a bias between the valuing of direct and indirect costs.[7,8] Since most direct costs in health care are labour costs, they should be reduced as well if opportunity costs do not reflect salaries. In periods with severe shortage of labour, the salaries can underestimate the cost of labour and thus the cost of diseases that affect labour force participation.

Costing in health care poses a number of problems. Compared to, for example, financial markets, there is a genuine lack of reliable data.

Future costs and discounting

Future costs, as well as the future health benefit of an intervention, have a different valuation due to time preferences and the return on investment if the use of resources is postponed.[9]

Discounting is a method for making costs and other effects comparable. A discount rate is used to calculate the present value. Present values can then be compared. There is an intense discussion about the choice of discount rate. In practice it is a convention to use either 3% or 5% for both costs and benefits. However, there are arguments for using a lower discount rate for health effects, as is the case in the UK. Today, with the use of computers, it is easy to undertake a sensitivity analysis to see the impact of different discount rates on the result.

Cost of illness—methodology and practice

The cost-of-illness method has a long history. It is possible to find references dating from as long ago as the seventeenth century where they calculated costs for specific diseases. However, the modern cost-of-illness methodology, based on the theory of human capital, dates back to the early 1960s.[10]

A cost-of-illness analysis is a descriptive type of study, relating all costs to a specific disease or event and not to administrative units. Cost-of-illness studies should not be categorized as economic evaluations, as they do not examine clinical outcomes, but they can still provide information on which to base resource allocation choices and also serve as a baseline for subsequent economic evaluations.[11] There is a debate on the value of undertaking such calculations (see, for example, refs 12–14). The criticism is that they do not directly inform about the costs and benefits of different opportunities for resource allocation. It has also been pointed out that cost-of-illness studies lead to circular arguments and confusion in priority-setting—if a disease is shown to be costly, does that mean that more or less resources should be spent on the disease? The use of the human-capital approach for valuing the loss of production has also been questioned. Although it is correct that cost-of-illness studies do not give direct evidence of the efficiency of allocation of resources, it is too strong to state that they have no policy relevance. In well-performed and complete cost-of-illness studies, all relevant costs to society are included, and one of the major advantages of cost-of-illness studies is that they give *information* about how resources are spent or lost in society due to a certain disease. Cost-of-illness studies can be seen as 'health accounts', which can complement national accounts that outline economic activities in the population.

Multiple sclerosis as an example

To illustrate two different cost-of-illness approaches, the results of two Swedish studies[15,16] on multiple sclerosis (MS) are shown in Table 37.1. As can be seen, the

Table 37.1   The cost of MS in Sweden as obtained by two different approaches

Type of cost	Cost (million SEK)	
	Top–down study for 1994 (ref. 15)	Bottom–up study for 1998 (ref. 16)
Total direct costs	370	3266
Institutional care	354*	649[†]
Ambulatory care	13	364
Drugs	3[‡]	533
Other direct costs	—	1720
Total indirect costs	1366	1602
Short-term sickness absence	183	87
Early retirement	1183	1515[§]
(Intangible costs)	—	(2702)
Total costs	1736	4868 (7570)

*In-patient care and nursing home care.
[†]In-patient care and rehabilitation.
[‡]No interferon drugs.
[§]Early retirement and long-term sickness absence.

two approaches give different results. The main reason for this is that different data sources have been used to perform the cost calculations.

Top–down studies are based on register data. The total cost for hospitalization, as an example, is separated according to the main diagnosis. The same can be done for physician visits or prescriptions when diagnosis-related data are available. All costs for a defined diagnosis are then added together. The same is done for indirect costs for morbidity, short-term sickness absence, and early retirement pensions.

The advantage of this approach is that it avoids double-counting and gets a total distribution of all costs. The disadvantage is that the costing is limited to what is in the registers. For MS, where many resources outside the health-care system are used, for example, in the municipalities, this approach underestimates the true cost, since there are normally no registers covering this consumption of resources. The coding of discharges, for example, the choice of main diagnosis, will have a significant impact on the result. Comorbidity can have a great impact that is not taken into account by this method. For MS this problem is of minor importance, since the degree of comorbidity is low.

In a bottom–up study, the total costs for a group of patients with a defined disease are estimated. This can be done in great detail, which is a big advantage. The disadvantage is that you have to extrapolate from a small group of patients to the whole population. A biased sample can give a very biased result when the sample estimate is multiplied by a population factor. The assessment as to which costs are due to a defined disease also poses problems. It is easier to estimate all costs for a group of patients, which was the method chosen in the second MS study presented above. But that means that epidemiological methods, the calculation of aetiological fraction,

Table 37.2 The effect of disease severity on annual total cost per patient and quality of life

Disability level*	Total cost (SEK)	Quality of life (scale: 0–1)
Mild (EDSS ≤3.0) (n=126)	156 120	0.68
Moderate (EDSS 3.5–6.0) (n=121)	303 072	0.52
Severe (EDSS ≥6.5) (n=162)	764 403	0.17

*EDSS, Expanded Standard Disability Status Scale (for MS).

must be used to assign specific costs to a defined disease. Thus, there is an important distinction between the costs of a disease and the costs for patients with that disease. For patients with MS, it is rather easy to separate the costs due to the disease at the individual level. But for a disease like diabetes it is almost impossible.

One advantage with individual data is that it is possible to study the determinants of costs. For example, in MS we can study how disease severity is related to costs and quality of life (Table 37.2). The annual total cost (direct and indirect costs) per patient increases by a factor of about 5 (from 156 120 SEK to 764 403 SEK) when comparing a patient with mild disability with one with severe disability. Table 37.2 also shows that quality of life declines substantially as MS progresses.

Individual data on costs and quality of life related to the severity of disease can be very useful for modelling interventions in chronic progressive diseases. In such cases it is necessary to supplement clinical trial data, which by necessity can only cover a short part of the disease span, in the analysis of the cost-effectiveness of interventions.

Conclusions

Disease-costing relates costs to a defined disease or group of patients with the disease. This provides relevant information about the resources used and lost due to the disease; information that is generally not available in the health-care system. It should, however, be remembered that cost-of-illness studies are not economic evaluations that show the cost and benefits of different resource allocations. They can at best be used as a basis for such studies, for example, modelling studies combining clinical, epidemiological, and economic data to assess the cost-effectiveness of alternative allocations of resources.

There are established methods for costing. But there are major problems with the data for such estimates. The sometimes very different estimates for the same disease are often due to the use of different data-sets.

The fact that there is a well-established method for costing does not mean that there are no remaining controversies. These relate to the valuation of non-market production, that is, informal care, valuation of indirect costs due to morbidity, the inclusion and valuation of intangible costs, and the valuation of mortality costs.

References

1. Johannesson M. *Theory and methods of economic evaluation of health care*. Dordrecht: Kluwer Academic Publishers, 1996.
2. Drummond MF, O'Brien B, Stoddart GL, Torrance GW. *Methods for the economic evaluation of health care programmes*, 2nd edn. Oxford: Oxford Medical Publications, 1997.
3. Meltzer D. Accounting for future costs in medical cost-effectiveness analysis. *J Hlth Econom* 1997; **16**: 33–64.
4. Luce B, Elixhauser A. Estimating costs in the economic evaluation of medical technologies. *Int J Technol Assess Hlth Care* 1990; **6**: 57–75.
5. Koopmanshap MA, Rutten FFH, van Ineveld BM. The friction cost method for measuring indirect costs of disease. *J Hlth Econom* 1995; **14**: 171–89.
6. Koopmanschap MA, Rutten FFH. A practical guide for calculating indirect costs of disease. *PharmacoEconomics* 1997; **10**: 460–6.
7. Johannesson M, Karlsson G. The friction cost method: a comment. *J Hlth Econom* 1997; **16**: 249–55.
8. Liljas B. How to calculate indirect costs in economic evaluations. *PharmacoEconomics* 1998; **13**: 1–7.
9. Krahn M, Gafni A. Discounting in economic evaluation of health care interventions. *Med Care* 1993; **31**: 403–18.
10. Weisbrod B. The valuation of human capital. *J Pol Econom* 1961; **69**: 425–36.
11. Davey PJ, Leeder SR. The cost of migraine: more than just a headache? *PharmacoEconomics* 1992; **9**: 5–7.
12. Hodgson TA. Cost of illness studies: no aid to decision making? Comments on the second opinion by Shiell *et al*. *Hlth Policy* 1989; **11**: 57–60.
13. Drummond M. Cost-of-illness studies. A major headache? *PharmacoEconomics* 1992; **2**: 1–4.
14. Jönsson B. Measuring the economic burden in asthma. In *Asthma's impact on society* (ed. Weiss KB, Buist AS, Sullivan SD). New York and Basel: Marcel Dekker Inc, 1999: 251–67.
15. Henriksson F, Jönsson B. The economic cost of multiple sclerosis in Sweden in 1994. *PharmacoEconomics* 1998; **13**: 597–606.
16. Henriksson F, Fredrikson S, Masterman T, Jönsson B. Costs, quality of life and disease severity in multiple sclerosis: a cross-sectional study in Sweden. *Eur J Neurol* 2001; **8**: 27–35.

38
The economic burden of headache

Jean François Dartigues, Philippe Michel, and Patrick Henry

Introduction

There have been several excellent recent reviews of the literature on the economic burden of headache[1-3] so it seems unnecessary to provide one here, especially as not enough new data have been published to justify a new review. Instead, in this chapter we wish to give an epidemiologist's perspective on several points related to the economic burden of headaches and to try to answer some questions that we think are important if one wishes to decrease this burden.

The first question is: why has the economic burden of migraine been so often studied, while the burden of other types of headache remains largely unknown? Migraine is a frequent and clear clinical entity with operational criteria, the International Headache Society (IHS) criteria, admitted by the international scientific community; with (probably) a specific (even multifactorial) aetiology; with (probably) a specific natural history; and with (probably) a specific treatment. Thus, from this perspective, migraine is a good disease for neurologists, epidemiologists, economists, drug companies, and health authorities. In contrast, other types of headache lack even one of these criteria. For instance, tension-type headaches are frequent, but don't have really operational diagnostic criteria and a specific aetiology. Cluster headache has operational diagnostic criteria but is not frequent enough to constitute a public health problem.

The rest of this chapter will deal with two further questions.

(1) In spite of the favourable criteria for the management of migraine, and for epidemiological or economic studies, is the relationship between migraine and cost really deterministic, and, if not, what is the effect on the validity of cost-of-illness studies?

(2) What are the consequences of the progress in the management of migraine on the burden of this disease?

Migraine and cost-of-illness studies

Cost-of-illness studies consist of three components:

(1) *direct cost*, incurred mainly by the health-care system in diagnosing and treating the disease;
(2) *indirect cost*, in term of lost production owing to lost working days, diminished productivity resulting from illness or disability, or losses incidental to premature death;
(3) *intangible costs* such as pain, suffering, or reduction in the quality of life of sufferers.

Cost-of-illnesses studies have estimated the direct and indirect cost of migraine in France as 6 billion French francs per year for 60 million inhabitants. That means that a French inhabitant pays on average 100 FF or 15 euros each year for migraine. Similar amounts of money have been estimated in other parts of the Western world. It is enormous, but is it true? Many factors interfere with the relationship between migraine and cost, even in the case of direct cost, which appears to be the most objective and easy to calculate cost (Fig. 38.1). The personalities of migraineurs and their beliefs as to the efficacy of the health-care system to treat migraine attacks contribute strongly to the coping strategies of migraineurs against migraine. All studies report that a large percentage of migraineurs never consult a physician for migraine (19–76%).[3] Many reasons could be given for that. Many migraineurs adopt effective coping strategies against pain and do not need care or use over-the-counter medications. In France (as also reported in other countries), 65% of migraineurs believe that migraine can never be cured, 43% think that nothing can be done against migraine,[4] and 52% believe that orthodox medicine is not effective against migraine.[5] The attitude of the primary care service physician and the efficacy of the first treatment given also influence the cost. After a first consultation, many

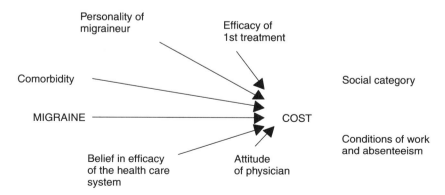

Fig. 38.1   Factors contributing to the economic cost of migraine.

patients do not return to their physician or neurologist. Edmeads[6] analysed the reasons for that in Canada. Edmeads found that 55% of patients were satisfied with the treatment and did not need consultation again, 17% did not return because of problems with medication, and 38% were turned-off by their doctors and felt that they were not taken seriously. In fact, 22 years ago Packard[7] showed that the main purpose of a consultation for a migraineur is to obtain explanation and reassurance, whereas the main purpose of the doctor is to bring about relief of pain.

Comorbidity and cost

Comorbidity, which refers to the coexistence of two medical conditions with a frequency greater than chance, could also interfere with cost. Psychiatric disorders, epilepsy, and stroke are the well known comorbidities of migraine.[8] But, in fact, many conditions are more frequent in migraineurs. In the French Mig-Access study,[4] conducted using a face-to-face interview in a French representative national sample, we have shown that backache, fatigue, depression, anxiety, abdominal pain, constipation, diarrhoea, and gynaecological and respiratory disorders are far more self-reported in migraineurs than in controls, and all these conditions justify resort to health care. Thus, it could be very difficult to attribute to a single motive a consultation of a general practitioner or aa hospitalization in patients with multiple comorbidities. In our opinion, these findings justify, in addition to cost-of-illnesses studies, an approach comparing migraineurs and non-headache subjects in order to better appreciate the incremental costs related to migraine.

This comparative approach give some surprising results. In the Mig-Access study, the comparison of the use of health-care services during a 6-month period showed that, in spite of multiple comorbidities, migraine sufferers used more consultations with general practitioners and complementary examinations, but did not use more of the other health-care services. Similarly, in the Gazel cohort, which is a French nationwide cohort of volunteers from EDF-GDF, the French power company that produces and supplies electricity and gas, we found no differences in absenteeism during 4 years of follow-up in migraineurs and in controls after adjustments for age, gender, and number of health impairments.[9] These results are certainly robust because the data collection on absenteeism is completely independent of the subject and the diagnostic procedure. In contrast, self-assessed performances at work were strongly impaired in migraineurs versus controls. The discrepancy between object-ive and subjective burden implies that the public health impact of migraine is lower than that on the individual person. Migraineurs may 'suffer silently' and work during migraine attacks. Another non-exclusive explanation could be that the migraineurs may adopt a compensatory coping strategy for health impairments other than migraine: since they miss work for their headaches, they may minimize their absences for other health impairments. The final explanation is that the conditions of work and of absenteeism might be peculiar to this study by virtue of the fact that the subjects are workers in a French public firm.

This latter explanation seems to be confirmed by the follow-up of the Mig-Access cohort, which comprised workers from different workplaces and in which we could separate absenteeism due to headache and absenteeism due to other conditions.[10] In this sample, there was an annual incremental absenteeism, defined as the mean annual absenteeism in the migraine sample minus that in the control group, estimated as 3.2 days. This absenteeism is the same for migraine attacks as for other medical reasons. We can conclude from these findings that the conditions of work and of absenteeism and also the social category are other important factors that partially explain the cost of migraine.

The effect of progress in management on the burden of migraine

During the past 10 years, many new treatments for migraine have become available, and the awareness of migraine has improved. In a disease with recurrent attacks, the efficacy of better treatment strategies could be associated with a decrease in the prevalence of migraine due to a decrease in the duration of the disease. In fact, some studies suggest, on the contrary, that the prevalence of migraine may be increasing,[11] but the authors admit that this apparent increase could be more related to better diagnostic management in primary care than to a true increase in prevalence. Two recent prevalence studies, in the USA[12] and in France,[13] conducted on national representative samples by telephone or face-to-face interviews, did not confirm this increase in prevalence and showed exactly the same rates at intervals of 10 years: 12.1% in 1989 and 12.6% in 1999 in the USA for migraines classified using the IHS criteria 1.1, 1.2, and 1.7;[14] 8.1% in 1990 and 7.9% in 2000 in France for migraines classified using the IHS criteria 1.1 and 1.2. In the same study, we introduced the Migraine Disability Assessment (MIDAS) score as a measure of the indirect cost of headache.[15] In 2000, the proportion of migraineurs with MIDAS grades III and IV was 12.4%. Migrainous disorders have the same magnitude of consequences in term of days lost due to headache (11.5% of grades III and IV), while other types of headache have far less consequences on this indicator (only 2.1% of grades III and IV). On the basis of these proportions, we can estimate the prevalence of migraine requiring medical attention at 1.6% which is enormous.

Conclusion

Thus, in spite of some progress in the management of headaches, migraine remains today a disease with a major economic burden. In the future, it will be crucial to take into account all factors influencing the economic burden of headache (Fig. 38.1) if we wish to really decrease this burden. In our opinion, an example of a good approach is the trial published by Lipton *et al.*[16] comparing stratified care versus step-care strategies for migraine, which controlled for several of these factors. They evaluated the cost-effectiveness of two treatment strategies, they standardized the attitude of the physician using the trial protocol, and they controlled for the other factors by randomization. Another important approach could be a more qualitative one, an anthropological approach to the relationship between migraineurs and their physicians in order to better understand the difficulties of communication.

References

1. Stang P, Cady R, Batenhorst A, Hoffman L. Workplace productivity. A review of the impact of migraine and its treatment. *PharmacoEconomics* 2001; **2001**: 231–44.
2. Lipton R, Stewart W, Reed M, Diamond S (2001) Migraine's impact today. Burden of illness, pattern of care. *Postgrad Med* 2001; **109**: 38–45.
3. Michel P. Socioeconomic costs of headache. In *The headache*, 2nd edn (ed. Olesen J, Tfelt-Hansen P, Welch K). Philadelphia: Lippincott Williams & Wilkins, 2000.
4. Michel P, Pariente P, Duru G, Dreyfus J, Chabriat H, Henry P Mig-Access: a population-based, nationwide, comparative survey of access to care in migraine in France. *Cephalalgia* 1996; **16**: 50–5.
5. Michel P, Auray J, Chicoye A, Dartigues J, Lamure M, Duru G, *et al*. Prise en charge des migraineux en France: coût et recours aux soins. *J Econom Med* 1993; **11**: 71–80.
6. Edmeads J. Why is migraine so common? *Cephalalgia* 1998; **18**: 2–7.
7. Packard R. What does the patient want? *Headache* 1979; **19**: 370–4.
8. Breslau N, Rasmussen B. The impact of migraine. Epidemiology, risk factors and co-morbidities. *Neurology* 2001; **56**: S4–S12.
9. Michel P, Dartigues J, Lindoulsi A, Heanry P. Loss of productivity and quality of life in migraine sufferers among French workers: results from the Gazel cohort. *Headache* 2001; **37**: 71–8.
10. Michel P, Dartigues J, Duru G, Moreau J, Salamon R, Henry P. Incremental absenteeism due to headaches in migraine: results from the Mig-Access French national cohort. *Cephalalgia* 1999; **19**: 503–10.
11. Rozen T, Swanson J, Stang P, SK. MD, Rocca W. Increasing incidence of medically recognized migraine headache in a United States population. *Neurology* 1999; **53**: 1468–73.
12. Lipton R, Stewart W, Diamond S, Diamond M, Reed M. Prevalence and burden of migraine in the United states: data from the American Migraine Study II. *Headache* 2001; **41**: 646–57.
13. Henry P, Auray J, Gaudin A, Dartigues J, Duru G, Lanteri-Minet M, *et al*. Prevalence and clinical characteristics of migraine disorders. GRIM 2000: a nationwide survey in France. Submitted.
14. Committee of Classification of the International Headache Society. Classification and diagnostic criteria for headache disorders, cranial neuralgia and facial pain. *Cephalalgia* 1988; **8**: 1–96.
15. Lipton R, Stewart W, Edmeas J, Sawyer J. Clinical utility of a new instrument assessing migraine disability: the migraine disability assessment score (MIDAS) score. *Headache* 1998; **38**: 390–1.
16. Lipton R, Stewart W, Stone A, Lainez M, Sawyer J. Stratified care vs step care strategies for migraine: results of the Disability Strategies of Care (DISC) study. *J Am Med Assoc* 2000; **284**: 2599–605.

39 Measuring the economic benefits of pharmacotherapy— general principles

Nicholas E.J. Wells

....

Introduction

Migraine and its management have been subject to increasing economic analysis over the past decade. This interest was stimulated in the first instance by the arrival of sumatriptan, the first of a new class of medicines (the selective serotonin 5-HT$_{1B/1D}$ agonists or 'triptans') for treating acute migraine attacks. Early economic studies concentrated on quantifying the burden migraine imposes on health-care systems, society as a whole, and individual sufferers. Subsequent investigations have sought to measure the effectiveness of antimigraine therapies in reducing these various burdens. For example, Lofland and colleagues[1] compared health-care resource utilization patterns in a managed care setting in the USA before and after the introduction of sumatriptan whilst Wells and Steiner[2] used a clinical trial to examine the effectiveness of eletriptan in reducing the amount of time over which sufferers are unable to perform their usual activities during a migraine attack.

The results of these and other studies represent a useful beginning to the more formal pharmacoeconomic evaluation of treatments for migraine. However, substantial variation is apparent with regard to, *inter alia*, the comprehensiveness of and objectives pursued by the studies, the methodologies, outcome measures, and investigational settings employed, as well as the inclusion of control and active comparator groups. Difficulties therefore confront comparisons of the results of different studies and this inevitably limits the usefulness of the information to clinicians and other decision-makers. This shortcoming is especially unfortunate as economic or 'value for money' considerations are playing an increasing role in informing choices between treatment options. The purpose of this chapter is therefore to help promote greater consistency in assessing the benefits and costs of pharmacotherapy by outlining the various approaches to economic evaluation and indicating their potential application specifically to acute migraine therapy. Preceding this discussion, it is relevant to explain the growing role of economics in the practice of medicine.

The need for economic evaluation

Economics is concerned with the scarcity of resources. People, money, time, and equipment are not in sufficient supply to enable the production or consumption of all the goods and services that society may desire. Choices have therefore to be made as to which activities will and will not be resourced. Such choices may, of course, be based on a variety of criteria but, from an economic perspective, the criterion of efficiency demands the selection of those activities that provide the best value for money. The latter is determined by comparing alternative courses of action in terms of their costs and outcomes. The economically efficient choice is that option that offers the greatest return from a given level of resource input or requires the smallest input to achieve a specified magnitude of output.

In the health-care arena, considerations of economic efficiency are increasingly entering the decision-making process. Constrained budgets in the face of escalating demands—fuelled by population ageing as well as growth, technological advance (leading not only to more expensive treatments but also to potentially greater numbers of sufferers being unable to benefit from intervention), rising public expectations regarding achievable health status, and the emergence of new diseases—are forcing providers towards the identification and selection of cost-effective treatments. One of the clearest examples of this trend is to be seen in the UK where the National Institute for Clinical Excellence (NICE) employs cost-effectiveness information to determine if medicines and other interventions should be available on the National Health Service (NHS).[3]

Headache does not lead to the consumption of substantial health-care resources. This does not mean, however, that treatments aimed at alleviating the disorder should be exempt from value-for-money scrutiny. Economic considerations are relevant to all interventions since opportunity costs accompany every resource allocation decision. And, in the specific case of migraine, technological progress in the form of the 'triptans' has not only led to higher episode treatment costs but is also encouraging larger numbers of sufferers to seek care.

Measuring the costs and outcome of pharmacotherapy

The different approaches to undertaking economic evaluation are summarized in Fig. 39.1. It is immediately clear that the scope for such analyses is broad, extending from a narrow focus on just the costs of a single intervention to a full economic appraisal comparing the costs and outcomes of one treatment with those of other options that might be employed.

As noted earlier, a significant number of the economic analyses undertaken in the field of migraine have examined the various costs generated by the disorder.

Are both costs and outcomes of the alternatives examined?

		No		Yes
		Examines only consequences	Examines only costs	Both
Is there comparison of two or more alternatives?	No	1A Partial evaluation 1B Outcome description	Cost description	2 Partial evaluation Cost-outcome description
	Yes	3A Partial evaluation 3B Efficacy or effectiveness evaluation	Cost analysis	4 Full economic Evaluation Cost-minimization analysis Cost-effectiveness analysis Cost-utility analysis Cost-benefit analysis

Fig. 39.1 Framework for evaluation (adapted from ref. 4).

Although cost-of-illness studies do not strictly fit into the framework shown in Fig. 39.1—because they are disease- rather than treatment-focused—it is worth clarifying their relevance to policy decision-making since it is widely believed that estimating the total societal cost of an illness is useful in this context.[5]

The methodology for conducting cost-of-illness studies was established by Rice in 1966.[6] The approach identifies three principal sources of cost: direct (medical) costs; indirect (productivity) costs; and personal suffering (intangible) costs. The first of these categories embraces expenditures in the relevant sectors of the health-care system on the prevention, detection, and treatment of disease. Thus, consultations and other contacts with health-care professionals, diagnostic procedures, medicines, and other interventions are included in this category. The costs are borne essentially by the health-care system, although some analyses also attempt to take account of expenditures made by patients themselves, for example, on over-the-counter medicines.

The second major category covers indirect costs and these comprise the production losses resulting from individuals being unable to work because of illness. Inability to work may simply take the form of short-term and very occasional absences resulting from temporary episodes of ill health. More severe disease and any associated disability may lead to longer absences whilst premature mortality obviously results in early permanent exit from the labour force. In addition to production losses resulting from sickness absence in this way, some studies seek to quantify the production values foregone where individuals persist in going to work whilst experiencing an episode of ill health but are unable to perform at their full potential.

This particular element of lost production has frequently been included in studies of the cost of illness for migraine and has sometimes been termed 'presenteeism'.

The remaining component of cost-of-illness studies consists of the costs of pain and suffering borne by patients as a consequence of disease. Although unequivocally an important part of a truly comprehensive cost-of-illness study, these burdens are frequently omitted because of the difficulties inherent in their quantification and subsequent valuation in monetary terms.

A common theme that has emerged from the migraine cost-of-illness research of the past decade is that the disorder is associated with substantial costs.[7] More specifically, the literature indicates that, whilst direct treatment costs are relatively modest (reflecting the fact that the condition is essentially managed in the primary care setting), costs attributable to migraine-related absence from, or reduced productivity at work are substantial.

Cost-of-illness analyses serve a number of useful purposes (Table 39.1), including raising awareness about the significance of diseases that tend to be rather neglected because they are not associated with high mortality rates. However, the observation of substantial costs, for example, is insufficient alone to indicate inefficiency and waste or a 'problem', the solution to which must be an input of yet further resources. In the absence of any information about the outcomes that are achieved through treatment it cannot be assumed that current spending patterns are efficient (that is, directed to those uses that offer maximum health returns) and it is not possible to determine whether additional resources should be allocated to the disease. Similarly, a low level of direct costs, as exemplified by migraine, cannot be taken to indicate an absence of 'problem'—indeed, a significant injection of additional resource may be warranted if the opportunity exists to generate better health outcomes.

Against this background, economists[8,9] maintain that cost-of-illness data cannot be employed in evaluating competing demands for scarce health-care resources and that allocation of the latter should depend on the availability of treatment options, their cost, and their efficacy.[10] This line of argument therefore identifies the approaches contained in cell 4 in Fig. 39.1 as the appropriate means of establishing which treatments represent value for money.

Table 39.1 Uses of cost-of-illness data

To provide a measure of the national resources potentially available to be regained

To identify the current economic costs of a given illness and their distribution across, for example, different sectors of health-care provision

To facilitate comparisons of these costs across different illnesses (assuming consistent costing methodologies have been employed)

To raise awareness about a given illness, especially where conventional mortality and morbidity data may understate its significance

To contribute to the determination of priorities for medical research

To provide information that can be used to forecast costs in future years

Cost-minimization analysis

The first and most straightforward of these techniques is cost-minimization analysis. Choice of this method predicates consensus regarding the appropriate outcome measure for assessing the effect of treatment and that available evidence shows that all options achieve the same level of outcome. Under these circumstances, the analysis requires a comprehensive assessment of the costs of using the different treatments, that is, a quantification not only of the price per dose or course but of all other health-care contacts and resource utilization linked to the use of the medicine in question. The economically efficient choice is then the treatment option that yields the common level of outcome at least cost.

This approach may be appropriate where simple analgesics can be employed to manage uncomplicated headaches. In migraine, however, it may have less relevance, especially in comparing the triptans where efficacy rates—headache response at 2 hours—are reported to range from 50% to 70%.[11] In such circumstances—where treatment alternatives differ in both their costs and outcomes—cost-effectiveness analysis may be the more appropriate analytical technique.

Cost-effectiveness analysis

Cost-effectiveness analysis relates costs to a single unit of effect or outcome that is relevant to the treatment/condition under consideration, for example, reductions in cholesterol levels or increases in peak expiratory flow rates in hypercholesterol-aemia and asthma, respectively. To provide a simple illustration, suppose headache response rate at 2 hours postdosing is the preferred outcome measure denoting successful treatment of a migraine attack and that with Medicine X 65% of patients obtain a positive response compared to 54% for those taking Medicine Y. If it is further assumed that the cost of treating a migraine attack with X is UK £8 compared with £7 for Y, then it may be calculated that the cost per successfully treated attack is £12.31 with X and £12.96 with Y. This example, in which X is revealed to offer the better value for money, emphasizes not only the importance of examining both costs and outcomes but also illustrates the point that the cheaper alternative may not always represent the most economically efficient choice.

Cost-effectiveness can provide a useful framework for comparing the value for money offered by different treatments for migraine attacks. The principal issue requiring attention concerns the choice of outcome measure. Clinical trials of migraine therapies have usually employed headache response at 2 hours after the first dose as the primary indicator of treatment efficacy. Specifically, assessment has centred on the proportion of attacks improving from severe or moderate headache at baseline to mild headache or no pain at 2 hours. By itself, however, this measure has limited precision and only partially reflects what may be important to migraineurs. It fails to differentiate, for example, between treatments generating a substantial improvement in migraine headache from severe at the start of treatment to pain-free 2 hours later and those only reducing the pain from moderate to mild over the same time period. In addition, effective treatment will embrace, from the patient's perspective, characteristics other than just headache response at 2 hours. The likelihood of recurrence, for example, is a relevant consideration as might also be the speed at which therapeutic benefit begins to be experienced. An early indication that the treatment is going to be effective will be important for patients in terms of planning their work and social activities. Consequently, a more complete outcome measure might also include the presence or otherwise of a headache response (severe or moderate pain moving to a minimum of mild) at 30 minutes or 1 hour.

Beyond considerations of recurrence and early therapeutic effect, a truly comprehensive measure would also accommodate the occurrence of side-effects, perhaps with a prespecified level of severity distinguishing treatment success from failure. In addition, account could be taken of the impact of treatment on other migraine symptoms (nausea, photophonia, photophobia, etc.) and on the speed of return to 'normal' functioning. Each such addition will add complexity to the outcome measure—especially if it is also deemed appropriate that the various elements noted above should be differentially weighted—and, with currently available treatments, will inevitably reduce the proportion of attacks defined as successfully treated. However, greater comprehensiveness is clearly necessary to yield an outcome measure that is a more valid indicator of patient benefit for use in cost-effectiveness analyses of migraine treatments than the conventional clinical trial measure of headache response at 2 hours. Against this background, the increasing interest being shown in, and the reporting of results for, the measure of 'sustained pain-free' (which requires complete freedom from headache by 2 hours, no recurrence of moderate or severe headache, and no use of rescue medication 2–24 hours postdose) is clearly an encouraging development.[12]

The strength of the cost-effectiveness approach is that it enables comparisons to be made of the value for money associated with different treatment options within a specific disease area such as migraine. Given a fixed budget, the selection of those treatments with the lowest 'cost per unit of health effect' will maximize the health output from the available resources.[13] However, the specific nature of the outcome measure is such that value for money comparisons cannot be drawn with different treatments employed in other disease areas. This inability to compare interventions with differing natural effects is a significant shortcoming if the cost-effective choice of migraine treatment means that additional funding would be required and that resources would have to be redirected from use in other diseases. The critical question raised in these circumstances is whether or not such a transfer of resources to migraine treatment would result in more health gain than that realized in their existing deployment. Simple cost-effectiveness analysis cannot answer this question.

Cost-utility analysis

One approach to addressing the issue lies in the use of cost-utility analysis, which employs an outcome measure that has universal application. The technique is an adaptation of cost-effectiveness analysis and relates the cost of an intervention to its effect on both the quantitative and qualitative aspects of health. The latter are reflected in a single utility (preference)-based measure such as the quality-adjusted life year (QALY), which brings together the impact of treatment on survival and the quality of life. (Quality is estimated on a scale from 0 (death) to 1 (perfect health) and is applied as an adjustment to each year of life remaining post-intervention.)

To illustrate the approach, suppose that without treatment an individual can expect to live for 5 years and that the quality of each of those years is rated at 0.5. Now suppose that an intervention costing UK £500 is administered that extends the life expectancy to 10 years with the quality of the first 5 of these years improved to 0.9 and that of the second 5 years to 0.6. From this information it may be calculated that the intervention results in an additional 5 QALYs at a cost of £100 per quality-adjusted life year gained.

In cost-utility analysis, the optimal decision rule involves ranking the incremental cost-utility ratios of different interventions (which by virtue of the universal outcome measure could span such diverse treatments as, for example, triptans for migraine, inhaled corticosteroids for asthma, hip replacements, and coronary bypass grafting) and selecting those with the lowest ratios (best value) until the budget is depleted.[14]

This approach is based on the principles of welfare economics and provides a sound theoretical basis for promoting efficiency in the use of available resources. Indeed, NICE in the UK, which assesses the clinical cost-effectiveness of interventions to determine if they should be publicly provided on the NHS, encourages the use of this analytical method. In reality, however, there is considerable debate about the robustness of the data (in particular, the quality weights, which may be derived in a number of different ways with sometimes inconsistent results), whether it is appropriate to combine quantity and quality together in a single measure (for example, is 7 years × 0.5 the same as 5 years × 0.7?), and the ethical implications inherent in the use of QALY data to guide health-care resource allocation.

The application of cost-utility analysis to migraine raises further, more specific questions. Effective migraine treatment will not impact on life expectancy, although it should result in quality of life gains. However, the episodic nature of migraine (on average 12 attacks a year each with a duration of 24 hours which in total is equivalent to less than 5% of a year) poses difficulties for assessing qualitative changes. In particular, can the improvements seen with current treatments and the way they have conventionally been gauged be meaningfully mapped on to the zero to one quality scale employed in cost-utility analysis? In other words, utility measures may be relatively insensitive to important improvements in health status for migraine sufferers.

Cost-benefit analysis

The final approach to economic evaluation identified in Fig. 39.1 is cost-benefit analysis. The technique seeks comprehensively to measure the costs and benefits associated with the use of a particular intervention in monetary terms. Cost-benefit analysis makes it possible to determine whether a particular intervention offers a net gain as well as how that gain compares with those achieved with other interventions (within and across disease areas). Selecting those interventions offering the greatest net gains will improve the efficiency of health-care resource utilization.

A major advantage of cost-benefit analysis compared to cost-effectiveness analysis is that it enables account to be taken of all the different outcomes that may be linked to the use of a particular treatment. Thus, gains accruing to patients in terms of, say, reduced pain or enhanced functioning in undertaking daily activities can be aggregated with those realized by society through reduced absenteeism from work. Both of these components would be relevant in the case of migraine. However, the use of the technique both in this specific disorder and more generally in health technology appraisal is severely constrained by the practical measurement difficulties of valuing such benefits in monetary terms. For this reason, the use of cost-benefit analysis in health care has been limited.

Conclusion

The economic benefits of pharmacotherapy are potentially wide-ranging and may be quantified from a number of different perspectives—those of the health-care system, the patient, and society as a whole. Such information may be gathered in formal controlled and blinded clinical trials or in observational or naturalistic studies undertaken in day-to-day medical practice and provide data that usefully build upon the conventional clinical markers of efficiency and effectiveness. However, as this chapter has made clear, benefit data must be combined with corresponding data on costs if information is to be provided that can help guide the efficient allocation of scarce health-care resources.

Several techniques of economic evaluation are available for bringing costs and outcomes together in this way. Whilst each method adopts common costing procedures, there are important differences in their approach to outcomes. In rather oversimplified terms, cost-minimization and cost-effectiveness analyses are used to assess the relative value for money of interventions with directly comparable outcomes (thus addressing *productive efficiency* or the maximization of health outcome for a given cost). Cost-utility and cost-benefit analyses facilitate broader comparisons of interventions with diverse outcomes (thereby addressing both productive efficiency and *allocative efficiency* or the distribution of resources across a mixture of health-care programmes in a way that maximizes the health benefit to society).

The conclusion of this chapter is that, whilst the latter two approaches constitute the theoretically correct routes to deriving an efficient use of resources, practical considerations suggest that, in the immediate future at least, cost-effectiveness analysis offers the most useful framework for assessing the value for money of competing migraine treatments, although further work is required to derive an appropriate and universally accepted measure of outcome.

References

1. Lofland JH, Johnson NE, Batenhorst AS, Nash DB. Changes in resource use and outcomes for patients treated with sumatriptan. *Arch Intern Med* 1999; **159**: 857–63.
2. Wells NEJ, Steiner TJ. Effectiveness of eletriptan in reducing the time loss caused by migraine attacks. *PharmacoEconomics* 2000; **18**: 557–66.
3. (UK) National Institute for Clinical Excellence. *Guide to the technology appraisal process*, 2001. www.nice.org.uk
4. Drummond MF, O'Brien B, Stoddart GL, Torrance W. *Methods for the economic evaluation of health care programmes*, 2nd edn. Oxford: Oxford University Press, 1997: 10.
5. Byford S, Torgerson DJ, Raftery J. Cost of illness studies. *Br Med J* 2000; **320**: 1335.
6. Rice DP. *Estimating the cost of illness*, PHS Publ. No. 947–6, Health economics series. Washington DC: US Government Printing Office, 1966.
7. Ferrari MD. The economic burden of migraine to society. *PharmacoEconomics* 1998; **13**: 667–76.
8. Shiell A, Gerard K, Donaldson C. Cost of illness studies: an aid to decision making? *Hlth Policy* 1987; **8**: 317–23.
9. Koopmanschap MA. Cost of illness studies—useful for health policy? *PharmacoEconomics* 1998; **14**: 143–8.
10. Drummond MF. Cost of illness studies: a major headache? *PharmacoEconomics* 1992; **2**: 1–4.
11. Tfelt-Hansen P, De Vries P, Saxena PR. Triptans in migraine. A comparative review of pharmacology, pharmacokinetics and efficacy. *Drugs* 2000; **90**: 1259–87.
12. Ferrari MD, Roon KI, Lipton RB, Goadsby PJ. Oral triptans (serotonin 5-HT$_{1B/1D}$ agonists) in acute migraine treatment: a meta-analysis of 53 trials. *Lancet* 2001; **358**: 1668–75.
13. Donaldson C. The (near) equivalence of cost-effectiveness and cost-benefit analyses. Fact or fallacy? In *Economic evaluation in healthcare* (ed. Mallarkey G). New Zealand: Adis International, 1999: 33–40.
14. Palmer S, Byford S, Raftery J. Types of economic evaluation. *Br Med J* 1999; **318**: 1349.

40
The economic cost and benefit of pharmacotherapy for headache

Michael T. Halpern

Introduction

Pharmacoeconomics is the field of evaluating the costs and benefits of health-care treatments, primarily treatment with medications. The basic goal of pharmaco-economics is to assess 'value for money', the benefits of a treatment relative to its costs. Pharmacoeconomics often involves assessment of a new therapy compared to the usual care or an older, standard therapy. These assessments can compare costs only or evaluate difference in costs relative to difference in outcomes (for example, cost-effectiveness analysis). Pharmacoeconomics is *part* of the decision-making process in the choice of therapy, not the single deciding factor. The decision as to whether a medication's benefits are 'worth' the cost varies among patient groups and societies.

Headache comprises a diverse range of conditions with differing effects and impacts. However, as discussed by Steiner,[1] '...the elements of burden are similar for all common headaches.' Among published studies evaluating the costs and benefits of pharmacotherapy for headache, almost all have focused on treatment for migraines; there are few (if any) published studies evaluating the pharmacoeconomics of other headache types. While migraines have certain differences from other head-ache disorders, these studies can be used as models for assessing the economics of pharmacotherapy for headaches in general.

Over the past several years, there has been a growing awareness of the importance of cost of care and cost-effectiveness in making treatment choices. This has included a focus on the overall economic impact of therapy, not just medication costs. This is especially important in migraine therapy, as the cost for drugs may vary substan-tially. Table 40.1 presents the average wholesale price (AWP) in US dollars per dose for a number of prescription and nonprescription migraine products (the price for products marked with an asterix were determined by an informal drug store survey). The price per dose of migraine medications varies by more than 100-fold. However,

Table 40.1   Average wholesale price (AWP, $US, 2000) per dose for migraine medications

Non-prescription medications
Excedrin Migraine*: $0.18 per 2 caps
Advil Migraine*: $0.30 per 2 caps
Motrin Migraine Pain: $0.16 per 2 caps
Prescription medications
APAP/dichloralphenazone/isometheptene: $0.34 to $0.98 per 2 caps
Caffeine/ergotamine: $1.45 to $1.84 per 2 tabs; $5.68 per suppository
Methysergide maleate: $4.91 per 4 mg
Dihydroergotamine: Injectable, $30.72 per 2 mg; Nasal spray, $39.34 per 2 mg (4 sprays)
Sumatriptan: oral, $16.01 per 50 mg; Injectable, $51.04 per 6 mg; Nasal spray, $21.85 per spray
Naratriptan: $17.58 per 2.5 mg
Rizatriptan: $14.86 per 10 mg
Zolmatriptan: $14.74 per 2.5 mg

*Prices for these medications are based on an information survey of drug stores.

pharmacoeconomic assessments cannot evaluate only the medication price; the overall cost of therapy (including other types of health-care resource utilization), indirect costs, and treatment outcomes must also be included in these assessments.

It is clear that patients are willing to pay substantial amounts for effective, fast-acting migraine therapy. In a study presented by Lenert and Minh,[2] the willingness to pay (WTP) for migraine medications was determined using an internet survey. The median WTP was 4.1% of monthly income, corresponding to US $130. However, this WTP was reduced for less than optimal medications. For example, the median WTP was $75 per month if the medication has a 50% chance of causing rebound headache; $50 per month if it has a 2-hour delay in effect; and $15 per month if it doesn't relieve nausea. Thus, while patients value effective migraine therapy, this valuation is highly dependent on the effectiveness and side-effects of the treatment.

Migraine prophylactic therapy

Migraine treatment can be classified as prophylactic (to prevent migraine attacks) or acute (to treat attacks once they occur). Prophylactic therapy is uncommon; the proportion of migraine patients receiving prophylactic medications has been reported as 13–20%.[3,4] At present, there are apparently no published complete pharmacoeconomic evaluations of migraine prophylactic therapy.

Adelman *et al.*[5] compared prophylactic and acute migraine drug prices. The basis of this comparison is 'cost-equivalent number' (CEN), the number of headaches per month for which the cost of prophylactic medication equals the cost saved from acute therapy medication avoided. The CEN is the 'break-even point' for the cost of prophylactic therapy based on migraine frequency: at migraine frequencies higher than the CEN, the cost of prophylactic medication is less than the cost of acute medications avoided, resulting in net savings in medication costs.

Adelman *et al.*[5] present CEN values for a hypothetical migraine treatment costing US $14 per dose. The CEN in this scenario ranges from 0.9 for amitriptyline (indicating that the cost of amitriptyline as a prophylactic medication would equal the cost saved from acute medication avoided if a patient experienced 0.9 attacks per month) to 25.8 for fluoxetine (indicating that fluoxetine costs break even with acute treatment costs avoided only for patients with almost daily migraines). The highest CEN value presented by Adelman *et al.* is for nimodipine, which is 95.1. All of these calculations assume that only one dose of the hypothetical acute treatment medication would be required to treat a migraine attack; if more doses are required, CEN values would be lower.

While the CEN is a useful measure for evaluating prophylactic medication costs, it is limited. This form of analysis does not take into account other medical care costs that may be avoided by prophylactic treatment (for example, physician's visits, diagnostic tests, etc.), indirect costs saved from avoiding migraine attacks, or differences in patient outcomes and patient preference. More complete pharmacoeconomic evaluations of migraine therapy are needed.

Acute migraine therapy

Published pharmacoeconomic studies involving acute migraine therapy may present information on direct costs, indirect costs, or total costs. Direct costs are primarily health-care costs, including medication, physician visits, emergency department visits, tests/procedures, and hospitalizations. Indirect costs are mainly costs associated with lost time due to migraines, including workplace absenteeism and decreased productivity while at work (also called presenteeism) as well as time away from usual non-work activities. Total costs are the sum of direct and indirect costs. Direct costs for migraine patients are lower than might be expected for a chronic and often debilitating disease. This, in part, reflects the low frequency of medical care received by many patients. Many migraineurs have not been accurately diagnosed by a physician. According to the American Migraine Study II,[6] only 48% of migraine patients have received such a diagnosis. Further, migraine patients do not routinely consult their physicians regarding their migraines. Also, most migraine patients receive only non-prescription medications.[6] Thus, the indirect economic burden of migraine tends to be substantially greater than the direct costs.

Almost all published evaluations of the costs (or costs and benefits) of acute migraine therapy have focused on the use of triptans. One exception is the study by Turkewitz *et al.*[7] assessing the impact of self-injected ketorolac on decreasing the number of emergency department visits. Among the published pharmacoeconomic studies, a majority has evaluated sumatriptan therapy. Sumatriptan was the first triptan introduced and is the most widely used product in this class.

Sumatriptan is available in oral, parenteral (subcutaneous), nasal, and suppository forms. Multiple economic studies have been published for subcutaneous and oral sumatriptan therapy. These are primarily open-label studies or models; a small number of these pharmacoeconomic analyses are based on randomized controlled trials (RCTs) or retrospective studies. These studies generally compare sumatriptan treatment to usual or customary therapy. Usual therapy is a diverse collection of prescription and non-prescription medications, representing the range of medication patients received prior to initiation of sumatriptan therapy. This results in limitations in being able to directly compare specific medications to sumatriptan. However, usual therapy is the most realistic comparison group, encompassing the medications commonly (and sometimes uncommonly) used by migraineurs.

Table 40.2 presents a summary of economic studies involving subcutaneous sumatriptan, while Table 40.3 provides similar information for oral sumatriptan. A number of general conclusions can be drawn from these studies. In general, all of

Table 40.2 Pharmacoeconomic studies of subcutaneous sumatriptan

Ref.	Comparator	Method*	Impact of treatment
8	Placebo	RCT	Decreased productivity loss, faster return to normal work performance, decreased use of rescue medication
9	Usual therapy	Markov model	Increased drug costs, decreased productivity loss, increased total costs
10	Usual therapy	Open label study	Decreased medical care visits
11	Usual therapy	Medical record review	Increased pharmacy utilization, decreased other medical resource utilization (including decreased telephone calls), decreased productivity loss, increased quality of life, increased satisfaction
12	Usual therapy	Open label study	Decreased productivity loss, decreased time away from normal activities
13	Usual therapy	Open, parallel-group study	Increased medical care costs, decreased indirect costs, increased total costs, decreased use of medications to treat adverse events, decreased productivity loss, decreased time away from usual activities, cost effectiveness of 132 Belgian Francs (direct only) or 53 Belgian Francs (total cost) per hour of relieved pain
14	Usual therapy	Open label study	Decreased productivity loss, decreased time away from normal activities
15	Subcutaneous dihydroergotamine mesylate	Decision analytic model	Incremental cost-effectiveness of $US4000 to $US6700 per year (1993 dollars) per additional successfully treated patient, depending on outcome measure
16	Placebo	RCT	Decreased productivity loss, decreased time to return to work

*RCT, Randomized controlled trial.

Table 40.3   Pharmacoeconomic studies of oral sumatriptan

Ref.	Comparator	Method	Impact of treatment
9	Usual therapy	Markov model	Increased drug costs, decreased productivity loss, net savings or offsets depending on formulation
17	Usual therapy	Prospective, observational study	Decreased absenteeism and productivity loss, decreased time away from normal activities, no change in resource utilization, improved quality of life and patient satisfaction
18	Usual therapy	Decision analytic model	Decreased costs
19	Oral sumatriptan— moderate/severe	Retrospective analysis	Decreased sumatriptan doses, decreased medication treatment costs
20	Oral caffeine/ ergotamine	Decision analytic model	Increased direct costs, decreased indirect costs, decreased total costs, cost-effectiveness of Can $98 per attack aborted, cost-utility of Can $29 366 per QALY
21	Usual therapy	Telephone survey/ retrospective study	Decreased absenteeism, decreased resource utilization, increased quality of life
22	Usual therapy	Open label study	Decreased absenteeism and productivity loss, net overall cost savings
23	Usual therapy	Telephone survey	Increased drug expenditures, decreased overall health-care utilization rates/costs, fewer migraine medications, decreased disability days
24	Usual therapy	Open label study	Decreased labour costs (based on absenteeism and productivity), benefit:cost ratio of 10:1 for labour:drug costs
25	Usual therapy	Open label study	Decreased medical care visits, decreased health-care costs
26	Usual therapy	Prospective, observational study	Decreased medical resource utilization, decreased productivity loss, decreased time away from usual activities, increased quality of life, increased satisfaction
27	Usual therapy	Clinical study	Decreased productivity loss, decreased time away from normal activities

these studies indicate increased medication costs after initiating sumatriptan therapy. Given the range of medication prices presented in Table 40.1, it is not surprising that sumatriptan costs more than usual therapy. However, patients receiving sumatriptan therapy generally have decreases in other direct medical care costs, such physician visits. Total health-care costs are often similar before and after initiation of sumatriptan therapy, with increased medication costs being offset (or partially offset) by decreases in other types of health-care resource utilization.

Table 40.4 Pharmacoeconomic studies of other triptan therapies

Ref.	Treatment	Comparator	Method*	Impact of treatment
28	Naratriptan	Usual therapy	Markov model	Increased medical care costs, decreased productivity loss, overall cost savings
29	Rizatriptan	Placebo	RCT	Decreased absenteeism and productivity loss
30	Rizatriptan	Placebo	RCT	Decreased productivity loss
31	Eletriptan	Placebo	RCT	Decreased time away from usual activities

*RCT, Randomized controlled trial.

Sumatriptan therapy generally results in decreased indirect costs, primarily assessed as decreased absenteeism and decreased productivity loss. Total costs (direct plus indirect costs) are also generally decreased following initiation of sumatriptan therapy.

Cost-effectiveness analysis (CEA) is a useful measure for assessing the incremental costs and benefits of a newer therapy relative to usual care or a specific comparator therapy. However, few of the sumatriptan economic studies have performed CEA. Further, those that included CEA have used a range of effectiveness outcome measures. These analyses include the cost per hour of relieved pain,[13] the cost per additional successfully treated patient,[15] and the cost per quality-adjusted life year (QALY).[20] The different effectiveness outcomes used for these analyses, and the lack of CEA for sumatriptan therapy in general, lead to difficulties in comparing results across migraine studies as well as with studies in other disease areas.

Beyond sumatriptan, there have been few published economic studies of other triptans. The identified published studies are presented in Table 40.4. One study of naratriptan by Caro *et al.*[28] used a model to evaluate direct and indirect costs compared to those associated with the usual therapy. The other published studies, for rizatriptan and eletriptan, were economic analyses based on RCTs with placebo comparisons. These studies evaluated only indirect costs.

Use of models in pharmacoeconomics

Many studies assessing the costs and outcomes of migraine therapy are based on models. In pharmacoeconomic analyses, models are required to address differences in objectives between clinical trials and pharmacoeconomic studies. In RCTs, the objective is to evaluate how safe and efficacious a medication is when used as prescribed. In contrast, the objective of pharmacoeconomic evaluations is to assess the net total costs and health consequences of the *decision* to use the medication. Further, RCTs often assess narrow endpoints (for example, response rate at 2 hours) and involve comparison to placebo. Pharmacoeconomic analyses focus on broader endpoints (for example, health-care resource utilization or disability) and involve comparison to an accepted therapy of usual care.

Several colleagues and I recently completed a model evaluating the costs and outcomes of early migraine treatment with oral sumatriptan (at onset of headache, when pain is mild) compared to delayed sumatriptan treatment. For delayed treatment, patients in the model waited 2 hours after migraine onset to treat their headaches. By this time, migraine pain might have spontaneously resolved (in which case, no treatment was taken), persisted as mild, or progressed to moderate/severe levels. Probabilities for the models were based on data from two recently published studies[32,33] and analysis of clinical trial diary data.[17] Results indicated that early sumatriptan treatment (either 50 mg or 100 mg) resulted in increased pain-free rates at 2 hours, 4 hours, and sustained (4–24 hours) compared to delayed treatment. Disability time was also reduced for patients with early treatment. The medical care costs for early versus delayed treatment were very similar, while the workplace costs (from absenteeism and decreased productivity) were lower for early treatment patients compared to those for delayed treatment patients. Consequently, the total cost (direct plus indirect) for early treatment was substantially lower than that for delayed treatment. These results suggest that, in certain migraine patient populations, early sumatriptan treatment may be an appropriate intervention to improve patient outcomes and decrease costs.

Assessment of workplace productivity loss

As discussed above, indirect costs (primarily workplace-related costs, absenteeism and productivity loss) are generally much greater than medical care costs for migraine patients. Most pharmacoeconomic studies have indicated that the use of migraine medications reduces workplace costs. The magnitude of the change in workplace costs following initiation of triptan therapy varies among published studies. Table 40.5 summarizes findings from these studies. Results are presented in terms of the impact of migraine therapy on productivity loss (time worked with migraine symptoms multiplied by the decreased efficiency at work) and on absenteeism. For these calculations, I assumed an average migraine frequency of 7.3 attacks per 3-month period, and 8 hours per workday. When productivity loss was not weighted by decreased work efficiency (that is, when only time worked with migraine was presented), I multiplied the time worked by the decreased efficiency if decreased efficiency data were presented.

The mean impact of triptan therapy on productivity loss time in the reviewed studies was 1.02 hours per attack, with a range of 0.08 to 3.0 hours per attack. Simi-larly, the mean impact of triptan therapy on absenteeism time in the reviewed studies was 0.80 hours per attack, with a range of 0.2 to 2.2 hours per attack. Converting these values to annual impacts based on the assumptions stated above, triptan therapy is projected to save an average of 3.7 days of productivity loss time and 2.9 days of absenteeism per year. One study[17] in Table 40.5 included values for improvement with sumatriptan therapy that were lower than those for any other study included in this table, particularly the productivity impact. The participants for this study were nurses and these results may reflect better migraine coping skills and/or reluctance to indicate that their workplace activities, predominantly patient

Table 40.5 Studies evaluating the impact of triptan therapy on workplace productivity and absenteeism

Ref.	Treatment	Comparator	Productivity impact (hours per attack)	Absenteeism (hours per attack)
8	Subcutaneous sumatriptan	Placebo	0.9	0.6
11	Subcutaneous sumatriptan	Usual therapy	3.0	2.2
12	Subcutaneous sumatriptan	Usual therapy	0.5	
13	Subcutaneous sumatriptan	Usual therapy	0.6	
14	Subcutaneous sumatriptan	Usual therapy	0.8	
16	Subcutaneous sumatriptan	Placebo	0.6	
17	Oral sumatriptan	Usual therapy	0.08	0.2
22	Oral sumatriptan	Usual therapy	0.9	0.3
26	Sumatriptan	Usual therapy	2.6	0.8
27	Sumatriptan	Usual therapy	0.8	
29	Rizatriptan	Placebo	0.4	0.7

	Productivity impact		Absenteeism	
	Mean	Range	Mean	Range
Impact per migraine attack (hours)	1.02	0.08–3.0	0.80	0.2–2.2
Impact per year (days)	3.7	0.3–11.0	2.9	0.7–8.0

care, were substantially compromised by migraine. If this study[17] were not included, the projected annual savings due to triptan therapy would be 4.1 days of productivity loss and 3.4 days of absenteeism.

The studies included in Table 40.5 represent a range of designs, settings, and comparator treatments, and are thus not truly comparable; determining a numerical average across these studies is not completely appropriate. Nonetheless, the values presented here provide a general overview regarding the impact of migraine therapy on the main determinant of indirect cost.

There are a number of problems associated with productivity assessment in most studies of migraine therapy. In general, the impact of migraine on workplace productivity is based on self-report, with migraineurs asked to state the amount of time they worked with a migraine and their average efficiency at work during this period. Questionnaires collecting these data have generally not been validated against most robust measures of productivity assessment, such as objective productivity measures or daily or hourly disability scores. In addition, productivity loss time and absenteeism are combined in a single value in a number of publications, preventing separate assessments of the different components of indirect cost. In some studies, productivity loss time is not weighted by decreased work effectiveness, thereby implying that no productive work occurred while the patient was experiencing migraine symptoms and equating time worked with migraine to time missed work due to migraine.

To make the impact of migraines on workplace productivity credible to employers, it is crucial to use robust measures of productivity loss. My colleagues and I recently published a study[34] assessing the impact of smoking status on workplace productivity. For this study, we selected a workplace population with multiple objective productivity measures, reservation agents at a major US-based airline. Data routinely collected on these reservation agents included telephone calls per minute, flights segments booked per minute, revenue (dollars) per minute hour, and unproductive time (time not available to answer the phone without a valid excuse). Most objective measures indicated higher productivity for former as compared to current smokers.

As part of this study[34] we also developed a new productivity instrument, the Health and Work Questions (HWQ), that was partially validated in comparison to the objective productivity measures. The HWQ consists of 24 questions in six subscales: productivity; impatience and irritability; concentration and focus; work satisfaction; satisfaction with supervisor; and personal life satisfaction. All questions consisted of 10-point likert scales. For the productivity subscale, respondents were asked to rate their work efficiency, quality, and amount of work from their supervisor's and their co-worker's perspective, as well as from their own perspective. That is, in addition to asking respondents to indicate directly their efficiency, quality, and amount of work, they were also asked to indicate how their co-workers and their supervisor would rate their work in these three categories. All responses were self-reported, but these additional questions asked respondents to provide self-report from a third-person perspective. The HWQ is available online at http://tc.bmjjournals.com/cgi/content/full/10/3/233/DC1. Copyright of the HWQ is owned by the GlaxoSmithKline Group of Companies ([©]2000).

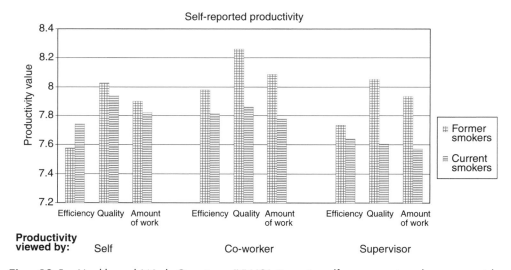

Fig. 40.1   Health and Work Questions (HWQ) items in self-assessment and assessment by others: productivity subscales by smoking status. (Reproduced from ref. 34 with permission from the BMJ Publishing Group.)

Mean results for current and former smokers from the productivity subscale questions are presented in Fig. 40.1. When asked to directly rate their workplace productivity, current and former smokers provided similar values. However, when asked to indicate how they believed their co-workers or supervisor would rate their productivity, former smokers provided substantially higher ratings than did current smokers. While the impact of smoking status on workplace productivity is likely to be quite different than the impact of migraine and migraine therapy, these results suggest that self-assessment of workplace productivity is not always straightforward. Simply asking migraineurs to self-report their time worked with migraine and work efficiency during this time is unlikely to provide credible results. More robust measures, including instruments validated in comparison to objective productivity measures or disability levels assessed at frequent time points, will be needed to convincingly demonstrate the impacts of migraine therapy on these important cost components.

Conclusions

Based on this summary of the literature evaluating the economics of migraine therapy, a number of conclusions can be drawn and suggestions for future work can be made.

(1) There are essentially no published economic studies of pharmacotherapy for headaches other than migraines. As preliminary work on the cost of illness for other headache types has indicated substantial burdens, economic studies on therapy for these other types of headache are needed. This will also provide information on how well the economic impacts of migraine therapy can serve as a model for the pharmacoeconomics of other headache types.

(2) The published economic literature on migraine treatment focuses almost exclusively on acute (abortive) migraine therapy. While prophylactic migraine therapy is not common, studies are needed to evaluate the economic impact of prophylactic therapy. Results from such studies could stimulate use of prophylactic therapy when appropriate.

(3) Most published studies of migraine therapy indicate similar or slightly increased medical care costs with newer medications, but decreased indirect costs. As indirect costs comprise the majority of the economic burden of migraine, assessment of the impact of migraine therapy on workplace productivity should be more robust and involve validated instruments.

(4) When a new therapy results in increased costs but improved outcomes, cost-effectiveness analysis should be performed to assess the treatment costs relative to the benefits in comparison to an older therapy or usual care. One or more standard effectiveness outcome measures should be used to permit comparisons among headache studies as well as across different disease conditions.

The literature evaluating the economic costs and benefits of migraine therapy has increased tremendously over the past few years. It is likely that the literature will continue to expand, both in terms of the types of headaches and treatments covered as well as in the quality and robustness of the study methodologies used.

References

1. Steiner TJ. Headache burdens and bearers. *Funct Neurol* 2000; **15** (Suppl. 3): 219–23.
2. Lenert L, Minh C. An internet study of patients' willingness to pay for migraine headache pharmacotherapies. *Value Hlth* 2001; **4**: 153.
3. Warshaw LJ, Burton WN. Cutting the cost of migraine: Role for the employee health unit. *J Occup Environ Med* 1998; **40**: 943–53.
4. Von Korff M, Black LK, Saunders K, Galer BS. Headache medication-use among primary care headache patients in a health maintenance organization. *Cephalalgia* 1999; **19**: 75–80.
5. Adelman JU, Brod A, Von Seggern RL, Mannix LK, Rapoport AM. Migraine preventive medications: a reappraisal. *Cephalalgia* 1998; **18**: 605–11.
6. Lipton RB, Diamond S, Reed M, Diamond ML, Stewart WF. Migraine diagnosis and treatment: results from the American Migraine Study II. *Headache* 2001; **41**: 638–45.
7. Turkewitz LJ, Casaly JS, Dawson GA, Wirth O, Hurst RJ, Gillette PL. Self-administration of parenteral ketorolac tromethamine for head pain. *Headache* 1992; **32**: 452–4.
8. Cady RC, Ryan R, Jhingran P, O'Quinn S, Pait DG. Sumatriptan injection reduces productivity loss during a migraine attack: results of a double-blind, placebo-controlled trial. *Arch Intern Med* 1998; **58**: 1013–18.
9. Caro G, Getsios D, Caro JJ, Raggio G, Burrows M, Black L. Sumatriptan: economic evidence for its use in the treatment of migraine, the Canadian comparative economic analysis. *Cephalalgia* 2001; **21**: 12–19.
10. Cohen JA, Beall DG, Miller DW, Beck A, Pait G, Clements BD. Subcutaneous sumatriptan for the treatment of migraine: humanistic, economic, and clinical consequences. *Fam Med* 1996; **28**: 171–7.
11. Cohen JA, Beall D, Beck A, *et al*. Sumatriptan treatment for migraine in a health maintenance organization: economic, humanistic, and clinical outcomes. *Clin Ther* 1999; **21**: 190–204.
12. Cortelli P, Dahlof C, Bouchard J, *et al*. A multinational investigation of the impact of subcutaneous sumatriptan. III: Workplace productivity and non-workplace activity. *PharmacoEconomics* 1997; **11** (Suppl. 1): 35–42.
13. Laloux P, Vakaet A, Monseu G, Jacquy J, Bourgeois P, van der Linden C. Subcutaneous sumatriptan compared with usual acute treatments for migraine: clinical and pharmaco-economic evaluation. *Acta Neurol Belg* 1998; **98**: 332–41.
14. Mushet GR, Miller D, Clements B, Pait G, Gutterman DL. Impact of sumatriptan on workplace productivity, nonwork activities, and health-related quality of life among hospital employees with migraine. *Headache* 1996; **36**: 137–43.
15. Payne K, Kozma CM, Lawrence BJ. Comparing dihydroergotamine mesylate and sumatriptan in the management of acute migraine. A retrospective cost-efficacy analysis. *PharmacoEconomics* 1996; **10**: 59–71.
16. Schulman EA, Cady RK, Henry D, *et al*. Effectiveness of sumatriptan in reducing productivity loss due to migraine: results of a randomized, double-blind, placebo-controlled clinical trial. *Mayo Clin Proc* 2000; **75**: 782–9.
17. Adelman JU, Sharfman M, Johnson R, *et al*. Impact of oral sumatriptan on workplace productivity, health-related quality of life, healthcare use, and patient satisfaction with medication in nurses with migraine. *Am J Man Care* 1996; **2**: 1407–16.

18. Biddle AK, Shih YC, Kwong WJ. Cost-benefit analysis of sumatriptan tablets versus usual therapy for treatment of migraine. *Pharmacotherapy* 2000; **20**: 1356–64.
19. Cady RK, Sheftell F, Lipton RB, Kwong WJ, O'Quinn S. Economic implications of early treatment of migraine with sumatriptan tables. *Clin Ther* 2001; **23**: 284–91.
20. Evans KW, Boan JA, Evans JL, Shuaib A. Economic evaluation of oral sumatriptan compared with oral caffeine/ergotamine for migraine. *PharmacoEconomics* 1997; **12**: 565–77.
21. Greiner DL, Addy SN. Sumatriptan use in a large group-model health maintenance organization. *Am J Hlth Syst Pharm* 1996; **53**: 633–8.
22. Gross MLP, Dowson AJ, Deavy L, Duthie T. Impact of oral sumatriptan 50 mg on work productivity and quality of life in migraineurs. *Br J Med Econom* 1996; **10**: 231–46.
23. Legg RF, Sclar DA, Nemec NL, Tarnai J, Mackowiak JI. Cost-effectiveness of sumatriptan in a managed care population. *Am J Man Care* 1997; **3**: 117–22.
24. Legg RF, Sclar DA, Nemec NL, Tarnai J, Mackowiak JI. Cost benefit of sumatriptan to an employer. *J Occup Environ Med* 1997; **39**: 652–7.
25. Litaker DG, Solomon GD, Genzen JR. Impact of sumatriptan on clinic utilization and costs of care in migraineurs. *Headache* 1996; **36**: 538–41.
26. Lofland JH, Johnson NE, Batenhorst AS, Nash DB. Changes in resource use and outcomes for patients with migraine treated with sumatriptan: a managed care perspective. *Arch Intern Med* 1999; **159**: 857–63.
27. Miller DW, Martin BC, Loo CM. Sumatriptan and lost productivity time: a time series analysis of diary data. *Clin Ther* 1996; **18**: 1263–75.
28. Caro JJ, Getsios D, Raggio G, Caro G, Black L. Treatment of migraine in Canada with naratriptan: a cost-effectiveness analysis. *Headache* 2001; **41**: 456–64.
29. Dasbach EJ, Carides GW, Gerth WC, Santanello NC, Pigeon JG, Kramer MS. Work and productivity loss in the rizatriptan multiple attack study. *Cephalalgia* 2000; **20**: 830–4.
30. Solomon GD, Santanello N. Impact of migraine and migraine therapy on productivity and quality of life. *Neurology* 2000; **55**: S29–35.
31. Wells NE, Steiner TJ. Effectiveness of eletriptan in reducing time loss caused by migraine attacks. *PharmacoEconomics* 2000; **18**: 557–66.
32. Cady RK, Sheftell F, Lipton RB, *et al*. Effect of early intervention with sumatriptan on migraine pain: retrospective analyses of data from three clinical trials. *Clin Ther* 2000; **22**: 1035–48.
33. Cady RK, Lipton RB, Hall C, Stewart WF, O'Quinn S, Gutterman D. Treatment of mild headache in disabled migraine sufferers: results of the Spectrum Study. *Headache* 2000; **40**: 792–7.
34. Halpern MT, Shikiar R, Rentz AM, Khan ZM. The impact of smoking status on workplace absenteeism and productivity. *Tobacco Control* 2001; **10**: 233–8.

41

A stratified approach to migraine management including zolmitriptan is clinically and economically superior to step care approaches: results from the Disability in Strategies of Care (DISC) study

B. Charlesworth, Richard B. Lipton, and Walter F. Stewart

Introduction

Acute treatment of migraine has traditionally followed a step care approach, whereby patients progress through a sequence of medications, ordered by a combination of perceived efficacy, safety, and cost, until pain relief is achieved.[1] This 'stepping up' may occur *across* a series of migraine attacks or *within* an individual attack. Either way, step care typically does not immediately address the full impact of migraine on the individual and can, therefore, leave patients inadequately treated. An alternative to step care is stratified care[1] where treatment choice is guided by disease severity from the outset. Patients with significant disability or need are given first-line therapy with a migraine-specific treatment, such as a triptan. Data from the Disability in Strategies of Care (DISC) study[2]—the first randomized trial in migraine specifically to compare stratified care with both step care approaches—are reviewed herein. A series of economic evaluations comparing stratified care with step care is also examined.[3,4]

Review of DISC

The DISC study was a controlled, open-label, randomized, parallel-group clinical trial involving 88 centres in 13 countries.[2] Of the 1109 migraine patients screened, 1062 were found to be suitable for trial entry. A total of 835 patients were analysed as the efficacy population. The Migraine Disability Assessment (MIDAS) questionnaire,[5-7] which assesses headache-related disability, was used to assign a disability grade to each patient. Patients with MIDAS grade II (mild disability) or grades III/IV (moderate to severe disability) were equally randomized to 1 of 3 treatment strategies (stratified, step care *across*, or step care *within*) for a series of 6 migraine attacks. An aspirin (800–1000 mg) plus metoclopramide (10 mg) combination (A + M) was used as nonmigraine-specific therapy, while oral zolmitriptan (2.5 mg; ZOMIG®) was used as migraine-specific therapy. In the stratified care group, MIDAS grade II patients received A + M and MIDAS grade III/IV patients received zolmitriptan for all six attacks. Patients whose treatment was stepped *across* attacks received A + M initially, but escalated to zolmitriptan for attacks 4–6 if treatment failed over attacks 1–3, that is, if insufficient headache response with A + M at 2 hours was experienced in 2 or more of the first 3 treated attacks. Similarly, patients whose treatment was stepped *within* attacks received A + M initially, but escalated to zolmitriptan if insufficient headache response was experienced 2 hours posttreatment. Primary endpoints included: (1) headache response at 2 hours (defined as an improvement from severe or moderate pain at baseline to mild or no pain at 2 hours); and (2) disability time per treated attack for the first 4 hours posttreatment (represented by the average area under the disability versus time curve; AUC). Disability was assessed using a visual analogue (0–100 mm) scale at 0, 1, 2, and 4 hours, and was measured in mm h (arbitrary units of disability time). Secondary endpoints included pain-free response at 2 hours and headache response at 1 and 4 hours.

Stratified care versus step care *across* attacks

Headache response (over all six attacks) was significantly better in the stratified care group compared with those receiving step care *across* attacks ($p < 0.001$ at 1, 2, and 4 hours; Fig. 41.1). The advantage of stratified care over step care *across* attacks was most evident within the first three attacks ($p < 0.001$). For attacks 4–6, the difference in headache response was not significant because in the step care group, patients inadequately managed over attacks 1–3 with A + M escalated to zolmitriptan 2.5 mg for attacks 4–6. Patients receiving stratified care reported significantly less disability time $p < 0.001$) over 4 hours compared with those in the step care group (AUC = 185 mm h versus 209.4 mm h). Similar results were reported for the pain-free endpoint—at 2 hours, a significantly greater ($p = 0.003$) proportion of attacks had achieved a pain-free response in the stratified care group compared with the step care *across* attacks group. Furthermore, in the step care group, the need to escalate to zolmitriptan after attacks 1–3 increased with MIDAS grade (56% for patients with MIDAS grade II to 74% for MIDAS grade IV), confirming that disability is a reliable predictor of treatment need.

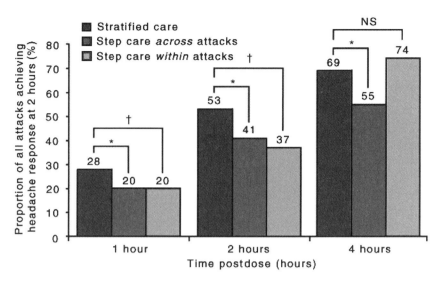

Fig. 41.1 Stratified care versus step care *across* and *within* attacks: headache response at 1, 2, and 4 hours (all attacks). *p<0.001 for stratified care versus step care *across* attacks. †p<0.001 for stratified care versus step care *within* attacks. NS, p=0.211. (Source: ref. 2.)

Stratified care versus step care *within* attacks

In terms of headache response (Fig. 41.1) and pain-free response, differences between the stratified care group and those who received step care *within* attacks diminished after 2 hours, when inadequately managed patients escalated to zolmitriptan. Moreover, significantly less disability (p<0.001) was reported in the stratified care group compared with the step care *within* attacks group (AUC=185 mm h versus 200 m h, respectively).

Economic analysis of stratified care versus step care

To determine the indirect societal costs incurred by using stratified care compared with step care *across* attacks, an economic analysis of the DISC data was undertaken.[3] The analysis considered: impairment of normal activities; lost work time (mean US hourly rate obtained from Bureau of Labor Statistics, USA, 1999); lost earnings plus drug acquisition costs; and total societal costs (including lost leisure time). The stratified care approach resulted in a saving of US $39 (~ UK £28) per patient over six attacks compared with a step care *across* attacks approach.

To compare the direct costs incurred using stratified care compared with step care *across* attacks, a decision analysis model was constructed to simulate a controlled clinical trial based on the design of the DISC study.[4] Migraineurs were randomly assigned to treat their attacks for 1 year with over-the-counter (OTC) analgesics,

Table 41.1 Estimated health service resource use and cost per patient per year (taken with permission from ref. 4)

	Step care *across* attacks	Stratified care	Difference (stratified – step)
Number of primary care consultations	4.90	3.65	–1.25
Cost of primary care consultations (UK £)	£78.44	£58.34	–£20.10
Number of specialist referrals/consultations	0.23	0.02	–0.21
Costs of specialist referrals/consultations (UK £)	£21.32	£1.68	–£19.64
Number of attacks treated with zolmitriptan	9.51	15.26	+5.75
Cost of zolmitriptan (UK £)	£57.06	£91.55	+£34.49
Total health service costs (UK £)	£156.82	£151.57	–£5.24

A + M, or zolmitriptan under a stratified care or step care *across* attacks approach. For the cost analysis, a health service perspective was adopted. Data inputs included: frequency and disability of migraine, derived from population-based studies; response rates specific to each MIDAS grade for each level of treatment, obtained from an international consensus opinion study; UK drug acquisition costs for zolmitriptan; and expected costs of primary and specialist care consultations (costs of OTC analgesics and A + M were considered negligible). Total health-care costs per patient per year, calculated by the economic model, were UK £151.57 for stratified care and £156.82 for step care, a difference of £5.25 (Table 41.1).[4] Health service costs per successfully treated attack were estimated at £12.60 for stratified care, compared with £23.43 for step care *across* attacks.[4]

To determine the cost-effectiveness of stratified care compared with step care (*within* and *across* attacks), an economic evaluation of the total costs associated with the three treatment strategies was undertaken,[8] adopting a societal perspective. The evaluation included acquisition costs for study and escape medications (based on UK 2000 market prices), costs of managing severe or serious adverse events (based on UK 1998–99 costs), and indirect costs due to lost time (either as reduced productivity at work or lost time in normal activities, that is, paid work, unpaid work, and leisure time). Both measures of lost time were valued equally. Reduced productivity at work was measured in lost working equivalents (LWE: lost working time + (working hours × ineffectiveness at work)). Overall mean costs per patient were highest using a step care *across* attacks approach, regardless of the measure of time (LWEs or lost normal activity) valued. When LWEs were valued, stratified care was also less costly than step care *within* attacks, primarily due to the lower mean LWEs per patient over six attacks in the stratified care group (Fig. 41.2). When lost normal activity time was valued, the mean costs of stratified care were marginally higher than those for step care *within* attacks (UK £432 versus £383 per patient over six attacks). However, stratified care is still cost-effective compared with step care *within* attacks, with a 1% increase in response rate to treatment having an incremental cost of only UK £0.34 direct and £2.86 indirect over six attacks.

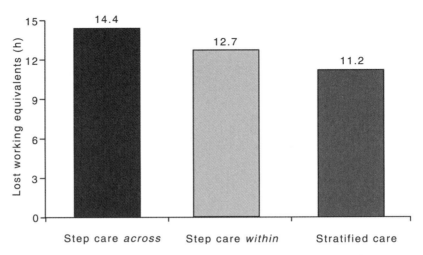

Fig. 41.2   Mean lost working equivalents (hours) per patient over six attacks. (Source: ref. 3).

Conclusions

A controlled, clinical trial using oral zolmitriptan (2.5 mg) as the migraine-specific therapy has shown that stratified care is superior to traditional step care approaches (*across* and *within* attacks), resulting in superior clinical outcomes and superior economic outcomes. In the DISC study, stratified care was clinically superior to both step care strategies in terms of headache response, pain-free response, and disability time. Compared with step care *across* attacks, the indirect societal costs are lower when a stratified approach is adopted. Furthermore, economic modelling suggests that stratified care results in lower direct medical costs compared with step care *across* attacks. When the overall costs of migraine are considered, stratified care is clinically superior and less costly than step care *across* attacks. Stratified care is also more cost-effective than step care *within* attacks, delivering greater clinical benefit per unit of cost. Based on these findings and the wider benefits to patients, physicians, and health-care payers, we recommend that stratified care should become the preferred approach for treating migraine in clinical practice, delivering the right treatment first time.

References

1. Lipton RB. Disability assessment as a basis for stratified care. *Cephalalgia* 1998; **18** (Suppl. 22): 40–6.
2. Lipton RB, Stewart WF, Stone AM, Lainez MJ, Sawyer JP. Stratified care is more effective than step care strategies for migraine: results of the Disability in Strategies of Care (DISC) study. *J Am Med Assoc* 2000; **284**: 2599–605.

3. Tepper SJ, Meddis D. Reducing the costs of impairment of normal activities due to migraine: a stratified-care approach. *Proceedings of the 42nd Annual Meeting of the American Headache Society*, Montreal, 2000: 223.
4. Williams P, Dowson AJ, Rapoport AM, Sawyer J (2001). The cost effectiveness of stratified care in the management of migraine. *PharmacoEconomics* 2001; **19**: 819–29.
5. Stewart WF, Lipton RB, Whyte J, *et al*. An international study to assess the reliability of the Migraine Disability Assessment (MIDAS) score. *Neurology* 1999; **53**: 988–94.
6. Stewart WF, Lipton RB, Kolodner KB, Sawyer J, Lee C, Liberman JM. Validity of the Migraine Disability Assessment (MIDAS) score in comparison to a diary-based measure in a population sample of migraine sufferers. *Pain* 2000; **88**: 41–52.
7. MIDAS Questionnaire. Accessed from: URL: http://www.migraine-disability.net/About_MIDAS/questionnaire5.pdf [accessed 21 November 2001].
8. Sculpher M, Millson D, Meddis D, Poole L. Cost-effectiveness analysis of stratified versus stepped care strategies for acute treatment of migraine: the Disability in Strategies for Care (DISC) study. *PharmacoEconomics* 2002; **20** (2): 91–100.

42

A comparative study of the effectiveness of eletriptan, Cafergot®, and sumatriptan in reducing the time loss associated with migraine attacks

Nicholas E.J. Wells

Introduction

In addition to increasing their understanding of the pathophysiology of migraine, researchers are also learning more about its social and economic impact. Several studies over the last decade have focused on these factors, as well as on the indirect costs attributable to them.[1-3] The overriding conclusion of such studies is that, while health-care utilization costs resulting from migraine are far from negligible, costs linked to reduced productivity are even more substantial. In fact, 75–90% of the total economic cost of migraine has been attributed to lost productivity.[4] A recent study from the USA suggests that these indirect costs—US $13.3 billion—account for an even greater proportion of the direct cost of migraine—US $1.03 billion.[2]

As new medications to treat migraine emerge, so does the potential for reducing the overall financial and social burden of migraine associated with time loss. The study of time loss reported here differs from some others in that it is based upon blinded, randomized, controlled trials, and it observes time lost from both work and non-work activities during a single migraine attack. Eletriptan (40 mg and 80 mg) was compared with Cafergot® (2 mg ergotamine tartrate plus 200 mg caffeine), sumatriptan (50 mg and 100 mg), and placebo. Total time loss and work time loss were determined from patient questionnaires.

Methods

This analysis was based upon two randomized, multicentre, double-blind, placebo-controlled studies, with similar patient populations.[5,6] Subjects were men and women 18 years of age who had a history of migraine and who were expected to suffer, on average, one migraine attack (with or without aura) every 6 weeks. To be eligible, subjects were required to demonstrate an ability to take the study medication as out-patients and to record its effects.

The first study (study A) compared eletriptan 40 mg and eletriptan 80 mg with Cafergot and placebo.[5] A total of 937 patients were randomized to seven treatment sequences. Study B compared eletriptan 40 mg and eletriptan 80 mg with two doses of sumatriptan, 50 mg and 100 mg, and placebo.[6] In this study, 1008 patients were randomized to seven different treatment groups whose members took different combinations of the active medications and placebo. In both studies, patients could take up to two doses of study medication for treating an attack. The time-loss analyses were confined to those study treatment arms in which active drug was available throughout the attack; treatment sequences in which study drug was preceded or followed by placebo were excluded. The first treatment was taken following onset of migraine headache of severe or moderate intensity; the second treatment in the sequence could be taken if symptoms were not alleviated 2 hours after the initial dose, or if the headache recurred within 24 hours of taking the first treatment.

Study endpoints, total time loss and work time loss associated with migraine, were assessed through entries in a headache diary that patients completed 24 hours after the last dose of medication. Grounds for exclusion were inappropriate or missing data, or inconsistent responses to relevant questions. Interpretation of the results was based on the medians and interquartile ranges; the data follow distributions that are non-normal (non-Gaussian), are sometimes highly skewed, and do not allow for means and standard deviation summaries. Statistical comparisons between different treatment groups were undertaken using the Wilcoxon Rank Sum test (two-sided alternative). Because no formal estimation of statistical power was made for the time-loss element of these two studies, a lack of statistical significance in a comparison does not necessarily imply an absence of actual effect.

Results

In study A (eletriptan versus Cafergot), time-loss questionnaires were completed by all 423 subjects, of whom 399 (94%) were evaluable for total time loss. However, only 142 (34%) were evaluable for work time loss, primarily because migraine attacks did not occur during usual work hours. Similarly, in study B (eletriptan versus sumatriptan versus placebo), 597 (98%) of the 611 subjects were evaluable for total time loss, reducing to 204 (33%) for work time loss.

Demographic profiles for both studies were consistent with the gender distribution of migraineurs observed in the general population—predominantly female.[7] In the Cafergot trial, 87% of the patients evaluable for total time loss were female, as were 88% in the sumatriptan study. A similar age distribution across the treatment arms occurred in both studies.

In the Cafergot study, 92% of the patients reported time loss from usual activities because of the migraine attack (Table 42.1), ranging from 88% of subjects in the eletriptan 80 mg treatment arm to 95% of those in the Cafergot study arm. Significantly less total time loss occurred with eletriptan 40 mg or 80 mg than with Cafergot. Median total time loss was 5 hours for eletriptan 40 mg and 4.3 hours for the 80 mg dose, as compared with 7 hours for Cafergot (eletriptan 40 mg versus Cafergot, $p=0.003$; eletriptan 80 mg versus Cafergot, $p<0.001$) (Fig. 42.1).

The second endpoint, work time loss, resulting from either absenteeism or reduced performance at work while experiencing illness, was reported by 98% of the evaluable patients. Patients treated with eletriptan experienced a median of 2 to 3 hours less work time loss than those treated with Cafergot. Statistical analysis indicates that the difference between eletriptan 80 mg and Cafergot was statistically significant ($p=0.022$). In the 40 mg eletriptan study arm, the difference in work time loss, when compared with Cafergot, approached statistical significance ($p=0.065$).

In the sumatriptan study (study B), 91% of the evaluable patients experienced a period of time when the migraine attack interfered with usual activities. Both doses of eletriptan performed significantly better than placebo: 4.0 to 4.3 hours of total time loss versus 8 hours ($p < 0.001$) (Fig. 42.2). For both doses of eletriptan the median total time loss was approximately 1 hour less than that observed for both doses of sumatriptan (5 hours), but this difference did not achieve statistical significance. Similarly, patients who received eletriptan recorded less interruption to their work activities than those who received sumatriptan or placebo, but the differences were not statistically significant. It should be noted that the sample size for these

Table 42.1 Comparison of total time loss and work time loss (hours) between eletriptan and Cafergot (reprint permission obtained from Brookwood Medical Publications)

Treatment group	Number of		Time loss (hours)				
	Evaluable patients	Patients with time loss*	Minimum	q25	Median	q75	Maximum
Total time loss							
Eletriptan 40 mg	106	97	0.0	2.0	5.0	9.0	60.0
Eletriptan 80 mg	104	92	0.0	2.0	4.3	8.0	72.0
Cafergot	189	180	0.0	4.0	7.0	12.0	48.0
Work time loss							
Eletriptan 40 mg	45	45	0.1	2.5	3.1	7.0	24.0
Eletriptan 80 mg	28	27	0.0	2.0	3.9	6.2	8.9
Cafergot	69	67	0.0	3.0	5.9	8.3	16.1

*The number of patients who reported total time loss or work time loss greater than zero.

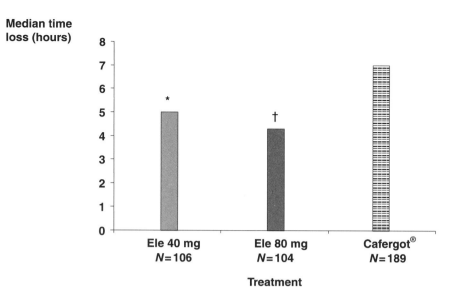

Fig. 42.1 Median total time loss for eletriptan (40 mg and 80 mg) compared with Cafergot®.
*Eletriptan 40 mg versus Cafergot® ($p < 0.003$). †Eletriptan 80 mg versus Cafergot® ($p < 0.001$).

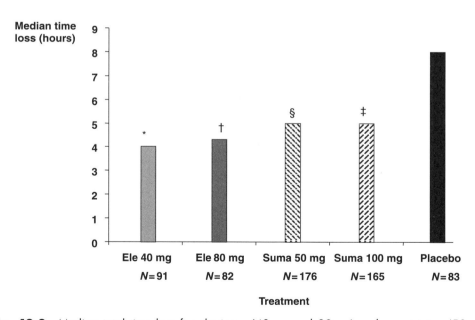

Fig. 42.2 Median total time loss for eletriptan (40 mg and 80 mg) and sumatriptan (50 mg
and 100 mg) compared with placebo. *Eletriptan 40 mg versus placebo ($p < 0.001$). †Eletriptan
80 mg versus placebo ($p < 0.001$). §Sumatriptan 50 mg versus placebo ($p < 0.001$). ‡Sumatriptan
100 mg versus placebo ($p < 0.001$).

two studies was not based on showing statistical differences between treatment for the time loss parameters.

Finally, it is important to note that the time-loss data reported here are consistent with the clinical endpoints observed in the host clinical studies, which reported superior efficacy of eletriptan over Cafergot, sumatriptan, and placebo 2 hours following the initial dose.[5,6] Moreover, time-loss results for the two doses of eletriptan and placebo are highly consistent with a larger study reported elsewhere.[8]

Conclusion

Patients treated with eletriptan had significantly less total time loss than those treated with Cafergot or placebo. Similarly, there was also a trend toward less total time loss for eletriptan patients in comparison with patients treated with either 50 mg or 100 mg doses of sumatriptan. Furthermore, eletriptan 80 mg patients also experienced less work time loss than those treated with Cafergot or sumatriptan, although the differences were statistically significant only versus Cafergot.

The time-loss data from this study correlate with the clinical endpoints observed in clinical studies, where eletriptan's efficacy rate at 2 hours after initial dosing is superior to those of Cafergot, sumatriptan, and placebo.[5,8] From these findings it can be concluded that eletriptan, when taken at the onset of symptoms, reduces the time during which patients suffering from a migraine are unable to participate in their usual activities. This implies benefits for both patient quality of life and workplace productivity.

References

1. Ferrari MD. The economic burden of migraine to society. *PharmacoEconomics* 1998; **13**: 667–76.
2. Hu XH, Markson LE, Lipton RB, Steward WF, Berger ML. Burden of migraine in the United States: disability and economic costs. *Arch Intern Med* 1999; **159** (8): 813–18.
3. Cull RE, Wells NEJ, Miocevich ML. The economic cost of migraine. *Br J Med Econom* 1992; **2**: 103–15.
4. Coukell AJ, Lamb HM. Sumatriptan: a pharmacoeconomic review of its use in migraine. *PharmacoEconomics* 1997; **11**: 473–90.
5. Diener HC, Reches A, Pascual J, Jansen J-P, Pitei D, Steiner TJ. Efficacy, tolerability and safety of oral eletriptan and ergotamine plus caffeine (Cafergot®) in the acute treatment of migraine: a multicentre, randomised, double-blind, placebo-controlled comparison. *Eur Neurol* 2002; **47** (2): 99–107.
6. Pryse-Phillips WEM. Comparison of oral eletriptan (40–80 mg) and oral sumatriptan (50–100 mg) for the treatment of acute migraine: a randomised, placebo-controlled trial in sumatriptan-naive patients. *Cephalalgia* 1999; **19**: 355–6.
7. Breslau N, Rasmussen BK. The impact of migraine: epidemiology, risk factors and co-morbidities. *Neurology* 2001; **56** (Suppl. 1): S4–S12.
8. Wells NEJ, Steiner TJ (2000). Effectiveness of eletriptan in reducing time loss caused by migraine attacks. *PharmacoEconomics* 2000; **18**: 557–66.

43
The socio-economic impact of migraine in Spain

M.J.A. Láinez, M.J. Monzón, and the Spanish Occupational
Migraine Study Group

Introduction

The introduction of International Headache Society (IHS) criteria has made possible epidemiological studies to consolidate the statistics on the prevalence of migraine. However, few studies have been made in the setting of the workplace, even though the prevalence of migraine peaks between the ages of 30 and 45 years, the time of peak activity and productivity in patients' lives.

Migraine is a common condition that negatively impacts on the quality of life of the affected individuals. It also carries a large social and economic burden, particularly in terms of lost work and productivity. The financial burden of migraine comprises direct costs, associated with medical care, and indirect costs, caused by absence from work and reduced productivity. In 1995 we carried out a study to determine the prevalence of migraine in the Spanish work setting, the associated use of health-care services by migraineurs, and the economic impact generated.

Material and methods

Eleven major companies representative of the different production sectors of the country (banking, services, steel industry, manufacturing, communication, etc.) were selected. All possess their own medical services and the study was channelled through the company health-care services in two stages. In the first stage, during a period of 4 months, every employee was asked during the annual check-up to complete a questionnaire based on IHS criteria for the detection of migraine. The answers were analysed centrally. In the second stage, those patients diagnosed with migraine received a second questionnaire consisting of a 12-item form (ML 95) evaluating health-care resource utilization and productivity related to migraine. The completed questionnaire was returned directly by the employees to the study coordinating centre. The financial costs generated were calculated from each company based on the salary reports of the different professional groups.

Results

A total of 7837 employees completed the first questionnaire. The global prevalence of migraine in the employees was 14.6%. The active Spanish population (1994) was 11.7 million, so we can estimate an active population with migraine of 1.7 million.

Of the 1118 migraine patients 577 (51.6%) responded to the second-stage questionnaire. Regarding health-care resources utilization, a remarkable 93.2% of patients had not visited the doctor during the last 12 months, because most of them (64%) used over-the-counter (OTC) medication to resolve the migraine. The second reason for not visiting a doctor was that they thought 'it would be of no help' (22.6%). The other causes for not visiting a doctor were that they could not pay for visit (0.4%), it was not convenient for them (5.4%), they didn't feel too bad (2.2%), they were afraid of what the doctor would tell them (0.7%), and other reasons (23.9%) (Table 43.1).

The annual number of working days lost due to migraine attacks was 0.8 for males and 1.1 for females. The number of days of work with migraine was 18.8 for males and 28 for females, with a mean level of effectiveness of 66.6% for those migraine-affected days. Adding up the number of working days lost due to absenteeism and reduced productivity, a combined grand total of 7.06 days for males and 10.5 days for females is arrived at (global mean, 8.5 days). Applying these findings to the whole Spanish working population we estimated a loss of 13.1 million of work days yearly at a cost of 162 000 million Spanish pesetas (975 million Euros) due to lost days of productivity related to migraine. We calculated also the direct cost related to the use of health-care services by migraineurs with a result of 8868 million Spanish pesetas (53 million euros) yearly.

Table 43.1 Reasons cited for not utilizing the health-care services for migraine in the last 12 months in response to the second questionnaire (ML 95). Of those filling out the questionnaire, 93.2 % had not visited the doctor for migraine in the last 12 months

Reason	Percentage
Used self-medication	64
It would be of no help	22.6
Could not pay for visit	0.4
It was not convenient for me	5.4
I did not feel too bad	2.2
I was afraid of what the doctor would tell me	0.7
Other reasons	23.9

Discussion

Since the introduction of IHS criteria,[1] it has been possible to carry out epidemi-ological studies in most Western countries, thereby contributing to the statistics on the prevalence of migraine.[2,3] However, few studies have been made in the work setting, where aspects such as prevalence in terms of socio-economic or professional groups remain a subject of controversy. In this sense, an alternative approach to the quantification of the problem of migraine is to investigate its economic costs; this would in turn allow us to develop intervention studies and evaluate the cost-efficacy relationship of the different treatment protocols.[4]

The prevalence of migraine in the workplace was at the level expected for this age group (between 18 and 65 years). The use of health-care services by subjects with migraine was found to be unexpectedly low and was due, in part, to a high rate of self-medication. Recent studies have revealed that the direct costs of migraine are generally lower in Europe than in the USA, probably because of the increased use of emergency department and specialist consultations for the treatment of migraine in the USA.[4] Several studies have investigated use of medication among patients with migraine showing that a high percentage of them rely solely on OTC agents. Two studies that directly compared the use of OTC medications with that of prescription medications showed that more patients used OTC preparations.[4]

When evaluating the indirect costs of migraine we found that our results for the number of lost days per year are similar to those of other population-based European studies and much lower than those of American studies (Fig. 43.1). In the European studies, estimates range from 1.8 to 7.1 days in men and 0.9 to 10.5 days in women.[5-7] Values obtained in the USA were much higher (6.3 to 8.7 days per month).[8] The subjective assessments by patients of work effectiveness for those migraine-affected days were remarkably similar to those in other studies (Fig. 43.2).[5-8]

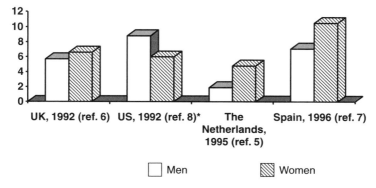

Fig. 43.1 Total annual work days lost by patients with migraine. *Days per month.

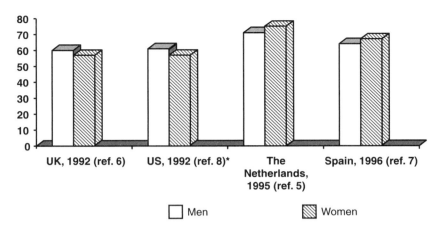

Fig. 43.2 Work-effectiveness (%) during migraine attacks as subjectively assessed by migraineurs.

Table 43.2 Estimated annual cost of lost productivity as result of migraine for the total population of individuals with migraine

Country	Year	Ref.	Cost (million UK£)
UK	1992	6	950
USA	1992	8	4306
Spain	1996	7	810
Canada	1994	9	232
Sweden	1991	10	21

The indirect costs are the most important in the total burden of migraine, representing more than 90% of the total cost in our country. Published estimates of the value of lost productivity in several countries are equivalent to several hundred million UK pounds per year (Table 43.2).[5–10]

References

1. Headache Classification Committee of the International Headache Society. Classification and diagnostic criteria for headache disorders, cranial neuralgias and facial pain. *Cephalalgia* 1988; **8** (Suppl. 7): 19–28.
2. Rasmussen BK, Jensen R, Schroll M, Olesen J. Epidemiology of headache in a general population—a prevalence study. *J Clin Epidemiol* 1991; **44**: 1147–57.
3. Lipton RB, Stewart WF. Migraine in the United States: a review of epidemiology and healthcare use. *Neurology* 1993; **43**: S6–S10.

4. Ferrari MD. The economic burden of migraine to society. *PharmacoEconomics* 1998; **13**: 667–76.

5. Van Roijen L, Essink-Bot ML, Koopmanschap MA, *et al*. Societal perspective on the burden of migraine in the Netherlands. *PharmacoEconomics* 1995; **7**: 170–9.

6. Cull RE, Wells NEJ, Miocevich ML. The economic cost of migraine. *Br J Med Econom* 1992; **2**: 103–15.

7. Láinez JM, Titus F, Cobaleda S, *et al*. Socioeconomic impact of migraine [abstract]. *Funct Neurol* 1996; **11**: 133.

8. Osterhaus JT, Gutterman DL, Plachetka JR. Healthcare resource and lost labour costs of migraine headache in US. *PharmacoEconomics* 1992; **2**: 67–76.

9. O'Brien B, Goeree R, Streiner D. Prevalence of migraine headache in Canada: a population-based survey. *Int J Epidemiol* 1994; **23**: 1020–6.

10. Björk S, Roos P. *Economic aspects of migraine in Sweden*. Lund: Institute for Health Economics, Working paper no. 8, 1991.

44 Reductions in medical and pharmacy resource utilization associated with the addition of preventive medication to the migraine management strategy

Stephen D. Silberstein, Paul K. Winner, and Joseph J. Chmiel

Introduction

Recent drug therapy advances have led to the development of effective new agents and new treatment strategies that make it possible to reduce the pain and disability associated with migraine headaches and to more effectively manage chronic migraine. The effect of preventive migraine therapy on the utilization of medical and pharmaceutical resources has not been extensively studied. The present investigation sought to determine the expected level of long-term (12-month) utilization reduction that can result from adding a preventive medication to a migraine management therapy that already includes acute medication. For this retrospective analysis, utilization information contained in the Lifelink™ Integrated Claims Database (IMS Health, Plymouth Meeting, PA)[1] was examined. Data were drawn from 40 indemnity and Preferred Provider Organization (PPO) health-care plans that covered members in 21 states. Most (75%) claims originated in the midwestern USA.

Acute medication claims were limited to those generated by patients who received the most prescribed[1] acute agent, sumatriptan (Imitrex® tablets or spray). Preventive medication claims data included all forms of divalproex sodium

(Depakote®), valproic acid (for example, Depakene®), propranolol (propranolol HCL, Inderal®, Inderal® LA), tricyclic antidepressants, and other beta-blockers not in the propranolol group.

For the acute+preventive cohort, statistical analyses of pharmaceutical use, out-patient office visits, visits to emergency rooms, and use of computerized tomography (CT) and magnetic resonance imaging (MRI) diagnostics after the initial preventive medication dispensement were compared to usage patterns during the 180 days prior to the initial preventive medication. Similar comparisons of the utilization of high-end diagnostic technology were made for the other two cohorts. Changes in acute medication dispensements were assessed using one-sample t-tests.

A mean of 42.7 units of sumatriptan were dispensed to patients in the acute+preventive cohort in the 180 days prior to the initial preventive medication. This decreased to 39.8 units during the 0–179 days following the initial preventive medication, a change of −2.9 units (−6.8%, $p = 0.189$), and further to 33.7 units during the 180–359 days after the initial preventive medication, a change of −9.0 units (−21.1%, $p = 0.0004$). The decline was also noted in three of the four baseline usage subgroups. During the final 6-month period, patients averaging 10 or more units of sumatriptan monthly during baseline reduced utilization by 37.6% ($p = 0.0001$); those taking 8 to 10 units monthly during baseline reduced utilization by 30.7% ($p = 0.008$); and those taking 6 to 7 units monthly during baseline reduced utilization by 2.6% ($p = 0.881$) (Fig. 44.1).

During the second 6 months after the initial preventive medication, as compared with the 6 months preceding preventive therapy, office and other out-patient visits with a migraine diagnosis decreased by 51.1%, emergency department visits with a migraine diagnosis decreased by 81.8%, CT scans with a migraine diagnosis decreased by 75.0%, MRIs with a migraine diagnosis decreased by 88.2%, and other

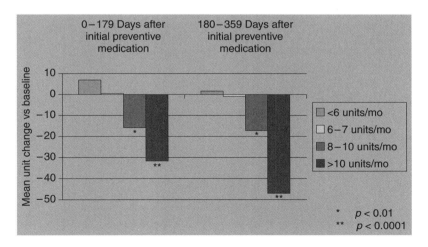

Fig. 44.1   Acute medication utilization changes from baseline among acute + preventive cohort subgroups.

migraine medication dispensements decreased by 14.1%. Patients in the untreated cohort had 6-month CT scan and MRI utilization rates of 6.7% and 1.2%, respectively. In contrast, CT scan utilization in the two treated cohorts was considerably lower (Fig. 44.2), and MRI utilization became lower after treatment (Fig. 44.3).

Comparing the two treated cohorts, the acute only group had lower CT scan and MRI utilization during baseline than the acute+preventive cohort, suggesting a difference in baseline headache severity and/or frequency. However, following initiation of treatment, these high-end diagnostic technology utilization rates for the two cohorts equalized.

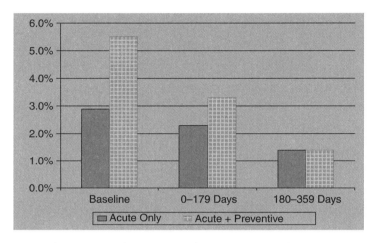

Fig. 44.2 Six-month CT scan utilization rates for acute only and acute + preventive cohorts. The 3-month CT scan utilization for the acute only cohort was adjusted to a 6-month rate.

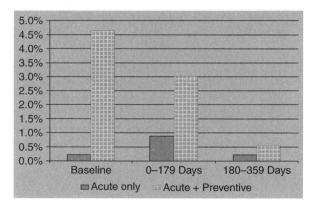

Fig. 44.3 Six-month MRI utilization rates for acute only and acute + preventive cohorts. The 3-month MRI scan utilization for the acute only cohort was adjusted to a 6-month rate.

Discussion

These utilization data from insurance claims support clinical findings that preventive medication reduces frequency and severity of attacks, as evidenced by data that showed a diminishing need for and use of acute medication. This is especially true of those patients most severely affected, that is, those taking 8 or more units of sumatriptan monthly. In the top three subgroups as segmented by sumatriptan use at baseline, utilization of acute medication, as well as associated medical services (office visits, emergencey department visits, and use of CT and MRI diagnostics), declined substantially following the initiation of preventive medication.

The resource utilization reductions found in this study support the current migraine management guidelines by showing that preventive therapy reduces pain and suffering, as evidenced by the need for fewer acute attack interventions. Reducing patients' pain and suffering has broader societal effects as well—a not insignificant one being the potential to raise worker productivity and lower the indirect costs incurred by employers. In the light of those possibilities, this study indicates that further investigations into the indirect cost impact of preventive migraine therapy are necessary. Study limitations exist in retrospective analyses of claims data. It is known that claims databases may contain coding errors and missing data.

Migraine preventive drug therapy was effective in reducing resource consumption when added to therapy consisting only of an acute medication (sumatriptan). The most pronounced reductions in the utilization of acute medication were observed at the highest levels of acute medication usage, but noteworthy reductions were seen in patients with lower levels of acute medication usage as well. However, substantial reductions in the consumption of physician's services following the initiation of preventive medication were observed fairly consistently across varying migraine severity subgroups. In addition, both acute and preventive medications were associated with lower utilization of high-end diagnostic technology.

Reference

1. Lifelink Integrated Claims Database, IMS Health, Plymouth Meeting, PA.

45 Utilization and price differentials of selective 5-HT$_1$-receptor agonists in the European countries

Pietro Folino-Gallo, Fabio Palazzo, Giuseppe Stirparo,
Sergio De Filippis, and Paolo Martelletti

Introduction

Migraine is a common condition and, according to several population-based surveys, its prevalence rate ranges from around 10% to 12% of the general population.[1–3] This high rate of prevalence suggests that migraine has an important social impact; however, wide variations in clinical phenotypes of the disease, that is, intensity, frequency, duration of the attacks, and related disability, make it difficult to estimate the whole burden of migraine.[4–6] Moreover, low-frequency migraine sufferers often reject any structured medical approach and escape from in-depth analysis of human, social, and economic costs caused by their disease.[7–9] Thus novel approaches are needed in order to integrate the traditional clinical evaluation of migraine with its socio-economic impact.[10–13]

A directory (EURO-Medicines) of all medicines available in the European countries was recently reported.[14] Such a directory can be helpful in estimating the impact of migraine therapy by analysing data about utilization and expenditure for pharmaceutical compounds selectively indicated for the treatment of migraine.

Since 1991 selective 5-HT$_1$-receptor agonists (triptans) have been introduced for the treatment of migraine attack and five different compounds (eletriptan, naratriptan, rizatriptan, sumatriptan, zolmitriptan) are presently available in several European markets. Almotriptan and frovatriptan are completing pre-registration procedures and will shortly reach the market. Triptans have radically improved migraine management because of their effectiveness, tolerability, and safety[11–13] and their use, despite the high cost, has greatly increased in the last few years. Comparison at a European level of their consumption and expenditure can thus provide useful information and represents a new methodological approach for a better understanding of migraine global burden. Moreover, large discrepancies between the European countries in both utilization and prices have been described for a variety of medicines but no data are available for either triptans or other antimigraine therapies. For all of these reasons we thought it was of interest to perform an international comparison of European countries in terms of utilization of and expenditure for triptans. The aim of the study was to survey prices, nation-wide utilization, and expenditure for triptans at a European level.

Materials and methods

Data were obtained from the EURO-Medicines database, a European Union-funded project to collect information about the available medicines in the European countries, whose data are now available on the internet (www.euromedicines.org). Details of the methodology and data sources used for collecting and analysing this data are provided elsewhere.[14] Triptan utilization was calculated in daily defined doses (DDD/1000 inhabitants/day) according to the WHO Anatomical Therapeutical Chemical (ATC) system, a hierarchical classification where medicines are divided into 14 main groups (first level), with three therapeutic/pharmacological/chemical subgroups (second, third, and fourth levels, respectively), and with a fifth level corresponding to the chemical substance. Each medicine can thus be identified by an alphanumeric code (for example, N-02-C-C-01 for sumatriptan, which means: neurologicals–analgesics–antimigraine–selective 5-HT$_1$-agonists–sumatriptan). The daily defined dose (DDD) is the assumed average maintenance dose per day for a drug used for its main indication in adults. It is only a unit of measurement and does not necessarily reflect the prescribed or recommended dose. The DDD for triptans corresponds to the recommended single dose (naratriptan 2.5 mg, rizatriptan 10 mg, sumatriptan 100 mg, and zolmitriptan 2.5 mg).

The cost per DDD was calculated by dividing the retail price of the pack by the number of DDDs contained in the pack. For price comparisons, when more pharmaceutical forms were available, oral forms only were taken in account.

Expenditure data and retail prices were calculated in the local currency and converted into euros using a fixed conversion rate (12 euros) or the October 2001 exchange rate. Index numbers with 1997 as baseline were used for historical comparisons.

Results

In 1999 utilization of triptans was around 1 DDD/1000 inhabitants/day in Denmark, Germany, Sweden, and Norway. Finnish consumption was lower (Table 45.1). The historical trend from 1997 to 1999 shows the greatest increase in Germany (+155%) and Norway (+71%). More modest increase are observed for Sweden

Table 45.1   Utilization of triptans (DDD/1000 inhabitants/day)

Country	1997	1998	1999
Denmark	0.80	0.90	1.00
Germany	0.42	0.82	1.07
Sweden	0.70	0.90	0.90
Norway	0.58	0.71	0.99
Finland	0.18	0.19	0.19

(+29%), Denmark (+25%), and Finland (+6%). Consumption of triptans in Germany in 1999 was sixfold greater than in Finland (1.07 versus 0.19 DDD/1000 inhabitants/day, respectively).

The widest increases from 1997 to 1999 in both utilization and expenditure happened in Germany (+155% and +99%, respectively). Utilization in Finland from 1997 to 1999 increased by 6% as compared with 25% in Denmark. At the same time expenditure for triptans increased in Finland by 43% versus only 6% in Denmark.

The price per DDD (100 mg for oral forms) of sumatriptan differs between countries by 400% (oral forms only); Austria has the highest prices and Denmark the lowest (Fig. 45.1). Large price differentials also exist within countries (Fig. 45.1) in relation to pack sizes and strengths of the products: lower strengths and smaller packs are more expensive than higher strengths and bigger packs. These national differentials are widest in Belgium (from 11.15 to 19.71 euros per DDD; 77%) and

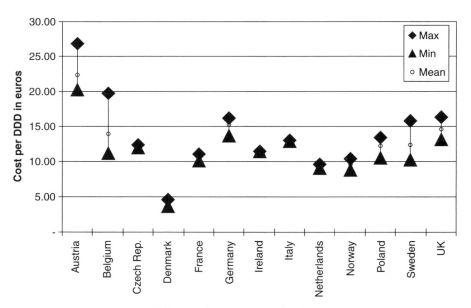

Fig. 45.1   Sumatriptan. Price differentials between and within countries.

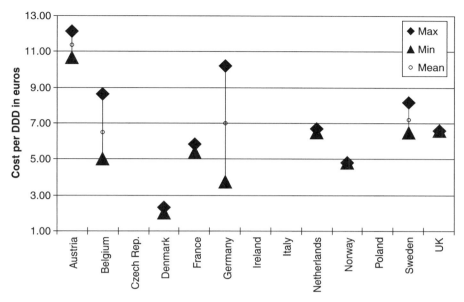

Fig. 45.2 Naratriptan. Price differentials between and within countries.

in Sweden (from 10.30 to 15.73 euros per DDD; 53%). The differences are smaller in the Czech Republic (3%) and Ireland (0%).

The price per DDD (2.5 mg) of naratriptan differs between countries by more than 400%; Austria has the highest prices and Denmark the lowest (Fig. 45.2). For naratriptan also large price differentials exist within countries related to the pack sizes and strengths of the products: national differentials are widest in Germany (from 3.75 to 10.23 euros per DDD; 173%) and in Belgium (from 5.00 to 8.64 euros per DDD; 73%). The differences are smallest in the Netherlands (3%) and in the UK and Norway (0%).

Large price differentials, greater than 400%, also exist for zolmitriptan (Fig. 45.3). Zolmitriptan-containing products are most expensive in Austria and Germany and cheapest in Denmark. The widest within-country differentials are in Norway (from 5.22 to 9.21 euros per DDD; 76%) and Belgium (from 5.58 to 9.32 euros per DDD; 67%). The lowest differentials for zolmitriptan are in the Netherlands (3%) and the UK and Ireland (0%).

Rizatriptan was in 1999 available in fewer countries and had lower price differentials (121% between countries; 45% within country; Italy) (Fig. 45.4).

Discussion

From our data it appears that utilization of triptans in 1999 was around 1 DDD/1000 inhabitants/day in most countries where utilization data were available except

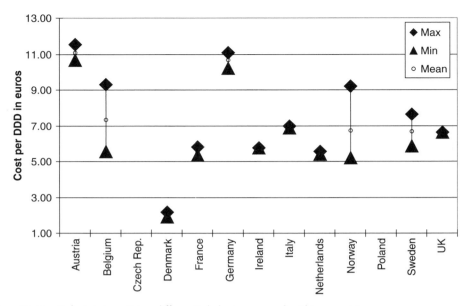

Fig. 45.3   Zolmitriptan. Price differentials between and within countries.

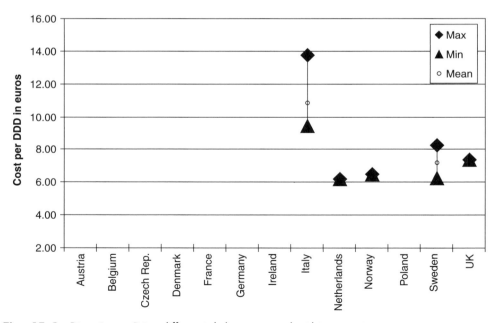

Fig. 45.4   Rizatriptan. Price differentials between and within countries.

for Finland whose consumption was about one-fifth that of the other countries. The analysis of the historical trends demonstrates that the increase in consumption from 1997 to 1999 was different between countries, ranging from +157% in Germany to +6% in Finland. Assuming that migraine incidence is not different between countries, these differences could be attributed to several causes: from a wider use of anti-migraine medicines other than triptans, to the utilization of lower dosages because of different clinical approaches or because patients were treated early in the attack when pain is still at a mild phase. Perhaps, these same reasons could alter the apparent homogeneity in triptan utilization, but no data are presently available to confirm or disprove this hypothesis.

The differences in the number of available triptans, together with the wide price differentials between and within countries, and differences in national reimbursement systems and organization of health care, add further variables in interpreting differences in overall triptan consumption and in the market share of the single compounds, which probably could find a partial explanation in their price differentials.

Conclusion and perspectives

Our data demonstrated the existence of a trend toward a similar level of triptan consumption (about 1 DDD/1000 inhabitants/day + 10%) except in Finland. No data are available to say if this similar nationwide consumption reflects similar clinical practice. Price differentials between and within countries still persist. A reduction of these price differentials can be the basis (and could be the starting point) of a wider European harmonization in triptan consumption and migraine management.

References

1. Rasmussen BK. Epidemiology and socio-economic impact of headache. *Cephalalgia* 1999; **19** (Suppl. 25): 20–3.
2. Stewart WF, Lipton RB, Celentano DD, Reed ML. Prevalence of migraine headache in the United States: relations to age, income, race and other sociodemographic factors. *J Am Med Assoc* 1992; **267**: 64–9.
3. Henry P. Migraine: epidemiological data, repercussions on daily life and socio-economics cost. *Pathol Biol* 2000; **48**: 608–12.
4. Hu XH, Markson LE, Lipton RB, Stewart WF, Berger ML. Burden of migraine in the Unites States. Disability and economic costs. *Arch Int Med* 1999; **159**: 813–81.
5. Steiner TJ. Headache burdens and bearers. *Funct Neurol* 2000; **15** (Suppl. 3): 213–19.
6. WHO. *Headache disorders and public health: education and management implications*. Geneva: WHO/MSD/MBD/00.9. 2001; pp. 1–12
7. Bigal ME, Moraes FA, Fernandes LC, Bordini CA, Speciali JG. Indirect costs of migraine in a public Brazilian hospital. *Headache* 2001; **41**: 503–8.
8. Holmes WF, MacGregor EA, Dodick D. Migraine-related disability: impact and implications for sufferers' lives and clinical issue. *Neurology* 2001; **56**: S13–S19.

9. Gerth WC, Carides GW, Dasbach EJ, Visser WH, Santanello NC. The multinational impact of migraine symptoms on healthcare utilisation and work loss. *PharmacoEconomics* 2001; **19**: 197–206.

10. Lipton RB, Stewart WF, Reed M, Diamond S. Migraine's impact today. Burden of illness, pattern of care. *Postgrad Med* 2001; **109**: 43–5.

11. Silberstein SD, Goadsby PJ, Lipton RB. Management of migraine: an algorithmic approach. *Neurology* 2000; **55** (Suppl. 2): S46–S52.

12. Colman SS, Brod MI, Krishnamurty A, Rowland CR, Jirgens KJ, Gomez-Manchilla B. Treatment satisfaction, functional status, and health-related quality of life of migraine patients treated with almotriptan or sumatriptan. *Clin Ther* 2001; **23**: 127–45.

13. Stang P, Cady R, Batenhorst A, Hoffman L. Workplace productivity. A review of the impact of migraine and its treatment. *PharmacoEconomics* 2001; **19**: 231–44.

14. Folino-Gallo P, Walley T, Frolich JC, Carvajal A, Edwards IR. Availability of medicines in the European Union: results from the EURO-Medicines project. *Eur J Clin Pharmacol* 2001; **57**: 441–6.

46 Regaining time lost during migraine attacks with eletriptan

Nicholas E.J. Wells

Background

During the last decade there has been an increasing awareness of the economic and social burdens of migraine.[1-4] Whilst medical management of migraine places a relatively small resource burden on the health-care system, productivity losses are substantial—estimates from the UK, for example, suggest annual costs of UK £600–£750 million.[5] Losses in the USA in 1997 have been estimated as US \$13 billion.[6] Although more difficult to value in monetary terms, migraine attacks also reduce the time sufferers would usually devote to non-work activities, thereby having a negative impact on quality of life.[7] This chapter examines the effectiveness of eletriptan in reducing both aspects of time loss associated with migraine attacks.

Methods

Male and female patients, aged 18 years or older, from Europe, Australia, and South Africa were enrolled in a phase III, randomized, double-blind, parallel-group study that compared the effectiveness and tolerability of oral eletriptan, a potent, selective 5-$HT_{1B/1D}$ agonist, with placebo.[8] Subjects had a history of at least one migraine attack every 6 weeks with or without an aura, according to diagnostic criteria defined by the International Headache Society (IHS).[9]

Patients were randomized to one of five treatment groups (eletriptan 40 mg/eletriptan 40 mg, eletriptan 40 mg/placebo, eletriptan 80 mg/eletriptan 80 mg, eletriptan 80 mg/placebo, placebo/placebo). Treatment consisted of an initial dose following the start of a migraine attack and a second dose if the first dose failed to diminish or completely resolve the headache in 2 hours or if headache recurred in 24 hours. Time loss comparisons were evaluated among patients who were randomized to receive eletriptan as a first and second dose and among those who could have received placebo both times (n=692). Although the clinical trial extended over three attacks, only the first attack was employed for the time loss study.

Patients were given a questionnaire requesting information about time loss from usual activities, whether at work, home, or elsewhere, to be completed 24 hours after the last dose taken. Questions were designed to elicit, to the nearest half-hour, the amount of time during which the patient was unable to undertake usual activities. Patients also noted additional time lost beyond the 24-hour period.

Analyses were limited to those patients who were randomized, treated, and had valid data. End points included total time and work time lost. Means and standard deviations were deemed inappropriate for statistical analysis because the data followed distributions that were non-normal (non-Gaussian). Instead, summary statistics, including medians and interquartile ranges, were employed on evaluable patients. The null hypothesis was that the distributions of time loss would be the same for all treatment groups. Comparisons between the groups was made using the Wilcoxon-rank sum test (2-sided alternative).

Results

In agreement with other studies of migraine, female patients comprised 84% of the study population compared to 16% of males. A majority of the patients were aged 30–45 years. Evaluable patients in the three treatment arms had similar demographic profiles. Results for the eletriptan 40 mg/eletriptan 40 mg, eletriptan 80 mg/eletriptan 80 mg, and placebo/placebo groups are abbreviated as E40/E40, E80/E80, PBO/PBO, respectively.

Overall, 92% of the patients experienced time loss from usual activities; this proportion ranged from 88% among those who received E40/E40 to 96% in the placebo group (Table 46.1). Placebo-treated patients reported the greatest amount of time loss (median 9 hours; interquartile range 4 to 22 hours). In contrast, patients in the E40/E40 and E80/E80 groups reported a median time loss of only 4 hours. Interquartile ranges were 2 to 6.3 hours and 2 to 8 hours, respectively. Thus, both eletriptan doses generated a time savings of 5 hours compared with placebo.

Distributions of individual assessments of time loss for patients receiving placebo, E40/E40, and E80/E80 are shown in Figs 46.1–46.3. Among the patients who received E40/E40, 37% lost 2 hours or less compared to 9% of those who received placebo. At the other end of the spectrum, just 8% of the E40/E40 group lost 24 hours or more versus 25% of the placebo group ($p < 0.001$).

A similar comparison between those who received E80/E80 or placebo revealed that 31% of the E80/E80 group lost 2 hours or less (placebo group, 10%). This difference was statistically significant ($p<0.001$). Furthermore, younger individuals (<30 years) in the placebo group tended to lose less time than those in the older age groups (>30 years). However, there were relatively few patients in the young group.

When time loss analysis focused on the workplace, 80% reported time loss among the three groups (Table 46.1). Placebo patients lost significantly more time

Table 46.1   Median number of hours lost during treated migraine attack (reprinted from ref. 10 with permission from Adis International Ltd)

| | | Median number of hours lost by | | | | | |
| | | | | | Patients aged (years) | | |
Treatment group	Subjects with time loss (%)	All patients	Male	Female	18–25	30–45	>45
Total time loss							
E40/E40	88.0	4.0	2.5	4.0	3.0	3.5	4.0
E80/E80	91.5	4.0	4.0	4.0	4.0	4.0	4.0
PBO/PBO	95.7	9.0	8.5	10.0	5.8	10.0	9.0
Work time loss							
E40/E40	76.0	2.5	1.3	3.8	2.5	3.0	1.5
E80/E80	77.0	3.0	3.0	3.0	4.0	2.0	4.0
PBO/PBO	84.2	4.0	6.0	4.0	3.0	5.0	4.0

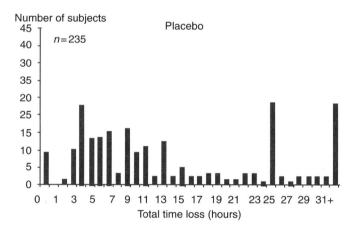

Fig. 46.1   Total time loss for migraine patients receiving placebo. (Reprinted from ref. 10 with permission from Adis International Ltd.)

(median 4 hours; interquartile range 2 to 8 hours) than E40/E40 (median 2.5 hours; interquartile range 1 to 6 hours, $p=0.013$) and E80/E80 (median 3 hours, interquartile range 1 to 6 hours, $p=0.013$).

Conclusion

Clinical trials of antimigraine agents have traditionally employed headache response 2 hours after treatment as an endpoint to evaluate efficacy. A cut-off of 2 hours,

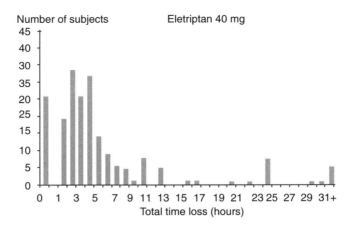

Fig. 46.2 Total time loss for migraine patients taking eletriptan 40 mg. (Reprinted from ref. 10 with permission from Adis International Ltd.)

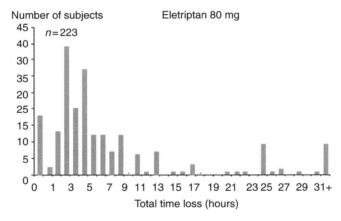

Fig. 46.3 Total time loss for migraine patients receiving eletriptan 80 mg. (Reprinted from ref. 10 with permission from Adis International Ltd.)

however, provides only partial information. Time loss from usual activities, as opposed to work time loss, has largely been ignored in the pharmacoeconomic literature. This present study shows that eletriptan, in doses of 40 mg and 80 mg, produces significant reductions in time loss from usual and work activities due to migraine headaches in comparison to that in placebo-treated patients. Eletriptan therefore has the potential to yield significant benefits for the quality of life of patients, as well as for the broader economy by reducing the personal and economic burden generated by the amount of time during which patients are unable to undertake their activities during migraine attacks.

References

1. Blau JN, Drummond, MF. *Migraine*. London: Office of Health Economics, 1991.
2. Björk S, Roos P. *Economic aspects of migraine in Sweden*, Working paper no. 8. Lund: Institute for Health Economics, 1991.
3. Van Roijen,L, Essink-Bot ML, Koopmanschap MA, *et al*. Societal perspectives on the burden of migraine in the Netherlands. *PharmacoEconomics* 1995; **7**: 170–9.
4. Clouse JC, Osterhaus JT. Healthcare resources and costs associated with migraine in a managed healthcare setting. *Ann Pharmacother* 1994; **28**: 659–64.
5. Cull RE, Wells NEJ, Miocevich ML. The economic cost of migraine. *Br J Med Econom* 1992; **11**: 103–15.
6. Hu HX, Markson LE, Lipion RB, *et al*. Burden of migraine in the United States, disability and economic costs. *Arch Intern Med* 1999; **159**: 813–18.
7. Solomon GD, Price KL. Burden of migraine, a review of its socioeconomic impact. *Pharmaco-Economics* 1997; **11** (Suppl. 1): 1–10.
8. Stark R, Dahlöf C, Haughie S, Hettiarachchi J, on behalf of the Eletriptan Steering Committee. Efficacy, safety and tolerability of oral eletriptan in the acute treatment of migraine: results of a phase III, multicentre, placebo-controlled study across three attacks. *Cephalalgia* 2002; **22** (1): 23–32.
9. International Headache Society. Classification and diagnostic criteria for headache disorders, cranial neuralgias and facial pain. *Cephalalgia* 1988; **8** (Suppl. 7): 19–28.
10. Wells NEJ, Steiner TJ. The effectiveness of eletriptan (Relpax) in reducing the time loss caused by migraine attacks. *PharmacoEconomics* 2000; **18** (6): 557–66.

47 Economics of headache: discussion summary

Jes Olesen

Since the major cost of migraine is in loss of working ability, it is crucial to have consensus about how to cost a lost work day. Bengt Jönsson stated that the simplest and most realistic costing is simply the salary for 1 day. It was suggested that a workday is not a workday. For example, if a train driver takes ill and the train does not leave, then hundreds of people may not get to work on time and hundreds of working hours may be lost. The answer to this is that in other situations patients may catch up with the lost working time and thus it may not cost anything. In all likelihood these factors average out when analysing the costs of large cohorts of affected people.

The next question was how to handle the situation when people are present at work but indicate that they work with decreased efficiency. One point of view is that this should not be costed at all because it is very subjective and because people may simply compensate for the lesser efficacy by being more efficient on other days. Opinions about this issue are somewhat divided but it was pointed out that everybody functions at varying efficiency from day to day and on average as much as they can. Therefore, it seems unlikely that decreased efficiency due to a disease can or will be compensated to any large degree. Overall, it must be reasonable to cost also days with decreased working efficiency in proportion to the estimated percentage decrease in working ability.

Two groups suggested that a triptan with lesser side-effects, in this instance cardiac side-effects, could save considerable amounts of money in comparison to another triptan with more such side-effects. It was calculated how much such side-effects might cost in terms of cardiological investigations. While this aspect is theoretically interesting and should be included to some extent in prospective comparative trials in the future, the data presented were considered to be very weak as there was statistically no documented difference in side-effects in head-to-head comparisons of the drugs in question.

Several chapters showed that the cost of modern acute migraine treatment is greatly outweighed by savings in terms of less use of medical services and less loss of working time. Taken together, these studies suggest an aggressive approach to migraine treatment that, in addition to saving costs, will also reduce the personal suffering and psychological burden of migraine. These softer parameters are difficult to translate into economic terms but nevertheless remain extremely important. They are probably best taken into account by using quality of life measures as discussed in a preceding section. Another interesting aspect is the demonstration of increased efficacy when people take the drugs early in the attack. The usual drug trial design, where people have to wait for treatment until migraine headache reaches medium or severe intensity, was originally created in order to assure that definite migraine attacks were being treated. Subsequently, it has been shown that most patients, given appropriate education, are able to distinguish fairly well between tension-type headache attacks and the early start of migraine. It was documented that it is significantly more cost-effective to treat early than to treat late. Early treatment has been clinical practice in most centres but apparently the previous trial design has in some centres resulted in instructions to patients not to treat until pain reaches medium to severe intensity.

Very little information has been available about the cost-effectiveness of prophylactic migraine treatment because prophylactic trials, with a few exceptions such as trials of valproate, were done more than 20 years ago. Chapter 44 presented a retrospective analysis of resource utilization in a large claims database. The results indicated that prophylactic treatment reduced the use of acute and other migraine medications as well as visits to physicians' offices and emergency departments. Also, the utilization of computerized tomography (CT) and magnetic resonance imaging (MRI) scans was reduced. These encouraging results should stimulate the collection of better economic and quality of life data in future prophylactic trials.

The wide variation in availability and pricing of migraine treatments throughout Europe was discussed in Chapter 45. It is very unsatisfactory that Europeans have differing availability of drugs and that costs vary so much from country to country. As Europe is coming more and more together efforts must be launched to create more equal opportunities for Europeans. The emerging patient organizations, such as The World Headache Alliance, are best suited to examine these issues and to claim equal rights for sufferers throughout the whole of Europe, since initiatives from physicians are often viewed with suspicion by news media and decision-makers.

It was advised that committee work is necessary to compile the large volume of information about the health economics of migraine. Data from such a report would probably be surprising to most decision-makers and would greatly support the World Health Organization's (WHO) documentation of migraine as a very costly disorder in terms of disability-adjusted life-years (DALYs). A suitable organization to initiate such a task would be the International Headache Society (IHS).

The fact that tension-type headache, particularly chronic tension-type headache, is even more prevalent and more costly than migraine has so far escaped notice. There are studies from Denmark indicating that tension-type headache may cost up to 3 times more than migraine in terms of lost working time, but much more information about tension-type headache is needed. Unfortunately, it seems that such studies are mostly done when drug companies become interested in a field because of the advent of new drugs. There is little public support for pharmacoeconomic studies of headache, but research groups dedicated to headache epidemiology and headache disability should initiate further projects in chronic tension-type headache as soon as possible. Again, it might be considered whether international bodies such as the IHS should actively encourage such studies in collaboration with the WHO.

Section
V

Guidelines and interventions

48 Evidence-based guidelines for migraine headache

Stephen D. Silberstein

This chapter summarizes the four evidence-based reviews on migraine management: acute, preventive, and non-pharmacological treatments, and the role of neuroimaging in patients with headache.[1–6] Duke University's Center for Clinical Health Policy Research (CCHPR), in collaboration with the American Academy of Neurology (AAN), completed four *Technical Reviews* on migraine sponsored by the US Agency for Health Care Policy and Research (AHCPR): self administered drug treatments for acute migraine;[7] parenteral (PR) drug treatments for acute migraine;[8] drug treatments for the prevention of migraine;[9] and behavioural and physical treatments for migraine.[10] Additional reports included diagnostic testing for headache patients, an update on sumatriptan and other 5-HT$_1$ agonists, and a report on butalbital-containing compounds for migraine and tension-type headache. A multidisciplinary panel (the US Headache Consortium) produced four treatment guidelines: diagnostic testing; pharmacological management of acute attacks; migraine-preventive drugs; and behavioural and physical treatments for migraine. Complete descriptions of the methodological details are described elsewhere.[4]

Neuroimaging

The following symptoms significantly increased the odds of finding a significant abnormality on neuroimaging of patients with non-acute headache: rapidly increasing headache frequency; a history of dizziness or lack of coordination; a history of localized neurological signs or a history of symptoms such as subjective numbness or tingling; and a history of headache causing awakening from sleep (although this can occur with migraine and cluster headache). The absence of these symptoms did not significantly lower the odds of finding a significant abnormality on neuroimaging.

Neuroimaging recommendations for nonacute headache

Consider neuroimaging for:

◆ patients who have an unexplained abnormal finding on the neurological examination (grade B);
◆ patients who have atypical headache features or headaches that do not fulfil the strict definition of migraine or another primary headache disorder (or have some additional risk factor, such as immune deficiency), when a lower threshold for neuroimaging may be applied (grade C[‡‡]).

Neuroimaging is not usually warranted when patients have migraine and a normal neurological examination. (Grade B[‡‡]).

Treatment of migraine

Migraine varies in frequency, duration, and disability among sufferers and between attacks. The intensity of care should be linked with the level of disability and symptoms such as nausea and vomiting for the acute treatment of symptoms of an ongoing attack (stratified care). It is not appropriate to continue ineffective or poorly tolerated medication in a sequential and arbitrary manner (step care). The goals of long-term migraine treatment are to: reduce attack frequency, severity, and disability; reduce reliance on poorly tolerated or ineffective acute pharmacotherapies; improve quality of life; avoid acute headache medication escalation; educate and enable patients to manage their disease; and reduce headache-related distress and psychological symptoms.

General principles of management

Establish a diagnosis. Educate migraine sufferers about their condition and its treatment. Discuss the rationale for a particular treatment, how to use it, and what adverse events are likely. Establish realistic patient expectations. Encourage patients to use diary cards or headache calendars to track days of disability or missed work, school, or family activities. Choose treatment depending on attack frequency and severity, the presence and degree of disability, and associated symptoms such as nausea and vomiting. Create a formal management plan and individualize management, which includes: considering the patient's response to, and tolerance for, specific medications; considering comorbidity/coexisting conditions; encouraging the patient to identify and avoid triggers.

Acute treatment

The goals of acute migraine treatment are to: treat attacks rapidly and consistently, without recurrence; restore the patient's ability to function; minimize the use of back-up and rescue medications; optimize self-care and reduce subsequent use of resources; be cost-effective for overall management; and have minimal or no adverse events.

To meet these goals:

- use migraine-specific agents (triptans, dihydroergotamine (DHE), ergotamine) when patients have moderate or severe migraine or when mild-to-moderate headaches respond poorly to nonsteroidal anti-inflammatory drugs (NSAIDs) or combinations such as aspirin plus acetaminophen plus caffeine;
- select a non-oral route of administration for patients whose migraine is associated with severe nausea or vomiting;
- consider a self-administered rescue medication when severe migraines do not respond to (or fail) other treatments;
- guard against medication-overuse headache. (Many experts limit acute therapy to *two headache days per week* on a regular basis.)

Evidence-based recommendations for acute treatment of migraine

Specific medications
Triptans (naratriptan, rizatriptan, sumatriptan, and zolmitriptan) are effective and relatively safe for the acute treatment of migraine headaches and are an appropriate initial treatment choice for patients who have moderate to severe migraine and no contraindications for their use (grade A). Initial treatment with any triptan is a reasonable choice when the headache is moderate to severe or in migraine of any severity when non-specific medication has failed to provide adequate relief in the past (grade C). Patients with nausea and vomiting may be given intranasal (IN) or subcutaneous (SC) sumatriptan (grade C).

Ergot alkaloids and derivatives
Ergotamine PO (oral)/PR (and caffeine combination) may be considered for selected patients with moderate to severe migraine (grade B). DHE nasal spray is safe and effective and should be considered for patients with moderate to severe migraine (grade A). DHE SC/IV (intravenous)/IM (intramuscular) and nasal spray may be given to patients who have nausea and vomiting (grade C). DHE SC, IM, and nasal spray are reasonable initial treatment choices when the headache is moderate to severe, or in migraine of any severity when non-specific medication has failed to provide adequate relief in the past (grade C). DHE IM, SC may be considered for patients with moderate to severe migraine (grade B). DHE IV plus antiemetics IV is an appropriate treatment choice for patients with severe migraine (grade B).

Non-specific medications

Antiemetics
Oral antiemetics are an adjunct to treat nausea associated with migraine (grade C). Metoclopramide IM/IV is an adjunct to control nausea (grade C) and may be

considered as IV monotherapy for migraine pain relief (grade B). Prochlorperazine IV, IM, and PR may be a therapeutic choice for migraine in the appropriate setting (grade B). Prochlorperazine PR is an adjunct in the treatment of acute migraine with nausea and vomiting (grade C). Chlorpromazine IV may be a therapeutic choice for migraine in the appropriate setting (grade B).

NSAIDs, non-opiate analgesics, and combination analgesics
Acetaminophen, alone, is not recommended for migraine (grade B). NSAIDs (oral) and combination analgesics containing caffeine are a reasonable first-line treatment choice for mild to moderate migraine attacks or severe attacks that have been responsive in the past to similar NSAIDs or non-opiate analgesics (grade A).

Butalbital-containing analgesics
Limit and carefully monitor their use with regard to overuse, medication-overuse headache, and withdrawal concerns (grade B).

Opiate analgesics
Parenteral opiates are a rescue therapy for acute migraine when sedation side-effects will not put the patient at risk and when the risk abuse has been addressed (grade B). Consider parenteral and oral combination use in acute migraine when the risk of abuse has been addressed and sedation will not put the patient at risk (grade A).

Other medications

- Isometheptene combinations may be a choice for patients with mild-to-moderate headache (grade B).
- Corticosteroids (dexamethasone or hydrocortisone) are a choice for rescue therapy for patients with status migrainosus (grade C).
- There is insufficient evidence to establish a role for IN or IV lidocaine (grade B).

Table 48.1 summarizes acute therapies for migraine.

Preventive treatment

The goals of migraine preventive therapy are to: (1) reduce attack frequency, severity, and duration; (2) improve responsiveness to treatment of acute attacks; and (3) improve function and reduce disability. One or more of the following helps guide management decisions on the use of preventive therapies: recurring migraines that, in the patients' opinion, significantly interfere with their daily routines, despite acute treatment; frequent headaches; contraindication to or failure or overuse of acute therapies; adverse events with acute therapies; the cost of both acute and preventive therapies; patient preference; and uncommon migraine conditions,

Table 48.1 Acute therapies for migraine

Group 1: Proven pronounced statistical and clinical benefit*	Group 2: Moderate statistical and clinical benefit†	Group 3: Statistically but not clinically proven or clinically but not statistically proven effective‡	Group 4: Proven to be statistically or clinically ineffective§	Group 5: Clinical and statistical benefits unknown¶
Specific DHE SC, IM, IV, IN DHE IV plus antiemetic Naratriptan PO Rizatriptan PO Sumatriptan SC, IN, PO Zolmitriptan PO *Non-specific* Acetaminophen, aspirin, plus caffeine PO Aspirin PO Butorphanol IN Ibuprofen PO Naproxen sodium PO Prochlorperazine IV	Acetaminophen+codeine PO Butalbital. aspirin, caffeine, +codeine PO Butorphanol IM Chlorpromazine IM, IV Diclofenac K, PO Ergotamine+caffeine+ pentobarbital+ Bellafoline® PO Flubriprofen PO Isometheptene CPD, PO Ketorolac IM Lidocaine IN Meperidine IM, IV Methadone IM Metoclopramide IV Naproxen PO Prochlorperazine IM, PR	Butalbital, aspirin, + caffeine PO Ergotamine PO Ergotamine+caffeine PO Metoclopramide IM, PR	Acetaminophen PO Chlorpromazine IM Granisetron IV Lidocaine IV	Dexamethasone IV Hydrocortisone IV

*At least 2 double-blind, placebo-controlled studies+clinical impression of effect.
†1 double-blind, placebo-controlled study+clinical impression of effect.
‡ Conflicting or inconsistent evidence.
§Failed efficacy versus placebo.
¶Insufficient evidence available.

including hemiplegic migraine, basilar migraine, migraine with prolonged aura, or migrainous infarction (to prevent neurological damage—as based on expert consensus).

The following consensus-based principles of care will enhance the success of preventive treatment. Consider non-pharmacological therapies and take patient preference into consideration.

(1) Medication use.
  ◆ Initiate therapy with the medication proven to be most effective.
  ◆ Initiate therapy with the lowest effective dose. Increase it slowly until clinical benefits are achieved in the absence of, or until limited by, adverse events.
  ◆ Give each drug an adequate trial (2–3 months).
  ◆ Avoid interfering medications (for example, overuse of acute medications).
  ◆ Use of a long-acting formulation may improve compliance.
(2) Evaluation.
  ◆ Monitor the patient's headaches with a headache diary.
  ◆ Re-evaluate therapy. If headaches are well controlled, consider discontinuing treatment.
(3) Take coexisting conditions into account.
  ◆ If possible, select a drug that will treat the coexistent condition and the migraine.
  ◆ Do not use a migraine drug that is contraindicated for the coexistent disease.
  ◆ Do not treat coexistent conditions with medications that exacerbate migraine.
  ◆ Beware of all drug interactions.
  ◆ Direct special attention to women who are or want to become pregnant.
(4) Behavioural treatments include: relaxation training, biofeedback therapy, and cognitive-behavioural training (stress-management). They are options when there is:
  ◆ patient preference for non-pharmacological interventions;
  ◆ poor tolerance to specific pharmacologic treatments;
  ◆ medical contraindications for specific pharmacological treatments;
  ◆ insufficient or no response to pharmacological treatment;
  ◆ pregnancy, planned pregnancy, or breast-feeding;
  ◆ history of acute medication overuse;
  ◆ significant stress or deficient stress-coping skills.

Cognitive and behavioural treatment recommendations

◆ Relaxation training, thermal biofeedback with relaxation training, electromyography (EMG) biofeedback, and cognitive-behavioural therapy are treatment options for migraine prevention (grade A).
◆ Behavioural therapy may be combined with preventive drug therapy to achieve additional clinical improvement for migraine relief (grade B).

Table 48.2 Preventive therapies for migraine

Group 1: Medium-to-high efficacy, good strength of evidence, and mild-to-moderate side-effects	Group 2: Lower efficacy than in group 1, or limited strength of evidence, and mild-to-moderate side-effects	Group 3: Clinically efficacious based on consensus and clinical experience, but no scientific evidence of efficacy	Group 4: Medium-to-efficacy, good strength of evidence, but with side-effect concerns	Group 5: Evidence indicating no efficacy over placebo
Amitriptyline	*β-blockers*	*Group 3a*	Methysergide	Acebutolol
Divalproex sodium	Atenolol/metoprolol/	*Antidepressants*		
Propranolol/	nadolol	Doxepin		Carbamazepine
timolol	*Ca-blockers*	Fluvoxamine		Clomipramine
	Nimodipine/verapamil	Imipramine		Clonazepam
	NSAIDs	Mirtazepine		Clonidine
	Aspirin/fenoprofen/	Nortriptyline		Indomethacin
	flurbiprofen	Paroxetine		
	Ketoprofen	Protriptyline		Nicardipine
	Mefenamic acid	Sertraline		Nifedipine
	Naproxen	Trazodone		Pindolol
	Naproxen sodium	Venlafaxine		
	Fluoxetine (racemic)	Cyproheptadine		
		Diltiazem		
	Gabapentin	Ibuprofen		
	Other	Tiagabine		
	Feverfew	Topiramate		
	Magnesium	*Group 3b**		
	Vitamin B$_2$	Methylergonovine		
		(methylergometrine)		
		Phenelzine		

*Side-effect concerns.

◆ Evidence-based treatment recommendations regarding the use of hypnosis, acupuncture, transcutaneous electrical nerve stimulation (TENS), chiropractic or osteopathic cervical manipulation, occlusal adjustment, and hyperbaric oxygen as preventive or acute therapy for migraine are not yet possible.

Pharmacological preventive therapy

Medications have been put into treatment groups (Table 48.2) based on their established clinical efficacy, significant adverse events (AEs), safety profiles, and the experience of the US Headache Consortium participants.

Group 1. Proven high efficacy and mild to moderate AEs.
Group 2. Lower efficacy (that is, limited number of studies, studies reporting conflicting results, efficacy suggesting only 'modest' improvement) and mild to moderate AEs.
Group 3. Use based on opinion, not randomized controlled trials: (a) low to moderate AEs; (b) frequent or severe AEs, safety concerns, or complex management.
Group 4. Proven efficacy; frequent or severe AEs (or safety concerns), or complex management.
Group 5. Proven to have limited or no efficacy.

Conclusion

The evidence-based analysis on the role of neuroimaging in migraine and the efficacy and safety of migraine therapies is one of the first and most extensive cooperative projects available for creating practice parameters across disciplines. These four evidence-based reviews reflect the high level of concern physicians have for the migraine patient, and the need for improving care across disciplines. These guidelines are intended to improve care and outcomes for all migraine sufferers. Hopefully, these evidence-based treatment guidelines for the migraine patient will be widely disseminated and provide a basis for future outcomes research.

References

1. Silberstein SD, Rosenberg J. Multispecialty consensus on diagnosis and treatment of headache. *Neurology* 2000; **54,** 1553.
2. Matchar DB, Young WB, Rosenberg JA, *et al.* (2000). Evidence-based guidelines for migraine headache in the primary care setting: pharmacological management of acute attacks. http://www.aan.com
3. Frishberg B, Rosenberg JH, Matchar DB, Pietrzak MP, Rozen TD (2000). Evidence-based guidelines in the primary care setting: neuroimaging in patients with nonacute headache. http://www.aan.com

4. McCrory DC, Matchar DB, Rosenberg JH, Silberstein SD (2000). Evidence-based guidelines for migraine headache: overview of program description and methodology. http://www.neurology.org

5. Campbell JK, Penzien D, Wall EM (2000). Evidence-based guidelines for migraine headache: behavioral and physical treatments. http://www.neurology.org

6. Ramadan NM, Silberstein SD, Freitag FG, Gilbert TT, Frishberg BM (2000). Evidence-based guidelines for migraine headache in the primary care setting: pharmacological management for prevention of migraine. http//www.neurology.org

7. Gray RN, McCrory DC, Eberlein K, Westman EC, Hasselblad V (1999). Self-administered drug treatments for acute migraine headache. Prepared for the Agency for Health Care Policy and Research, Contract No. 290–94–2025 (Technical Review 2.4, February). Available from the National Technical Information Service, Accession No. 127854.

8. Gray RN, McCrory DC, Eberlein K, Westman EC, Hasselblad V (1999). Parenteral drug treatments for acute migraine headache. Prepared for the Agency for Health Care Policy and Research, Contract No. 290–94–2025 (Technical Review 2.5, February). Available from the National Technical Information Service, Accession No. 127862.

9. Gray RN, Goslin RE, McCrory DC, Eberlein K, Tulsky J, Hasselblad V (1999). Drug treatments for the prevention of migraine headache. Prepared for the Agency for Health Care Policy and Research, Contract No. 290–94–2025 (Technical Review 2.3, February). Available from the National Technical Information Service, Accession No. 127953.

10. Goslin RE, Gray RN, McCrory DC, Penzien D, Rains J, Hasselblad V (1999). Behavioral and physical treatments for migraine headache. Agency for Health Care Policy and Research Contract No. 290–94–2025. National Technical Information Service Accession No. 127946.

49 Model interventions to improve headache outcomes in health-care systems

Morris Maizels

Introduction

Migraine afflicts over 10% of the population annually,[1] causing significant disability to the individual as well as to society. Direct health-care costs of migraine in the USA have been estimated to approximate US $1 billion, with indirect costs of $13 billion.[2]

Despite its high prevalence, impact on quality of life, and economic impact, migraine remains underdiagnosed and undertreated. In a population-based survey, only 50% of individuals who met International Headache Society (IHS) criteria for migraine had been diagnosed—an increase compared to 40% a decade earlier.[3] Similarly, only about 50% of patients who fulfil IHS criteria for migraine and see a physician for headache are accurately diagnosed.[4]

While migraine remains underdiagnosed and undertreated, other potentially life-threatening conditions share a similar fate. Fewer than 25% of hypertensives are well-controlled,[5] and 40% of diabetics do not have regular testing of glycohaemoglobin levels.[6] Several studies confirm that primary care physicians identify less than half of patients who meet criteria for major depressive disorder, and adequately treat only a portion of those.[7]

Traditional attempts to improve physician adherence to recommended standards have focused on education, promotion of guidelines, and, in hospital settings, critical care pathways. While guidelines do tend to lead to change in the desired direction, the amount of change is variable. Physicians who reported familiarity with Joint National Commission guidelines were consistently more likely to report lower blood pressure thresholds for treatment.[8] In general, however, guidelines from consensus development conferences are unlikely to influence care unless other factors promoting change are present.[9] Factors that increase the probability that a guideline will be effective include: internal development, dissemination as part of a specific educational intervention, and an implementation strategy using a patient-specific reminder at the time of consultation.[10]

One important barrier to appropriate primary care for any given condition is the multiplicity of concerns that a patient may raise at a single clinical visit. Klinkman attempts to explain the undertreatment of psychological disorders by examining the 'competing demands in primary care'.[7] In this model, numerous factors influence the recognition of the presenting problem. After making a risk assessment, the clinician may choose to treat, refer, temporize, or ignore the problem. For headache, it has been shown that an assessment of disability increases the likelihood that the problem will be evaluated, rather than ignored.[11]

Two possible approaches to improve headache care are: (1) organized programmes within health-care systems; and (2) improved methods for primary care physicians to treat headache patients.

Headache and managed care

Managed care organizations (MCOs) in the USA have the ability both to systematically organize and improve care, as well as to attempt to control costs by influencing or controlling physician behaviour. However, recent publicity for MCOs has focused on the withholding or restricting of services. In regard to migraine, some managed care plans limit the number of doses per month of triptan for which they will pay, or require patients to fail non-triptan therapy before covering triptan therapy (failure of step-care).

The 'competing demands' model for primary care (above) may be a useful model with which to explain managed care behaviour as well. Because numerous conditions are undertreated, MCOs also may decide to 'treat, temporize, refer, or ignore'. Conditions that receive priority are those: (1) that can be treated more cost-efficiently (for example, reducing hospital days for chest pain admissions); (2) where outside regulatory agencies (government and industry) demand demonstration of care (for example, mammography rates, use of beta-blockers after myocardial infarction); or (3) where the public demands certain services even though they are not national priorities (for example, teenage clinics).

In an attempt to improve care systematically for certain 'sentinel' conditions, MCOs have embraced the model of disease management. Disease management has been integrated into the health-care system for costly and life-threatening conditions such as diabetes mellitus, congestive heart failure, and coronary artery disease. One study of a health maintenance organization (HMO) documented that migraineurs generated nearly twice the number of medical claims, 2.5 times the number of pharmacy claims, and had an increased overall cost of 50% per member.[12] However, migraine has not yet been widely recognized as a condition whose care merits systematic attention.

Triptans are not disease management

Much of the published literature involving managed care has focused on the phar-macoeconomics of triptans. However, the use of triptans should not be confused with disease management for migraine. Further, while the use of sumatriptan and other triptans has clearly been shown to be cost-effective for restoring work pro-ductivity,[13-15] their impact on health resource utilization and cost is less clear. Proponents of triptans enthusiastically cite studies purporting to show a claimed bene-ficial impact of sumatriptan on health resource utilization and cost.[16] These studies have several limitations, including open-label design, failure to account for other factors that impact on outcome, reliance on patient recall, and indirect measures of cost.[17-21] A careful review of these studies by this author found little documentation to sub-stantiate actual overall cost savings resulting from the use of triptans.

Disease management

Disease management refers to the use of an explicit systematic population-based approach to identify persons at risk, intervene proactively, and measure out-comes.[22] Another definition of disease management is '...the continuous process of identifying and delivering the most efficient combination of resources for the treat-ment or prevention of disease, within a selected patient population'.[23] Disease management implies two important paradigm shifts away from the classic medical model: from acute care to chronic care, and from the model of one physician/one patient to a multidisciplinary team caring for a population of patients.

Principles of evidence-based medicine may be applied to the development of a disease management programme. From this perspective, four components are required: an integrated health-care delivery system; a comprehensive knowledge base regarding the condition; sophisticated information systems; and continuous quality improvement methods.[24] Solomon has reviewed the principles of disease management as applied to migraine (Table 49.1).[25]

Group models of care

Group models of medical care are well-suited for disease management programmes. Group models are based on the fact that patients with similar conditions (for example, diabetes) or similar demographics and needs (for example, the elderly) may receive both education and support in a group setting. Group models are widely used for psychological therapies. Johnson and Thorn reported that outcomes in patients with chronic headaches who received cognitive behavioural therapy in a group were similar to those in patients who received individual therapy.[26]

Scharff and Marcus reported on 35 patients with refractory headache who parti-cipated in an integrated, interdisciplinary approach.[27] The programme involved 5 weekly 3-hour sessions. The first hour was education led by a neurologist, the

Table 49.1 Key concepts to develop a disease management programme for migraine. (Adapted with permission from ref. 25)

Set appropriate goals:
Reduce overall costs
◆ reduce ED visits
◆ reduce pharmacy costs
Improve patient quality-of-life
Reduce workplace loss

Identify target populations:
ED records
Pharmacy profiles
Computer diagnostic coding
Disability rosters
General population

Components of care—proactive interventions
Algorithms
◆ diagnostic
◆ therapeutic
Quality of life/disability instruments
Education
◆ patients
◆ physicians
◆ staff
Multidisciplinary team
Referral guidelines

Continuous quality improvement
Outcomes measures (goals)
Patient/physician satisfaction

second by a physical therapist, and in the third, a psychologist taught progressive muscle relaxation or autogenic training, as well as principles of cognitive therapy. Over 70% of treated patients experienced a 50% or greater reduction in headaches at 6-month follow-up, and there was an average reduction in medication use of 71%. In a comparable group of patients who declined group treatment, only 26% had 50% or greater improvement.

The medical group model has been developed and integrated within Kaiser Permanente, an HMO with approximately 9 million members, mostly in the western USA. The model, known as the Cooperative Health Care Clinic (CHCC), initially targeted geriatric patients who were high utilizers of health care. Based on the model's success, it has expanded to become the foundation for high-risk patient management programmes, including programmes for diabetes mellitus, asthma, hypertension, hyperlipidaemia, congestive heart failure, depression, anxiety, irritable bowel syndrome, chronic fatigue syndrome, fibromyalgia, and now headache and others.[28] Outcomes of improved function and quality of life and fewer hospital days and emergency department visits are consistently shown.

Several group models for headache care have been developed within Kaiser Permanente. A description of the author's programme, as well as outcomes data, is detailed below.

The Woodland Hills Headache Clinic

The Woodland Hills facility serves a population of 160 000 members. All patients referred for headache (excepting cluster headache, acute headaches, young children, and patients where there is a concern for secondary causes) are first evaluated and educated in a group format. In addition to physician referrals, headache patients are recruited from emergency department (ED) rosters, and triptan over-utilizers are identified by the pharmacy. Up to 20 patients are scheduled and about 15 patients attend each group, which is held every other week. The model is efficient in terms of reducing the impact of 'no show' patients, a particular problem with patients who are narcotic-dependent. It also allows the delivery of education with group interaction, which appears more effective than an individual model, in particular for patients with chronic headache and medication overuse.

At the group, patients first complete a headache history as well as psychological screening forms. A registered nurse practitioner (RNP) then leads the group. Patients are asked to introduce themselves, and make some brief comment about their headaches. The didactic session covers migraine pathophysiology, triggers, and medication use, but focuses on medication overuse. Follow-up consultations are scheduled with the RNP or with a physician.

The results of the first 13 months of the Woodland Hills Headache Clinic are summarized in ref. 29. Two hundred and sixty-four patients attended 25 Headache Clinic classes between April 1999 and April 2000, and 233 had follow-up consultations (95 with the RNP and 138 with the physician). Pharmacy profiles were reviewed for 264 patients, and charts were available for review on 250.

The cost of triptans (and dihydroergotamine (DHE)) increased US $5423 (19%) for the 6-month follow-up period, while headache-related visits were reduced by 193/606 (32%), and headache-related emergency department (ED) visits were reduced by 126/256 (49%) (Fig. 49.1). Nearly all of the increase in triptan cost was accounted for by those patients who were not previously receiving triptans ($n = 44$, $10 359, mean $235, approximately 4 doses of triptan/month). High triptan utilizers had savings of $5198 ($n = 24$, mean $236).

Comparing patients by frequency of clinic visits, the greatest reduction in clinic visits was in the 75 patients who had made more than 2 visits in the previous 6 months (total 427 visits, mean 5.7), whose visits decreased by 46% in the following 6 months. This group also had the highest mean triptan costs ($124) at baseline, which rose (mean $20) 6 months later.

ED visits were reduced from 256 to 130 (49%). The proportion of headache-related visits to the ED fell from 256/606 (42%) visits to 130/413 (31%).

One hundred and thirty patients did not receive any triptan prescription before or after the clinic consultation. Compared to patients who received triptans, even reater reductions in headache-related visits (124/318, 39%) and ED visits (77/127, 61%) were seen.

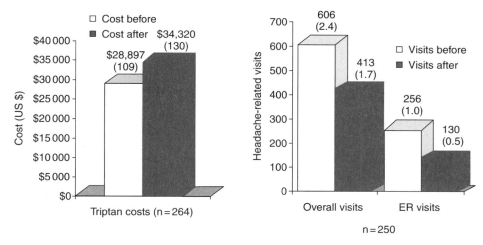

Fig. 49.1   Change in triptan costs and headache-related visits 6 months before and after headache group visit and consultation.

Table 49.2   Brief Headache Screen (BHS)

Please answer the following questions about your headaches:

1. How often do you get *severe* headaches (difficult or unable to continue normal function)?
   daily or   3–4 days/   2/week–   1/month   almost
   near daily   week   2/month   or less   never

2. How often do you get mild or less severe headaches?
   daily or   3–4 days/   2/week–   1/month   almost
   near daily   week   2/month   or less   never

3. How often do you take pain relievers, or any medication to relieve headache symptoms?
   daily or   3–4 days/   2/week–   1/month   almost
   near daily   week   2/month   or less   never

4. How often do you miss some work or leisure time because of headache?
   daily or   3–4 days/   2/week–   1/month   almost
   near daily   week   2/month   or less   never

5. Are you satisfied with the current medication you use to relieve your headaches?
   yes   no

6. Are you taking daily prescription medication to prevent headaches?
   yes   no

   If no, do your headaches trouble you enough to take daily preventive medication?
   yes   no

Thank you for answering these questions.

Clinical outcomes were measured categorically with the Brief Headache Screen (BHS; Table 49.2). Of 91 patients reporting severe headaches 3–7 days/week at baseline, 6-month follow-up data were received from 72(73%): 62(86%) reported less frequent severe headaches, with 55 (76%) reporting 2 days/week or less and 27(37.5%) having severe headaches once/month or less.

Patients recruited from the ED represented 21% of the Headache Clinic cohort, but accounted for $8392/$26787 (31%) of the group's triptan costs and 276/606 (46%) of headache-related visits at intake. At 6-month follow-up, triptan costs rose $2253 (27%, mean $43), with a decrease of 83 (45%) ED visits.

Within this HMO, there is no assigned cost for office or ED visits. An estimated cost of $60 for office visits and $100 for ED visits was derived. Based on these estimates, reduced visits to the clinic ($11 580) and ED ($12 600) yielded savings of $24 180. With the increase of triptan costs of $5423, the programme overall generated estimated savings of $18 757.

Primary care—'the last frontier'

Despite the success of the group model, it is unlikely that health resources would ever expand to allow specialist care for most headache patients, who comprise over 15% of the general population. Therefore, improving the care at a primary care level, as well as improving patient self-care, remain important mandates. Attempts to improve primary care for headache must account for the 'competing demands' in primary care (above).

The author recently reviewed care given to headache patients at an ED staffed by primary care physicians.[30] Only 33% of patients discharged with nonmigraine diagnoses had enough information documented to exclude migraine as the diagnosis. Eighty-six patients of the total cohort received follow-up telephone interviews. Of 59 patients recognized by ED physicians as having migraine, 20 (34%) had chronic or transformed migraine, of whom 18 (31%) were associated with medication overuse. Of 27 patients not diagnosed as migraine, 18 (67%) fulfilled IHS criteria for migraine, and 6 had chronic headache with migraine—only 3 had nonmigraine diagnoses.

It appears then that many primary care physicians are not familiar with the criteria for the diagnosis of migraine developed by the IHS. Simpler paradigms have been suggested. Solomon found that by requiring three of the following criteria—unilateral, throbbing, nausea, or light and noise sensitivity—one would have a sensitivity of 79% and specificity of 95%.[31]

A Brief Headache Screen (BHS) has been developed by the author (Table 49.2). The tool was initially developed to aid in population management programmes, but is being explored as a new paradigm for primary care diagnosis of migraine. The diagnostic portion of the BHS relies on the frequency of severe headaches (question 1), mild headaches (question 2), and medication use (question 3) to generate diagnoses. Patients with episodic severe headache are labelled as migraine. Patients with severe and/or mild headaches ≥ 3 days/week are labelled as having chronic daily headache; patients identified by question 1 as having migraine are labelled as chronic headache

Table 49.3 Relative contribution of each of three screening questions to: (1) identify migraine (question 1); (2) distinguish chronic migraine from episodic migraine (combination of questions 1 and 2); and (3) correctly label migraine with or without medication overuse (questions 1–3). The positive predictive value of episodic severe headache for migraine is 290/(290+19)=19% and that of episodic or daily severe headache for migraine is 337(337+36) 90%. The negative predictive value of episodic severe headache for migraine is 32/(32+53)=38% and that of episodic or daily severe headache for migraine is 15/(15+6)=71%

| | Number (%) correctly identified | | | |
| | Question 1 | | | |
	Severe 1–3	Severe 1–4	Questions 1+2	Questions 1+2+3
Any migraine (n=343)	290 (86)	337 (98)		
Episodic migraine (n=146)	—	—	78 (53)	62 (42)
Chronic migraine (n=197)*	—	—	184 (93)	168 (85)
Chronic migraine*†				
With medication overuse (n=169)	—	—	—	146 (86)
Without medication overuse (n=28)	—	—	—	22 (79)
Not migraine (n=51)	32 (63)	15 (29)	—	—

*Patients who have severe or mild headache 3 or more days/week are labelled as: chronic migraine if question 1 indicates migraine.
†Medication overuse is defined as symptomatic medication use 3 or more days/week.

with migraine. Medication overuse is recognized by use of symptomatic medication ≥ 3 days/week.

The BHS has been evaluated in 399 patients in three settings: an ED, a Family Practice department, and a Headache Clinic (Table 49.3).[32] The criterion of episodic disabling headache correctly identified migraine in 136/146 (94%) of patients with episodic migraine, and 154/197 (78%) of patients with chronic headache with migraine, with a specificity of 32/51 (63%). The combination of episodic or daily severe headache identified migraine in 100% of patients with chronic migraine. Only 7/343 (1.7%) of patients with migraine were not identified by disabling headache. The combination of severe and mild headache frequency was sensitive to daily headache syndromes in 218/232 (94%) with specificity of 87/162 (54%). Medication overuse was correctly identified in 164/182 (90%) with specificity of 129/207 (62%).

The BHS may serve as a useful paradigm for primary care physicians. Migraine is rapidly recognized as an episodic disabling headache. Daily headache syndromes are recognized but require further evaluation. All headache patients are rapidly screened for medication overuse.

The patient as the primary care provider

Ultimately, it is the patient who has the most to gain from proper treatment of headache. Education has long been considered a foundation of care for chronic disease. Computer-based technology and the internet make possible new approaches for diagnosis and treatment. The author is currently exploring the use of an internet-based headache assessment tool (a demonstration of the program may be seen at: http://www.allwebsoft.com/povss/laptop_demos/headache_expert). Patients may go on-line independently or complete the questionnaire by calling headache clinic personnel who read the questions over the phone. The diagnostic algorithm recognizes migraine and 'migrainous', transformed migraine; medication overuse; chronic and episodic tension-type headache; chronic, episodic, and atypical cluster headache; and various brief headache syndromes.

The program is designed to offer headache assessments, which are later reviewed by medical personnel. Non-physician personnel could readily be trained in its use. The program offers patients a significant opportunity to obtain an accurate headache diagnosis, and is a useful aid for disease management programmes. An ongoing research protocol uses the program to screen ED headache patients. Patients who receive a new diagnosis, such as migraine or medication overuse, are referred either to their primary care physician or to the headache clinic. Copies of the computer assessment are included.

Discussion

Managed care organizations have a unique opportunity to improve the care of headache patients. Programmes that are designed to reduce costs, such as by identifying triptan overutilizers, can improve the care of headache patients as well, if done in a clinically relevant manner. The two populations of headache patients who are most likely to benefit from proactive intervention are triptan overutilizers and ED headache patients.

The group appointment model has become the 'engine' for disease management programmes that might otherwise place an unacceptable burden on health system resources. Patients who are referred, or identified by proactive screening, can be educated and screened in a group environment, and then seen in follow-up consultation. Similar programmes would be difficult to implement without a group process.

Attempts to understand the 'healing' nature of the group process have yielded interesting findings. In an arthritis group, all subjects showed an increase in knowledge and desired behaviours compared to a control group, but improvement in health status did not correlate with either of these variables.[33] All patients who improved said that they felt they had more control over their symptoms. The psychological theory of self-efficacy has been explored as the basis for this finding.

Limitations of the group model should be mentioned. A group appointment would be difficult to initiate for an individual physician who is not part of a larger

Table 49.4 Multiaxial behavioural assessment of the headache patient (from ref. 34)

I	Headache diagnosis, frequency, severity
II	Analgesic or abortive use, overuse, and abuse
III	Behavioural and stress-related risk factors (triggers, aggravators)
IV	Comorbid psychiatric disorders
V	Functional impact and disability

medical group. Not all patients wish to participate in a group. However, nearly all patients who attend express high satisfaction with the programme. A certain amount of start-up effort is required to initiate a group, with administrative support. Finally, reimbursement issues for group visits remain. On the other hand, health plans that reimburse for actual ED costs would probably save substantially more than the amount calculated in the study quoted.

Because of competing demands, primary care physicians require more than conventional education in order to provide improved care for headache patients. Guidelines and paradigms should be expressly designed for these physicians and their practice environments. Field testing of these paradigms is important to document their utility.

Even when physicians recognize migraine, they frequently do not recognize reasons for refractory or difficult headache. A multiaxial assessment format, analogous to the psychiatric diagnostic system of the American Psychiatric Association *Diagnostic and statistical manual of mental disorders* (DSM-IV), has been proposed (Table 49.4).[34]

Conclusion

Migraine remains underdiagnosed and undertreated, despite advances in classification systems and treatment approaches. Principles of disease management can be applied to populations of patients with headache, with positive economic impact on the health-care system. Attempts to improve diagnosis and treatment also require paradigms that address the unique challenges of the primary care environment. Headache patient themselves may prove to be the ultimate resource for improving their own care.

Acknowledgement

The author's research cited in this manuscript was supported by educational grants as well as consultation from the Disease Management division of Merck & Co.

References

1. Breslau N, Rasmussen BK. The impact of migraine. Epidemiology, risk factors, and co-morbidities. *Neurology* 2001; **56** (Suppl. 1): S4–S12.
2. Hu HX, Markson LE, Lipton RB, Stewart WF, Berger ML. Burden of migraine in the United States: disability and economic costs. *Arch Intern Med* 1999; **159**: 813–18.
3. Lipton RB, Diamond S, Reed M, Diamond ML, Stewart WF. Migraine diagnosis and treatment: results from the American Migraine study II. *Headache* 2001; **41**: 638–45.
4. Stang PE, Osterhaus JT, Celentano DD. Migraine: Patterns of healthcare use. *Neurology* 1994; **44** (Suppl. 4): S47–S55.
5. Stockwell DH, Madhavan S, Cohen H, Gibson G, Alderman MH. The determinants of hypertensions awareness, treatment, and control in an insured population. *Am J Public Hlth* 1994; **84**: 1768–74.
6. Anderson D. Managed care meets the diabetes-management challenge. *Bus Hlth* 1996; **14** (1, Suppl. A): 19–21.
7. Klinkman MS. Competing demands in psychosocial care: a model for the identification and treatment of depressive disorders in primary care. *Gen Hosp Psychiatry* 1997; **19**: 98–111.
8. Hyman DJ, Pavlik VN. Self-reported hypertension treatment practices among primary care physicians: blood pressure thresholds, drug choices, and the role of guidelines and evidence-based medicine. *Arch Intern Med* 2000; **160**: 2281–6.
9. Haines A, Feder G. Guidance on guidelines: writing them is easier than making them work. *Br Med J* 1992; **305**: 785–6.
10. Grimshaw JM, Russell IT. Effect of clinical guidelines on medical practice: a systematic review of rigorous evaluations. *Lancet* 1993; **342**: 1317–22.
11. Holmes WF, MacGregor A, Dodick D. Migraine-related disability: impact and implications for sufferers' lives and clinical issues. *Neurology* 2001; **56** (Suppl. 1): S13–S19.
12. Clouse JC, Osterhaus JT. Healthcare resource use and costs associated with migraine in a managed healthcare setting. *Ann Pharmacother* 1994; **28**: 659–64.
13. Schulman EA, Cady RK, Henry D, *et al.* Effectiveness of sumatriptan in reducing productivity loss due to migraine: results of a randomized, double-blind, placebo-controlled clinical trial. *Mayo Clin Proc* 2000; **75**: 782–9.
14. Cady RK, Ryan R, Jhingran P, O'Quinn S, Pait DG. Sumatriptan injection reduces productivity loss during a migraine attack: results of a double-blind, placebo-controlled trial. *Arch Intern Med* 1998; **158**: 1013–18.
15. Legg R, Sclar D, Nemec NL, Tarnai J, Mackowiak, JI. Cost benefit of sumatriptan to an employer. *J Occup Environ Med* 1997; **39**: 652–7.
16. Warshaw LJ, Burton WN, Silberstein SD, Lipton RB. Migraine: a problem for employers and managed care plans. *Am J Man Care* 1997; **3**: 1515–23.
17. Legg RL, Sclar DA, Nemec NL, Tarnai J, Mackowiak JI. Cost-effectiveness of sumatriptan in a managed care population. *Am J Man Care* 1997; **3**: 117–22.
18. Greiner DL, Addy SN. Sumatriptan use in a large group-model health maintenance organization. *Am J Hlth-Syst Pharm* 1996; **53**: 633–8.
19. Streator SE, Shearer SW. Pharmacoeconomic impact of injectable sumatriptan on migraine-associated healthcare costs. *Am J Man Care* 1996; **2**: 139–43.
20. Cohen JA, Beall D, Beck A, *et al.* Sumatriptan treatment for migraine in a health maintenance organization: economic, humanistic, and clinical outcomes. *Clin Therapeut* 1999; **21**: 190–204.
21. Lofland JH, Johnson NE, Batenhorst AS, Nash DB. Changes in resource use and outcomes for patients with migraine treated with sumatriptan: a managed care perspective. *Arch Intern Med* 1999; **159**: 857–63.

22. Epstein RS, Sherwood LM. From outcomes research to disease management: a guide for the perplexed. *Ann Intern Med* 1996; **124**: 832–7.
23. Kozma CM, Kaa KA, Reeder CE. A model for comprehensive disease state management. *J Outcomes Manage* 1977; 4–8.
24. Ellrodt G, Cook DJ, Lee J, Cho M, Hunt D, Weingarten S. Evidence-based disease management. *J Am Med Assoc* 1997; **278**: 1687–92.
25. Solomon GD. Interventions and outcomes management in migraine. *Dis Manage Hlth Outcomes* 1998; **3**: 183–90.
26. Johnson PR, Thorn BE. Cognitive behavioral treatment of chronic headache: group versus individual treatment format. *Headache* 1989; **29**: 358–65.
27. Scharff L, Marcus DA. Interdisciplinary outpatient group treatment of intractable headache. *Headache* 1994; **34**: 73–8.
28. Noffsinger EB, Scott JC. Understanding today's group visit models. *Group Practice J* 2000; **49**: 46–58.
29. Maizels M, Saenz V, Wirjo J. Impact of a group-based model of disease management for headache. Manuscript submitted.
30. Maizels M. Evaluation and treatment of headache patients by primary care physicians in an emergency department in the era of triptans. *Arch Intern Med* 2001; **161**: 1969–73.
31. Solomon S. Criteria for the diagnosis of migraine in clinical practice. *Headache* 1991; **31**: 384–7.
32. Maizels M, Burchette R. A rapid and sensitive paradigm for screening headache patients in primary care settings. Manuscript submitted.
33. Lorig K, Gonzalez V. The integration of theory with practice: a 12-year study. *Hlth Educ Quart* 1992; **19**: 355–68.
34. Lake AE. Behavioral and nonpharmacologic treatments of headache. *Med Clin N Am* 2001; **85**: 1055–75.

50 Model interventions to improve headache outcomes in the workplace

Walter F. Stewart and Richard B. Lipton

Introduction

There is growing evidence and recognition that migraine and a host of other conditions cost employers in lost work time. In a phrase, health is related to productivity. In this chapter, we address the challenging issue of what employers can do to reduce lost work time from illnesses in general, and specifically from migraine. We begin by defining what the term 'intervention' means since this encompasses any effort that is made to alter the course of an illness in a population. Work-related interventions do not emerge in a vacuum. We consider what motivates such programmes and how headache, as a health problem, measures up. To frame a model intervention, we next consider what employers and employees need and then describe the elements of a programme that addresses these needs. Throughout the discussion it is important to recognize that over 80% of individuals who work for pay throughout the world, including most Western countries, work in a setting or complex with fewer than 500 employees. As such, most workplaces do not have an on-site nurse, physician, or other allied health professional. Recognizing this fact, we consider a model intervention programme that addresses the broad interest of those who work for pay, rather than confine ourselves to work settings where there are substantial on-site health resources that can be brought to bear.

Work-related intervention: what does it mean?

In this chapter the term 'work-related intervention' is used to mean the implementation of a programme designed to reduce the impact of illnesses on ability to work. Those who work for pay are the target population of interest and the goal is to reduce lost productive time from illness. Model interventions may be deployed inside or outside of the workplace. The focus on lost productive time as an endpoint does not necessarily imply that the intervention is confined to a workplace setting. Other factors dictate what is optimal and include the receptivity of the target population, logistics, and costs. For this reason, we use the term 'work-related' intervention, not 'workplace' intervention. The latter implies that the intervention is focused on the employee's worksite. Finally, a work-related intervention pro-gramme is not an experiment where employees are provided with atypical incentives (for example, financial remuneration to participate as is typical of clinical trials) or where unusual efforts are made to influence outcomes. An intervention must be pragmatic to be successful.

Why implement work-related interventions?

Employers bear a majority of the cost of health care used by employees, either in the form of insurance, taxes (for example, where government is the direct payer but the employer covers costs indirectly through taxes), or both. Health-care coverage for the employer can be viewed as both a cost that needs to be controlled and as an investment that needs to be effectively managed to gain a return. To view health care as an investment it is essential to look at both direct medical costs and indirect costs in the form of lost productive time. As an investment, employers are looking for cost-effective approaches to the use of health care to improve the outcomes of employees. In particular, health problems that interfere with ability to work (that is, either time lost from work or reduced performance at work) are sensible targets for re-directing health-care resources. If lost productive time is reduced, then employ-ers are the economic beneficiary. The conditions and illnesses that have an impact on work are also likely to be important candidates for improving the efficacy of medical care, since interference with ability to perform activities is often a strong motivation for seeking care. The challenge to employers is to redirect health care and deploy programmes that mitigate the impact that selected health conditions have on work.

In this context, the workplace itself does not define the nature of the interven-tion, nor should an intervention be confined in this way. A focus on work does, however, afford an unique opportunity to communicate with and redirect health care to a targeted and captured population in a manner that may not be feasible in the general population. A 'work-related' intervention makes the best use of direct cost expenditures in order to reduce indirect costs. How this is achieved depends on the clinical conditions, work culture, local medical care system, and available sup-plementary resources (for example, on-site medical staff, information technology, etc.), but is not dependent on deployment through on-site clinics. A work-related intervention programme encompasses awareness and education campaigns with the intention of improving efficacy of care and access to the most effective care as soon as possible.

Selecting conditions for intervention: does migraine measure up?

A number of conditions are known to cause lost time from work and to reduce performance at work. It is not feasible or sensible for an employer or health plan to simultaneously launch interventions for all such conditions. Ultimately, the employer bears most of the cost of any intervention, either directly or indirectly, and must be convinced that there are tangible benefits from such an investment. What criteria drive employer interests?

Use of medical care is often motivated by the extent to which a health problem interferes with the ability of individuals to function in their primary roles (that is, work, household, social, etc.) of interest. Functioning in the work role is of direct interest to employers. When impaired function persists due to illness, an employer loses revenues. For a specific illness, two factors drive employer interest: the overall indirect cost burden of the illness in an employed population and the opportunity to successfully reduce the burden.

Prevalence of illness, frequency and duration of episodes of decreased functioning, and the average amount of lost work time per episode drive the indirect cost of illness. It is not surprising, therefore, that the more common conditions are those with the highest indirect costs. Using data from a recent US national survey, the American Productivity Audit, a number of chronic episodic[1] illnesses are both common and associated with a significant number of hours per week of lost work time (see Fig. 50.1; chronic illnesses such as diabetes and congestive heart failure are associated with persistent progressive changes and pose a significant direct and indirect cost burden to employers; data on these and other conditions are not displayed

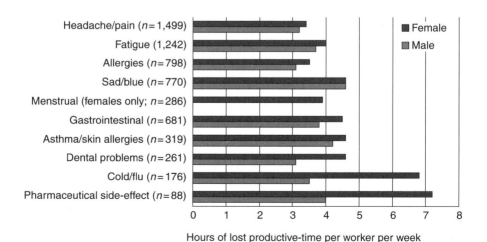

Hours of lost productive-time per worker per week

Fig. 50.1   Mean hours of lost productive-time per worker per week among those reporting specific health conditions in The American Productivity Audit, 2001.

in Fig. 50.1). Whether a specific condition poses a cost burden to an employer will depend, in part, on the demographic profile of the workforce. Medical conditions are not uniformly distributed in the population and, for example, may predominate in one or the other gender (for example, migraine) or younger or older populations (for example, arthritis).

Indirect cost burden alone is not sufficient to consider whether an intervention is worthwhile. Even in defined working populations where specific conditions pose a significant cost burden, it may not be possible to influence patient outcomes in a cost-effective manner. Finally, conditions that are the best candidate for intervention will also depend on the following factors.

♦ There is a substantial opportunity gap, that is, the size of the gap between what employees currently experience (for example, effectiveness of care, probability of a successful outcome) and what they can practically achieve. The larger the gap, the greater is the opportunity to use direct costs expenditures to reduce indirect costs. In general, only a portion of the lost work-time associated with an illness can be recovered. Data from clinical trials provides the most credible proof of what can be recovered.
♦ There is a good likelihood that low-cost interventions can be developed to fill the gap.
♦ Interventions can be successfully implemented.
♦ Interventions are acceptable. Some conditions, for example, depression, pose significant challenges because of stigma and privacy and confidentiality concerns.

How does headache measure up (Table 50.1)? In this context it is worth considering migraine headache specifically, since a substantial share of the indirect cost of illness from headache is caused by migraine. Migraine headache is very common with a prevalence of 12% in the population, 17% among women and 6% among men.[1] Migraine is more prevalent between the ages of 25 and 50 years, the age band when people are likely to be most productive at work. Migraine attacks are frequent. The median episode rate among studies is about one attack per month.[2] In addition, lost work time per episode is high. Among those with migraine, about 1.5 hours are lost per week from headache. Approximately, 40% of the migraine sufferers who work for pay account for 75% of the lost work time.[3] The indirect cost burden from migraine is substantial (US $13 billion in the USA) compared to the direct cost of care.[4] Finally, there is substantial evidence from population-based studies to indicate that migraine headache is undertreated, even for those who are disabled by their attacks,[5] and, as with most conditions, patient are likely to benefit from education on the development of self-management skills. The contrast in relative cost burden combined with evidence on the existing gap in care opens opportunities for success. Evidence from clinical trials suggest that the use of triptans reduces the impact of migraine on work (see Chapter 40, this volume). While rigorous measures of lost time or productivity were not used in most work-related studies of triptans, the evidence consistently supports an indirect cost treatment benefit. Recent evidence suggests that the benefits from triptans may be

Table 50.1 Evaluation of migraine headache as a candidate for work-related intervention

Criteria	Evaluation of migraine
Condition must be sufficiently prevalent in a working population to pose a burden and opportunity	Migraine affects approximately 17% of women and 6% of men. It is most prevalent at ages of peak productivity
Condition must cause substantial lost productive time and related indirect costs	Migraine attacks are frequent (median of 1/month) and on average cause 1.5 hours of lost work time per week. In the US alone, migraine is estimated to cost employers US$13 billion dollars a year in lost productive time
There must be an opportunity gap	It is well established that migraine is underdiagnosed and undertreated even among individuals who are incapacitated by attacks. Even among those who seek care, individuals often lapse from care because it is ineffective
Effective and low-cost interventions can be devised to fill the gap	There are four points of influence for migraine: consumer education; behavioural self-management; acute treatment; and preventive treatment. Patient education and behavioural management strategies are well developed. While individuals vary in their response to specific treatments, there are a broad range of acute and preventive treatments available for migraine. Treatments consistently reduce the impact of headaches on functioning and reduce the frequency of attacks. Growing evidence indicates that they reduce lost productive time. In addition, patients are likely to benefit from systematic education
Successful solutions can be implemented, including acceptability and use of solutions	To be determined
The aggregate benefits of the intervention programme as measured in reduced lost productive time must outweigh any increase in direct costs	To be determined

underestimated, especially if the treatment is taken when the headache is mild in contrast to what is usual, when the headache is moderate to severe.[6] This type of evidence represents only one aspect of the benefit of any intervention. A work-related programme must provide treatment management as part of a larger programme that encompasses patient education and acquisition of self-management skills.

Migraine headache certainly measures up in terms of the indirect cost burden that it poses to employers and the benefits of treatment. Whether there is a substantial gap in care and opportunity depends on local health-care conditions and the demographics of an employer's workforce. Work-related interventions for migraine will favour working populations who are female or younger (that is, <45 years of age).

What do employers need?

Employers are in the business of producing goods and services. In so doing, they *measure and manage* processes to ensure that production quality and deadlines are met. This is done to use resources in the most effective manner to achieve short- and long-term production and profit goals. Successful employers develop and use metrics, since they recognize that quality measurements are the foundation of good management. While most employers recognize that health problems have an impact on ability to work, they choose to do nothing. This is the rational response since employers do not have the means to measure the impact that health problems have on lost productive time.

To define the impact of health problems on work and to measure the benefits of intervention, employers need a clearly defined metric. For this purpose, we recommend lost productive time as the metric of choice, instead of productivity. Productivity and productive work time are related (Fig. 50.2). Productivity, the amount of goods and services generated per unit paid time, is influenced by both the amount of productive time available and a host of business factors that are outside the control

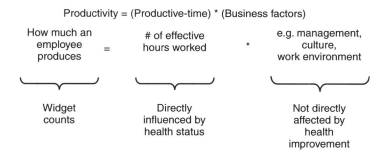

Fig. 50.2   Relation between productivity and productive work time.

of a worker (for example, work environment, scheduled demand, management style and procedures, compensation, etc.). These business factors are not influenced by health problems. Moreover, interventions designed to improve health outcomes do not influence these business factors; productivity *per se* is therefore a poor measure of the benefits of a health intervention. Interventions directly influence how much time a worker is available to produce. Whether this time is effectively managed is the responsibility of the employer and managers, not the health-care system. For this reason, productive-time and its complement, lost productive-time, are metrics that directly measure the impact of health on work. Lost productive-time, has two components: missed time (that is, missed days or missed hours during a day of work) from work and effective lost time while at work from reduced ability to perform, often referred to as 'presenteeism'. For most health problems, present-eeism is usually the dominant source of lost time and the most challenging to measure.

Employers also need convincing evidence that an intervention programme will be cost-effective. In brief, the evidence that is essential can often be boiled down to two important statistics. The cost of the intervention programme per employee per month and the reduction in lost work time (translated into a monetary figure) per employee per month that is achieved from the intervention. Employers want to know that the cost per month is less than the return in reduced lost time. In this framework, the cost per employee per month includes the cost of the intervention itself and the impact that the intervention has on short- and long-term direct costs (that is, use of health-care services).

It is likely that lost work-time among employees will be driven by more than one dominant illness and that more than one of these illnesses can be influenced by interventions. Employers will favour intervention strategies that address needs for multiple illnesses, rather than a single illness. Fragmented programmes increase the intervention cost per illness and do not take advantage of logistical factors that are common to any intervention (for example, communication costs). Moreover, the common illnesses that affect working populations are often comorbid. For example, migraine and depression are strongly comorbid.[7] These two conditions are among the most costly to employers and, together, have the greatest impact on health status and ability to function.[8] Interventions that address both illnesses offer the advantage of improving management and self-care among those who suffer from the comorbidity, individuals who are likely to account for a disproportionate share of both the direct and indirect costs. Interventions that are targeted to these individuals offer the greatest opportunity for gains. Moreover, these individuals warrant the most attention.

Finally, monitoring is critical to quality management. Employers need quantitative information to determine if the intervention is having any impact on costs. Specifically, employers need to know how direct costs are changing, the cost of the intervention, and if lost-work time from illnesses is declining. This information is an essential part of the ongoing cycle of the management process that is required to fully adapt any intervention to a non-experimental setting and the peculiarities of any defined working population.

What do employees need?

Ultimately, work-related intervention programmes must be designed to meet the needs of employees. Two very basic questions need to be answered. What do employees need and want and what will employees actually use? Meeting the needs and interests of employers is important but not sufficient for success. Meeting the needs of employees is both necessary and sufficient for an intervention to be successful. Defining what an employee wants is a 'two-way street'. It depends, in part, on what employees tell us and, in part, on their reaction to what is being offered. The intersection of the two is likely to be the optimal starting point for defining what the intervention should be.

One approach to defining what employees need is to evaluate the challenges they face in navigating the health-care system and in making effective use of services. There are a number of ways to define these challenges. One approach is to frame needs in terms of a 'barriers-to-medical-care' model (that is, the barriers that employees face in the health-care arena that interfere with successful health outcomes). An advantage of this approach is that it leads to tangible *points of influence* and intervention targets, namely, problems that need to be solved on behalf of an employee in using the health-care system. A model-based needs assessment is incomplete unless it is validated in some way. Focus groups and surveys of employees offer a direct means of validation. This type of supplementary information is useful in understanding what employees want from the health-care system, to measure their reaction to what is being offered by an intervention, and to understand their broader interests in health beyond what is currently offered by traditional care (for example, complementary medicine).

Individuals with migraine headache face three common barriers to achieving a successful outcome: they do not seek care; the care they seek is ineffective; or there is inadequate follow-up by the physician or follow-through by the patient (see Table 50.2 for details). Employees often face a somewhat invisible barrier to seeking care for a condition like migraine that is known to interfere with their ability to function. This barrier can occur because of:

♦   accommodation (that is, assumptions that the condition and state are normal);
♦   a perception that there is no solution;
♦   diminished motivation because of lack of success from past experience;
♦   inability to navigate the health-care system.

In part, the need for solutions to these barriers is defined by the gap between the health status of an employee (for example, diminished ability to function) and the opportunities for a successful health outcome. The opportunity for success begins with tools that motivate consumers to effectively seek care for their condition. On the face of it, tools such as MIDAS (Migraine Disability Assessment)[9] that motivate individuals in need to seek care will initially increase direct costs and may not serve an employer's interest in the short term. Whether or not this is a concern depends on a number of factors. First, employers will tolerate some increase in direct costs if

Table 50.2 Barriers-to-care and points of influence and intervention in migraine management

Description of barrier	Solution options	Success defined by
Barrier: Migraine sufferer is in need of care and should seek care		
Patient does not recognize the symptom or impact as abnormal	Severity tools (e.g., MIDAS) Personalized Health Risk assessment Targeted education	Self-awareness: patient is aware of illness and consequences
Patient does not recognize that there is a solution for the health problem	Targeted education	Patient recognizes needs and benefits of care
Patient is not motivated to seek care due to general (e.g. views of medical care) and specific (e.g. bad medical encounters) barriers	Personalized Health Risk assessment (MyBody™) Targeted education Comprehensive patient history tool that captures biopsychosocial factors (WeListen™)	Patient is motivated to seek care
Patient does not understand health-care system (e.g. insurance coverage) and how to navigate through the health-care system	Personalized insurance guide Health system Q&A	Patient identifies a care-provider and seeks care
Barrier: patient has an ineffective medical encounter		
Patient lacks skills to be an effective communicator in the medical setting	Health risk assessment linked to personalized notes on how to talk to and manage doctor Physician training on migraine diagnosis	Patient effectively communicates needs Patient has control over medical decision-making process
Patient receives inadequate or inappropriate care due to poor medical management	Patient education re: treatment options, expectations Targeted physician training on use of acute and preventative treatments and patient education	Care provider delivers optimal care
Patient receives care, but does not understand implications of care and his or her own role	Targeted efforts to improve self-efficacy	Patient feels empowered to care for self and understands optimal care regimen
Patient does not engage in appropriate self-management	Education and skill building through web-based tools	
Barrier: Poor follow-up by the physician or poor follow-through by the patient		
Patient receives quality care with understandable instructions, but fails to adhere to instructions	Proactive adherence tools	Patient adheres to treatment and plan for care
Patient does not follow-up with provider to ensure successful outcome	Targeted self-efficacy tools Personalized education retreatment regimen	Patient seeks follow-up as needed and achieves optimal care

they see results in reducing lost productive-time. Second, employees are more likely to be valued in tight labour markets and the notion that health care is an investment in labour is more acceptable to employers. Third, the time frame for assessing direct costs is important. While direct costs may increase in the short term, early intervention may both reduce the future direct cost of illness (for example, if migraines become more severe as care is delayed) and reduce indirect costs.

Even if employees use the health-care system, they face a number of challenges in achieving a successful outcome. Navigating the medical care system is complex, even for a sophisticated and well-informed consumer. Employees will be more successful if they are well equipped to use medical care services. For migraine specifically, physicians are not always aware of what migraine sufferers want.[10] Patients need to be educated on what to say to their doctor, what is appropriate care, and what to expect. Patients also need to be informed that they should take more control of their own care by acquiring knowledge and self-management skills to ultimately play a more active role. In general, interventions that make employees more effective are an asset to employers because they are likely to both decrease the need for care and increase satisfaction with care. Physicians need to be effectively educated about the elements of treatment guidelines[11] for headache and proven[12] and cost-effective methods[13] of patient management.

Up to this point, we have framed patient need in a barriers-to-care model. This is a starting point. The solutions that address employee needs must be validated. Specifically, this means ensuring that what will be offered is what employees want and, more importantly, will use. We need to avoid the pitfall of the 'if we build it they will come' philosophy and ensure that the priorities that are addressed are shaped by what employees want.

Conclusions

Implementing a model work-related intervention programme for migraine headache is challenging. Research over the last 10 years has led to substantial advances in improving migraine management and in devising solutions for a number of the barriers that migraine patients face in achieving more successful outcomes. However, substantial gaps remain in translating research into practice and, in particular, in making practice relevant to employer and employee needs. Model work-related intervention programmes are likely to emerge by first addressing the needs of all stake-holders and from the testing of pragmatic and cost-effective solutions.

References

1. Stewart WF, Lipton RB, Celentano DD, Reed ML. Prevalence of migraine headache in the United States. *J Am Med Assoc* 1992; **267** (1): 64–9.
2. Stewart WF, Shechter A, Lipton RB. Migraine heterogeneity: disability, pain intensity, and attack frequency and duration. *Neurology* 1994; **44** (Suppl. 4): S24–S39.

3. Von Korff M, Stewart WF, Simon D, Lipton RB. Migraine and reduced work perform-ance: a population-based diary study. *Neurology* 1998; **50**: 1741–5.

4. Hu HX, Markson LE, Lipton RB, Stewart WF, Berger ML. Disability and economic costs of migraine in the United States: a population-based approach. *Arch Intern Med* 1999; **159**: 813–18.

5. Lipton, RB, Stewart WF, Simon D. Medical consultation for migraine: results from the American Migraine Study. *Headache* 1998; **38**: 87–96.

6. Cady RK, Sheftell F, Lipton RB, *et al*. Effect of early intervention with sumatriptan on migraine pain: Retrospective analyses of data from three trials. *Clin Ther* 2000; **22**: 1035–48.

7. Breslau N, Schultz LR, Stewart WF, Lipton RB, Lucia V, Welch KMA. Headache and major depression: Is the association specific to migraine? *Neurology* 2000; **54**: 308–13.

8. Lipton RB, Hamelsky SW, Kolodner K, Steiner TJ, Stewart WF. Migraine, quality of life and depression: a population-based case-control study. *Neurology* 2000; **55** (5): 629–35.

9. Stewart WF, Lipton RB, Kolodner KB, Sawyer J, Lee C, Liberman J. Validity of the Migraine Disability Assessment (MIDAS) score in comparison to a diary-based measure in a population sample of migraine sufferers. *Pain* 2000; **88** (1): 41–52.

10. Lipton RB, Stewart WF. Do doctors know what migraine patients want from their treatment? *Headache* 1998; **39** (Suppl. 2): S20–S26.

11. Silberstein SD. Practice parameter: evidence-based guidelines for migraine headache (an evidence-based review): report of the Quality Standards Subcommittee of the American Academy of Neurology. *Neurology* 2000; **55**: 754–62.

12. Lipton RB, Stewart WF, Stone AM, *et al*. Stratified care vs step care strategies for migraine: the Disabilities in Strategies of Care (DISC) study: a randomized trial. *J Am Med Assoc* 2000; **284** (20): 2599–605.

13. Rapoport A, Lipton RB, Williams P, Sawyer J. Cost-effectiveness of stratified care in the management of migraine. *Value Hlth* 2000; **3** (2): 80.

51 Analysis of headache patients' behaviour in the pharmacy: results of a French multicentre study

Bruno Mihout, Michel Lantéri-Minet, Alain Slama, and Fatima Nachit-Ouinekh

Introduction

Migraine remains an underdiagnosed pathology. Many migraineurs are not currently treated within the health-care system and are therefore not treated with effective prescription drugs. Most migraineurs are treated with self-medication.[1-2] Within this context, pharmacists can play an important role in the management of migraine. The study described in this chapter was undertaken to determine the characteristics of the headache patients who go to a pharmacy and to analyse their behaviour and expectations and the response of the pharmacist.

Methods and results

A prospective national study was conducted in France with 770 pharmacies from April to June 2000. Those pharmacies were recruited during national encounters, organized in 70 sites scattered around France, and chosen in accordance with the local density of pharmacies.

Each pharmacy was asked to include in the survey the first 10 persons who corresponded to one of the following criteria.

(1) The patient presented with headache symptoms and requested advice for his/her headache.
(2) The patient presented a prescription specifying headache treatment.
(3) The patient requested, of his or her own accord, a specific analgesic to relieve migraines or headaches.

The diagnosis of migraine was made according to International Headache Society (IHS) criteria using a self-administered patient questionnaire.[3] The statistical analysis was mainly descriptive. The test performed to compare the migraineurs and the non-migraineurs was the Pearson's chi-squared test, and it was interpreted with a 0.01 level of significance.

A total of 770 pharmacies agreed to participate in the study. Those 770 pharmacies include 7264 headache patients. Among the 7264 headache patients included in the study, one-third came to the pharmacy during a pain attack and 71% suffered from migraine headache; in 71% of cases a practitioner had not yet confirmed this diagnosis. Women were significantly more represented among the migraineurs than among the non-migraineurs (84% versus 73%). The migraineurs were slightly older than the non-migraineurs.

The IHS criteria that best discriminated between migraineurs and non-migraineurs were the pain duration, the aggravating factors (light and noise), and the associated digestive symptoms (nausea and vomiting) (Fig. 51.1).

The characteristics of the patients' management of headache are presented in Table 51.1. Ninety-four per cent of the migraineurs had told a doctor about their migraine, 55% within the last year. Sixty per cent of people suffering from migraine had prescriptions (versus 45% in non-migraineurs), 24% sought self-medication (versus 34%), and 12% came for advice (versus 18%). The drugs delivered for all patients are presented in Fig. 51.2.

Eighty-two per cent of the prescriptions were made by general practitioners. The main drugs delivered by the pharmacist to the migraineurs who had a medical prescription were triptans (45% of patients). A combination of analgesics plus

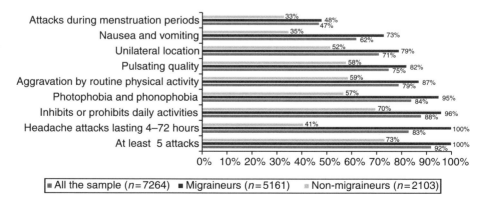

Fig. 51.1 Symptoms experienced.

Table 51.1   Management of the headaches (%)

	Percentage of		
	Migraineurs (n=5161)	Non-migraineurs (n=2103)	Entire sample (n=7264)
Patient asks the pharmacist			
To fill a prescription	60*	45	56
For a specific treatment	24	34*	27
For advice	12	18	13
Answer unknown	4	3	4
Has the patient told the doctor about his/her headache			
Yes, <1 year ago	55*	48	53
Yes, 1 to 3 years ago	12	12	12
Yes, more than 3 years ago	27*	17	24
No, never	6	21*	10
Answer unknown	1	2	1
Information about the patient held by the pharmacist			
Known for his/her headache	68	48	62
Known but not for his/her headache	19	34	24
New patient	11	16	13
Answer unknown	2	2	1
When did the patient come to the pharmacy?			
Outside the attack	58*	48	55
During the attack	32	39*	34
End of the attack	5	6	5
Answer unknown	5	7	6

*Significantly different.

nonsteroidal anti-inflammatory drugs (NSAIDs) was given to 72% of migraineurs who spontaneously requested a specific treatment and 45% of migraineurs who had asked the pharmacist's advice. The others drugs delivered are shown in Table 51.2. Fifteen per cent of the patients bought two drugs and 3% three or more. When the drug delivered was a repeat request, 75% of the headache patients declared that they were 'very' or 'quite' satisfied with their treatment.

Pharmacists encouraged 39% of the migraineurs who came for advice to consult a doctor and provided lifestyle and diet advice to 35%.

Discussion and conclusion

This research complements the studies conducted with medical practitioners or population-based studies.[4–5] Indeed, it permits us to focus on the population who is self-medicated and not managed (10% of patients had never told a doctor about

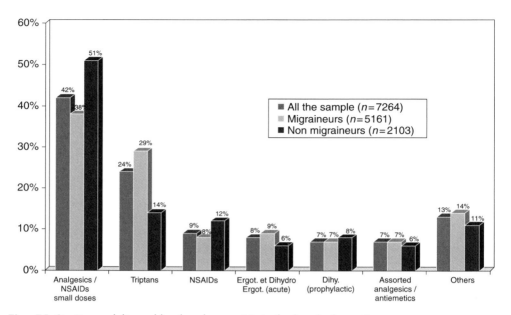

Fig. 51.2 Drugs delivered by the pharmacists to the headache patients.

Table 51.2 Drugs delivered to the migraineurs according to their request

Drug	Percentage of migraineurs receiving drug as a result of		
	Prescription (n=3091)	Specific request (n=1233)	Pharmacist's advice (n=594)
Analgesics+NSAIDs, small doses	25	72	45
NSAIDs	7	12	12
Analgesics+antiemetics	9	4	4
Ergotamine			
As symptomatic medication	14	2	2
As preventive medication	11	1	1.5
Triptans	45	3	4
Others	16	7.9	15.8

their headache). This research confirms that there is a need to encourage sufferers to consult a doctor in order to ensure access to appropriate medication and highlights the important role that pharmacists can play in improving the management of migraine and headache through advice and encouragement to consult medical practitioners.

References

1. Expertise Collective de L'Inserm (1998). *La Migraine: connaissances descriptives, traitements et prévention*. Paris: Inserm, 1998.
2. Stang P, Cady R, Batenhorst A, *et al*. Workplace productivity: a review of the impact of migraine and its treatment. *PharmacoEconomics* 2001; **19** (3): 231–44.
3. Headache Classification Committee of the International Headache Society. Classification and diagnosis criteria for headache disorders, cranial neuralgia and facial pain. *Cephalalgia* 1988; **8** (Suppl. 7): 1–96.
4. Lipton RB, Diamond S, Redd M, *et al*. Migraine diagnosis and treatment: results from the American Migraine Study II. *Headache* 2001; **41**: 638–45.
5. Dowson A, Jagger S. The UK Migraine Patient Survey. *Curr Med Res Opin* 1999; **15** (4): 241–53.

52 Comparison of the efficacy of self-medication and medical prescriptions in reducing the burden of headache

Hartmut Göbel, Marianne Petersen-Braun, and Axel Heinze

Introduction

Representative studies show that, for migraine and headaches, general practitioners (GPs) or primary care physicians (PCPs) are consulted most often (56%), while 16% of patients have consulted specialists in the previous year.[1] Forty-nine per cent of migraineurs had taken medication in the previous year to treat their migraine.[1] Twice as many over-the-counter drugs as prescription medicines were taken.[2] Emergency treatments were necessary for 13% of migraine patients,[3] and 7% of migraine patients had undergone in-patient treatment for their headaches.[6] In the preceding year, supplementary diagnostic techniques, such as computerized tomography (CT) or magnetic resonance imaging (MRI), had been used for 3% of migraineurs, and 2% of migraineurs required in-patient treatment for their headaches.[1] Because approximately one in 10 persons suffers from migraine, the health-care utilization by migraineurs can be expensive. During consultation migraine is often underdiagnosed. Nearly two-thirds of patients who satisfy the International Headache Society (IHS) diagnostic criteria for migraine were not identified as migraine patients. Migraine was most often diagnosed correctly by neurologists (35%), followed by internists (32%), GPs/PCPs (27%), anaesthetists (18%), and orthopaedists (16%).[4] A Canadian study showed that only one-third of headache patients returned after the first consultation, while 65% never returned. Of these, 55% were satisfied with the treatment first recommended and did not require any further consultation. However, 17% said they did not come back because they could not tolerate the medicine prescribed. Thirty-eight per cent indicated that they did not feel they were being taken seriously.[2] Together, these data clearly indicate that headache patients are not receiving adequate care under the existing health-care systems in various countries around the world. Therefore, the majority of patients with primary headaches treat their headache attacks themselves with self-medication. According to figures published by the German association of salaried staffs' health insurance funds, some 60 million packs of painkillers and migraine preparations were prescribed in Germany per year. The cost to the statutory health insurance funds came to DM 720 million. Including self-medication, sales of painkillers totalled around 200 million packs with an estimated total value of DM 1.4 billion. The German airline Lufthansa alone hands out 1.2 million headache tablets a year to its passengers. The total quantity of analgesics consumed in Germany is sufficient to provide up to 6% of the population with a continuous daily supply of painkillers for a whole year. The purpose of the population-based study reported in this chapter was to investigate the extent to which self-medication can help reduce the burden of headache in comparison to medication prescribed by a doctor.

Methods

Information about the efficacy of self-medication with over-the-counter drugs was collected from 470 patients fulfilling the IHS criteria for migraine with and without aura and from 321 patients fulfilling the IHS criteria for episodic tension-type headache. The patients were selected in a population-based nationwide study on the epidemiology of headaches in Germany.[4] Five thousand persons who were representatively selected for the purpose were asked to answer a standardized headache questionnaire about the existence, symptoms, and treatment of headaches. Of these, 4061 persons, or 81.2%, completed a questionnaire and sent it back. These 4061 respondents remained representative of the overall population of Germany in terms of sex, age, education, size of town, and region. The questionnaire was based on the 'Kiel Headache Questionnaire',[5] which contains the operationalized headache classification criteria as defined by the IHS. The respondents were asked standardized questions about the effect of self-medication on their incapacity due to migraine and tension-type headache. In addition, the treatment results of self-medication and medical prescription were compared. Persons fulfilling the IHS criteria for migraine or tension-type headache were requested to fill in a separate second questionnaire. In it they were asked whether they had started any medical treatment for their headaches. One hundred and seventy-seven of the 470 migraine patients (32%) and 207 of the 321 patients suffering from tension-type headache (64%) indicated that they had never consulted a doctor about their headaches. Consulting patients and non-consulting patients were divided into two groups and requested to fill in a second standardized questionnaire in which they were extensively asked about the efficacy of the drugs taken for headache treatment. Of the patients who had never consulted a doctor about their headache, 68% treated their headaches with drugs. To make direct comparison between the answers possible, only those patients who had taken the same preparation either on prescription or as self-medication were included in the analysis.

Results

The response rates for the same headache preparations are significantly dependent on the individual user group. Patients who use self-medication to treat their headaches display markedly higher response rates after 2 hours. In the case of the preparations used for self-medication, 60–80% of the respondents say that after 2 hours their headaches are either hardly noticeable or completely gone. Among patients who obtained their medicine on a medical prescription, the response rates are much lower. The percentage of patients whose headaches are hardly noticeable or completely gone after 2 hours is only between 30% and 53%, depending on the medication taken. The responder rates for acetylsalicylic acid used in self-medication versus prescription for either migraine or episodic tension-type headache are shown in Fig. 52.1.

The respondents display significant differences in dosage habits, depending on whether a drug used was obtained for self-medication or on a doctor's prescription. Patients who practice self-medication report a decisively lower dosage than patients who have had their medicine prescribed by a doctor. As a rule, self-medication respondents use one dosage unit of the medicine, that is, a coated or uncoated tablet. Fifty to 80% of all users, depending on the preparation, confine themselves to administering this one dosage unit. Considerably more dosage units are used in the case of prescribed preparations. As a rule, two dosage units are used here.

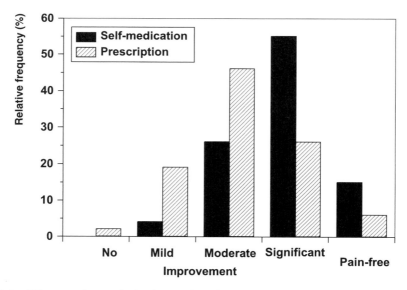

Fig. 52.1 Efficacy of acetylsalicylic acid 2 hours postdose in patients using the same preparation either on prescription or as self-medication.

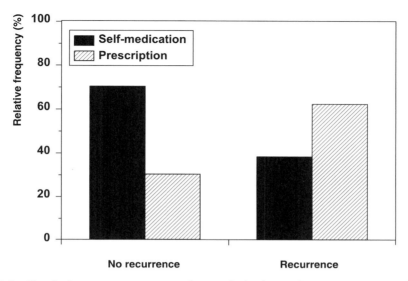

Fig. 52.2 Headache recurrence rate with acetylsalicylic acid in patients using the same preparation either on prescription or as self-medication.

In patients who practice self-medication the rate of recurrence of headaches requiring further intake of a medicine lies between 10% and 31%. For preparations prescribed by a doctor, however, the probability of a recurrence of the headache following initially adequate reduction lies between 25% and 80%. Furthermore, the time until headache recurs is significantly longer for drugs used in self-medication compared to prescription. The headache recurrence rates for acetylsalicylic acid used in self-medication versus prescription for either migraine or episodic tension-type headache are shown in Fig. 52.2.

The great majority of users of combination preparations are increasingly dissatisfied with a self-medication product as the number of combination partners increases. Whereas acetylsalicylic acid in an effervescent formulation is rated positively by 60% of the patients, this number drops to 46% for a combination of acetylsalicylic acid and paracetamol and to 25% for a combination of acetylsalicylic acid, paracetamol, and caffeine (Fig. 52.3).

Discussion

Self-medication is becoming an increasingly important area within headache treatment. Self-medication also has advantages for health-care systems. It facilitates adequate use of clinical skills, increases access to medication, and may contribute to reducing prescribed drug costs. However, self-medication may also be associated with risks such as misdiagnosis, drug interactions, polypharmacy, use of excessive drug dosage, and prolonged duration of use. This population-based study shows

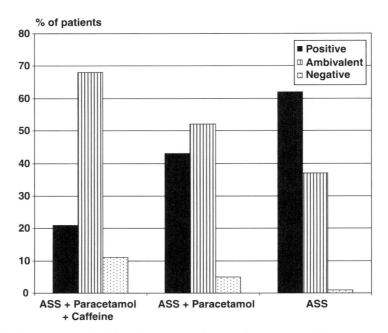

Fig. 52.3 Assessment of self-medication analgesics by patients. The majority of users of combination preparations are increasingly dissatisfied with the self-medication product as the number of combination partners increases. This is especially true for the combination of three active compounds, acetylsalicylic acid (ASS), paracetamol, and caffeine.

that patients who can treat their headaches with self-medication without needing to consult a doctor achieve a significant reduction in headache-induced incapacity with such therapy. The drugs taken in the setting of self-medication are more effective, the headache recurrence rates are lower, and the time to recurrence is longer. By contrast, sufferers who need to consult a doctor bear a considerably heavier headache burden and the therapeutic results with over-the-counter drugs are less satisfactory. Optimal therapy with an over-the-counter drug requires that the patient diagnose the headache condition correctly and use the drug in a manner that minimizes risk. The widespread use of over-the-counter products for headache treatment illustrates the potential value of increased drug availability for the health-care system.

References

1. Rasmussen BK, Olesen J. Symptomatic and nonsymptomatic headaches in a general population. *Neurology* 1992; **42** (6): 1225–31.
2. Edmeads J, Findlay H, Tugwell P, Pryse-Phillips W, Nelson RF, Murray TJ. Impact of migraine and tension-type headache on life-style, consulting behaviour, and medication use: a Canadian population survey. *Can J Neurol Sci* 1993; **20** (2): 131–7.

3. Celentano DD, Stewart WF, Lipton RB, Reed ML. Medication use and disability among migraineurs: a national probability sample. *Headache* 1992; **32**: 223–8.
4. Göbel H, Petersen-Braun M, Soyka D. The epidemiology of headache in Germany: a nationwide survey of a representative sample on the basis of the headache classification of the International Headache Society. *Cephalalgia* 1994; **14** (2): 97–106.
5. Göbel H. *Die Kopfschmerzen*. Berlin: Springer Verlag, 1997: 353–4.
6. Stang P, Osterhaus J. Impact of migraine in the United States: data from the National Health Interview Survey. *Headache* 1993; **33**: 29–35.

53
Evaluation of migraine in the workplace

S. Finkelstein, E. Berndt, G. Pransky, and J. Mackell

Background

The economic burden of migraine on society is both direct, that is, associated with the costs of medical care, and indirect, through absence from work and loss of productivity. Both the headache pain and associated symptoms of a migraine attack cause significant functional disability, which results in absence from work and reduced productivity while at work. Several recent studies attribute most of the economic impact of migraine to absenteeism and diminished productivity while at work.[1–4] While absenteeism has been used to measure the impact of migraine in the workplace, it has not been established as a valid surrogate for decreased productivity while at work.

Previous studies have been conducted to measure the effect of migraine on workplace productivity. These studies utilized different instruments, including the Migraine Work and Productivity Loss Questionnaire (MWPLQ) and the Migraine Disability Assessment (MIDAS).[1,5–6] However, the instruments used in studies to date have involved *self-reported* measures without objective validation.

In order to validate the use of subjective measures alone in evaluating the impact of migraine on physical function and work productivity, it must be possible to correlate subjective and objective data. This prospective study, reporting on individuals diagnosed with migraine, was conducted to examine the effect of migraine on productivity using both objective and self-reported data.

Methods

The study enrolled data entry workers located at three geographically diverse US sites. Eligible employees (full-time, employed a minimum of 3 months, not in the third trimester of pregnancy) who gave informed consent completed a screening questionnaire. Enrollees answered daily questions about headache and work productivity over 12 weeks. As part of the routine tracking, the employer collected a variety of daily productivity measures electronically. These productivity measures were used as the objective measures correlated with self-report. Following the 12-week period, participants underwent a diagnostic interview by a headache specialist to determine the presence of migraine.

Results

There was a high level of study participation (95%), compliance (total completing daily questions, 90%), and study completion (completing daily questions and follow-up diagnostic interview, 87%) among eligible employees. Of the eligible data-entry employees (mean age, 34.7 years; 97% female) who signed the informed consent form and completed the screening questionnaire, 13% reported that they had previously received a diagnosis of migraine.

All individuals diagnosed at study completion as migraine patients ($n=57$) were female. The racial composition of these patients was 78.9% White, 10.5% African-American, 0% Asian, and 10.5% other. Nearly 16% held an advanced degree beyond a high school diploma (Table 53.1).

Those participants who were diagnosed with migraine experienced an average of 11.5 headache days over the 12-week period. More than half of the migraine sufferers

Table 53.1 Demographic profile of migraine patients ($n=57$)

Variable	Value
Age, years	
Mean	33.9
Standard deviation	9.2
Minimum	19
Maximum	54
Gender, number (%)	
Male	0 (0)
Female	57 (100)
Race, number (%)	
White	45 (78.9)
African-American	6 (10.5)
Asian	0 (0)
Other	6 (10.5)
Education, number (%)	
Not a high school graduate	1 (1.8)
High school graduate	28 (49.1)
Some college, no degree	19 (33.3)
Associate's degree	6 (10.5)
Bachelor's degree	2 (3.5)
Some graduate education	1 (1.8)
Graduate degree	0 (0)

reported a headache frequency of more than 3 headaches per month and 23.2% of them were diagnosed with aura.

Migraine patients reported taking headache medication on 72.9% of total headache days. Of the types of medication available, over-the-counter medication, which was used on 54.2% of headache days, was the headache treatment used most frequently. Only 12% ($n=7$) of the migraine patients reported using triptans, and triptans were utilized on only 5.8% of total headache days experienced (Table 53.2).

A comparison of self-reported speed and electronically collected total daily output indicated that there was a significant positive correlation between self-reported and objective productivity measures for those with a diagnosis of migraine ($r = 0.2157$; $p < 0.0001$ for 2688 daily observations) (Table 53.3).

Table 53.2 Medication utilization for headache episodes in migraine patients ($n=57$)

Migraine-diagnosed cohort	Total number of headache days	Percentage of total headache days
No treatment	178	27.1
OTC medication	356	54.2
Triptan	38	5.8
Other migraine medication	82	12.5
Other nonpharmaceutical treatment	3	0.5
Total	657	100

*OTC, Over-the-counter.

Table 53.3 Relationship between daily subjective and objective output measures in migraine patients ($n=57$)

Subjective productivity scale	Objective productivity metric	Person-days reporting
0	163.6	5
1	—	0
2	121.9	9
3	132.0	28
4	148.3	49
5	163.5	137
6	175.1	233
7	183.2	625
8	201.7	832
9	220.5	581
10	222.0	189

Conclusions

Data from recent studies have demonstrated the substantial economic and societal impact of migraine, stimulating further research into the most effective diagnostic and treatment options. Migraine affects 2 to 3 times more women than men.[7] This study, conducted in a predominantly female work setting, compared both self-reported and objective data to evaluate the validity of subjective measures used alone to assess the burden of migraine in the workplace. Initial examination of the data showed a significant positive correlation between self-reported functioning and objective productivity output. Further examination of this correlation is warranted in different workplace environments.

It was also noted in this study that employees with migraine experienced frequent headaches. The relatively low overall treatment rates and the low rate of triptan utilization observed suggest that migraine often may be undertreated resulting in unnecessary disability and cost to employer and employee.[5]

References

1. Davies GM, Santanello N, Gerth W, Lerner D, Block GA. Validation of a migraine work and productivity loss questionnaire for use in migraine studies. *Cephalalgia* 1999; **19**: 497–502.
2. Osterhaus JT, Gutterman DL, Plachetka JR. Healthcare resource and lost labor costs of migraine headache in the US. *PharmacoEconomics* 1992; **2**: 67–76.
3. Solomon GD, Price KL. Burden of migraine. *PharmacoEconomics* 1997; **11** (Suppl. 1): 1–10.
4. Von Korff M, Stewart WF, Simon DJ, Lipton RB. Migraine and reduced work performance: a population-based diary study. *Neurology* 1998; **50**: 1741–5.
5. Ferrari MD. The economic burden of migraine to society. *PharmacoEconomics* 1998; **13** (6): 667–76.
6. Cady RC, Ryan R, Jhingran P, O'Quinn S, Pait DG. Sumatriptan injection reduces productivity loss during a migraine attack. *Arch Intern Med* 1999; **158** (9): 1103–8.
7. Breslau N, Rasmussen BK (2001). The impact of migraine: epidemiology, risk factors, and co-morbidities. *Neurology* 2001; **56** (Suppl. 1): S4–S12.

54 Headache patient management in 21 Italian headache centres

Paola Torelli and Gian Camillo Manzoni for the Headache
Study Group of the Italian Society of Neurology

Introduction

Primary headaches have a large social and economic impact on a country's population. Over the last few years, several studies have been conducted in order to identify those areas in a patient's personal and social life that are more heavily affected.[1] Of even greater topical interest are the surveys aimed at assessing management of headache patients in order to improve the outcome of the disorder.[2] Current diagnostic and therapeutic approaches in Italy vary widely between the different headache centres (HCs). In particular, there appears to be a total lack of consistent guidelines in this field.

The purpose of our study was to obtain accurate information about: (1) the administrative procedures related to the organizational management of patients requesting treatment at a specialized HC in Italy; and (2) the therapeutic and diagnostic approaches followed by physicians before admission of patients to the HC and by the HC neurologists.

Material and methods

Our study consisted of two different stages: a retrospective stage and a prospective stage. In the retrospective stage operators at each HC were asked to use a specially designed form to record all diagnoses made for first referrals seen at the HC between September 2000 and March 2001, as well as the relevant codes corresponding to the diagnostic criteria of the International Headache Society (IHS) classification. The aim at this stage was an 'epidemiological' evaluation of the primary or secondary headache forms diagnosed over a period of about 6 months. In the prospective stage operators at each HC were asked to fill in a special form for each of the 50 consecutive patients who showed up for the first visit at the HC from the time of their agreement to participate in the study (1 March 2001) until the end of June 2001. The form comprised four different sections. The patient's personal data (that is, sex, school level, and place of residence) and the duration of the disease were recorded in section 1. The various steps taken by the patient to be admitted to the HC for the first visit (that is, application, booking, and waiting time) were summarized in section 2. Finally, the patient's status (that is, diagnosis, examinations, and treatments taken before and after the visit to the HC) was reported in sections 3 and 4. The forms used in the two stages of the study for data collection were sent to all major Italian HCs, equally distributed in the Italian territory, after the centres confirmed their participation in the study. Data were analysed as a whole, without separating them according to the different participating centres, because centre selection was based in the first place on comparable characteristics of referral areas, patient 'flows', staff qualifications, and available technologies.

Results

Of the 28 HCs originally selected for the study 21 (75%) agreed to participate, providing data on 4020 patients in the retrospective stage and 884 patients in the prospective stage.

Retrospective stage

Of the patients investigated in the retrospective stage, 51.4% (2067 of 4020) were found to have migraine without aura (MO), 8.4% (339/4020) migraine with aura (MA), 9.4% (378/4020) and 9.1% (365/4020) episodic (ETTH) and chronic (CTTH) tension-type headache, respectively, and 3.1% (123/4020) cluster headache (CH). The patients with headache forms that could be coded to the 5–13 groups of the IHS classification numbered 383 out of 4020 (9.5%), including 138 (3.4%) with headaches associated with substance use or withdrawal.

Prospective stage

The patients seeking treatments at the HCs under study were 653 women (73.9%) and 231 men (26.1%). The mean age at the first visit was 37.6 years (37.9 years for females and 36.7 years for males). School level was a junior high school certificate for 297 patients (33.6%), a senior high school certificate for 365 (41.6%), and a university degree for 97 (11.0%); the remaining 13.8% had attended only primary school.

A proportion of 64.1% of patients (567 of 884) were living in the same munici-pality or the same province as the HC at which they were seeking treatment, 17.8% (157/884) in the same region, and 18.0% (160/884) in a different region. Slightly fewer than half of patients had been referred to the HC by their general practitioners (GPs) (401/884, 45.4%), 39.3% (348/884) had sought treatment at the HC independently, while only 4.5% (40/884) had been advised to seek treatment at a specialized headache centre by a neurologist and 10.8% (95/884) by a medical specialist other than a neurologist. The appointment for the HC visit was made by phone in 64.5% of cases (570/884), and by a personal request at the centre in 35.5% (314/884). More than half of patients (495/884, or 56.0%) were able to make the reservation directly with the HC, 31.2% (276/884) had to apply to local units of Italy's National Health Service, and 12.8% (113/884) arranged the visit through personal acquaintances in the medical field. The average waiting time for a visit at the HC was 77.5 days, and over half of patients (53.8%) had to wait 1 to 4 months. About half of patients (462/884, or 52.3%) presented at the HC with a previous diagnosis of headache. Of these diagnoses, 312 of 462 (67.5%) were found to be correct by the HC specialist, while 150 (32.5%) were not consistent with the diagnosis made at the end of the first visit. Upon admission to the HC, 24.4% (50/205) of MO cases, 27.7% (13/47) of MA cases, 16.9% (4/25) of ETTH cases, as much as 71.4% (15/21) of CTTH cases, and 48.0% (12/25) of CH cases were judged by the HC specialist not to have been properly diagnosed. Of the 172 diagnoses made by GPs, 72 (41.9%) were not consistent with those of the HC specialist; nor were 32 of 66 diagnoses (48.5%) made by specialists other than neurologists and 38 of 205 diagnoses (18.5%) made by neurologists. Overall, 366 out of 884 patients (41.4%) had had an examination prior to their first visit. Almost all patients under study (867/884, or 98.1%) had taken antiheadache drugs, but only 237 (26.8%) had had their headache treated with molecules exhibiting a preventive action. Data about 'postvisit' procedures showed that HC specialists requested a total of 173 neuroimaging examinations: electroencephalograms (EEGs) were prescribed in 121 cases, blood tests in 91 cases, and colour-flow Doppler sonography of the supra-aortic trunks in 48 cases. Preventive therapy was recommended in 549 of 884 patients (62.1%), whereas non-pharmacological treatments were recommended only in 28 patients (3.2%). The diagnoses made at the HCs were consistent with data from the retrospective stage of our study: 400 patients (45.2%) were found to have MO, 65 (7.4%) MA, 71 (8.3%) ETTH, 58 (6.6%) CTTH, and 30 (3.4%) CH. In 16 cases (1.8%), the headache could only be coded to group 13 of the IHS classification (headache not classifiable), and in 60 (6.8%) the headache did not fall into any of the groups of the existing classification. Only in 25 cases of 884 (2.8%)ws there a diagnosis of secondary headache.

Discussion

Defining the administrative procedures and the diagnostic and therapeutic approaches followed in the management of headache patients is an essential first step enabling investigators: first, to focus on behaviours that are not adequate to ensure good management of headache patients; and, second, to find similarities and differences with other organizational models that are adopted abroad. The main purpose of this study was to provide an accurate description of the current situation and was prompted by the need to identify trends at major Italian HCs, accounting for data that so far have been totally neglected by the medical literature.

The first remark that should be made about the data from our study is the role played in Italy by GPs in the diagnosis and treatment of headache: almost half the diagnoses made by GPs were not consistent with those of HC specialists, and about 40% of patients reported that they had sought treatment at a specialized headache centre independently. These findings appear to confirm the observations of the British Association for the Study of Headache,[3] which found that only a very small minority of GPs demonstrate a professional interest in management of headache disorders. They are also in agreement with data from a population-based survey in England in which, of people with migraine, only 49% had consulted their GPs for their headache while large numbers self-treated with over-the-counter medication. In light of the recommendations of the Task Force of the IHS,[4] every GP should have a broad knowledge of all types of headache, of how to manage the vast majority of cases, and of which cases to refer to a specialist. Moreover, every health-care system should be basically committed to the provision of educational programmes for patients aimed at increasing their basic knowledge of different headache types and their correct treatment.

The second point to note about our data is the high number of examinations taken under the instructions of either GPs or HC specialists, in spite of the fact that, based on a comprehensive review of the literature, EEGs are not indicated in the routine evaluation of patients presenting with headache[5] and available data indicate a very low rate of intracranial pathology in patients with headache when their neurological examinations are normal.[6]

Finally, the last thing to be noted is the limited use of non-pharmacological treatments in the preventive management of headache. In spite of the fact that it is difficult to apply a placebo-controlled design to non-pharmacological treatment studies and in many cases the reported trials are uncontrolled and unblinded, the existing evidence suggests the efficacy of certain behavioural and physical treatments, particularly in the management of migraine and TTH.[7,8] The activity of a few European HCs—notably, in Denmark and Germany—that use an integrated, multi-disciplinary approach to headache management may eventually provide interesting practical and scientific indications in the near future.

Conclusion

In Italy, the diagnosis of primary headache is still a problem for GPs and medical specialists other than neurologists. Therefore, it can be assumed that, as in other European countries, headache disorders are underdiagnosed and undertreated. Moreover, the number of examinations requested before and after the first visit at an HC is still very high, if we consider that the diagnosis of primary headache must essentially be based on the patient's past medical history and on the demonstration of the lack of abnormalities verifiable at the neurological examination. Finally, non-pharmacological treatments are very rarely prescribed in Italy.

References

1. Rasmussen B. Epidemiology of headache. *Cephalalgia* 2001; **21**: 774–7.
2. Danish Neurological Society and the Danish Headache Society. Guidelines for the management of headache. *Cephalalgia* 1998; **18**: 9–22.
3. British Association for the Study of Headache. *Review of the organisation of headache services in primary care and recommendations for change*, 1st edn. British Association for the Study of Headache, September 2000.
4. Task Force of the International Headache Society. Organization and delivery of services to headache patients. *Cephalalgia* 1997; **17**: 702–10.
5. Gronseth GS, Greenberg MK. The utility of the electroencephalogram in the evaluation of patients presenting with headache: a review of the literature. *Neurology* 1995; **45**: 1263–7.
6. Frishberg BM. The utility of neuroimaging in the evaluation of headache in patients with normal neurologic examinations. *Neurology* 1994; **44**: 1191–7.
7. Silberstein SD for the US Headache Consortium. Practice parameter: evidence-based guidelines for migraine headache (an evidence-based review). Report of the Quality Standards Subcommittee of the American Academy of Neurology. *Neurology* 2000; **55**: 754–63.
8. Lake AE 3rd. Behavioral and nonpharmacologic treatments of headache. *Med Clin North Am* 2001; **85**: 1055–75.

55

Migraine and chronic idiopathic headache in the French workforce: detection and management. The **NOEMIE** study protocol

Fatima Nachit-Ouinekh, Mohamed El Amrani, Abdelkader El Hasnaoui, and the National Orientation Committee

Background

In most employee health units, chronic idiopathic forms of headaches (migraine, chronic daily headache (CDH), and cluster headache (CH)) rank among the most frequently reported complaints. The highest prevalence rates are essentially observed among young adult professionals. Headaches are accompanied by a significant loss of productivity,[1,2] and the factors that set off headache symptoms are sometimes related to the professional activity itself. Employee health units would thus appear to play a particularly important health-care role in the field of chronic idiopathic headaches.[3]

The main goal of this project is to give the employee health unit a central role in the management of headaches in the French workplace by means of research/training action. In this context, the employee health unit would be involved in providing information, education, and prevention techniques, as well as detection and directing of patients to health-care circuits. The NOEMIE study is the main tool set up to support this research/training operation in the French workplace.

The objectives of this study are to:

◆ identify idiopathic headaches in the workplace and estimate respective prevalence rates;
◆ measure the psychopathological state (anxiety and/or depression) and quality of life of patients suffering from idiopathic headaches (migraine, CDH, and CH);
◆ describe the various health-care networks used by newly diagnosed patients and measure the impact of detection in terms of quality of life after 6 months.

Methods

This is a cross-sectional, observational, national, multicentre study with follow-up for 6 months.

The *study population* consists of patients suffering from chronic idiopathic headaches (migraine, CDH, and CH). Patients will be recruited from existing employee health units. The diagnosis of headache will be established according to an *algorithm* based on International Headache Society (IHS) criteria[4] (see Figs 55.1 and 55.2). The algorithm divides headache patients into three categories: migraine headache, CH, and

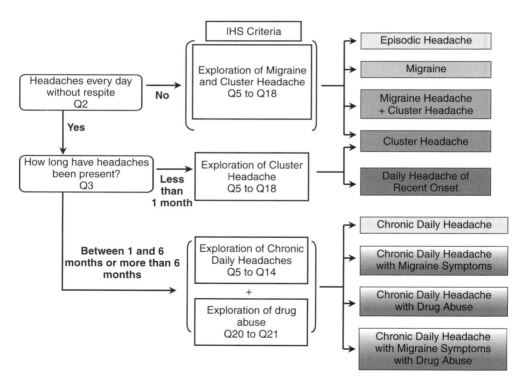

Fig. 55.1 Algorithm for the NOEMIE study.

Q1: Do you suffer from headaches?

Q2 : Do you suffer from headaches every day without respite?

Q3 : For how long have you been having headaches every day without respite?
- less than one month
- between 1 and 6 months
- more than 6 months

Q4 : Your headache:
- is constant
- occurs as attacks, between which you no longer suffer any pain

Q5 : How long do your headaches usually last without medication?
- less than 4 hours
- between 4 and 72 hours
- more than 72 hours
- don't know

Q6 : How long do your headaches usually last with medication?
- less than 4 hours
- between 4 and 72 hours
- more than 72 hours
- don't know

Q7 : Where is your headache usually located?
- on the right or left side of the head only
- sometimes on the right, sometimes on the left side of the head
- on both sides
- don't know

Q8 : Are your headaches pulsating?

Q9 : When you have a headache, do you experience pressure or tightening in your head?

Q10 : When you have a headache, do you suffer from:
- nausea
- vomiting
- both
- neither or don't know

Q11 : When you have a headache, does light bother you?

Q12 : When you have a headache, does noise bother you?

Q13 : Does your pain inhibit your usual activities or force you to lie down?

Q14 : Is your pain made worse by daily physical activities?

Q15 : How many attacks do you suffer per day?
- 1 to 8
- more than 8
- don't know

Q16 : Is the pain severe or excruciating?

Q17 : During an attack, is the pain accompanied by any of the following symptoms?
- Injection of the conjunctiva (bloodshot eyes)
- Nasal congection (blocked nose)
- Rhinorrhoea (runny nose)
- Miosis(contraction of the pupil)
- Shrinking of the palpebral fissure (opening between the eyelids)
- Oedema (swelling) of the eyelids

Q18 : Have you had more than four headache attacks in your life?

Q19 : Do you take medication to relieve your headaches?

Q20 : What medication have you taken in the last fortnight?
- On average, how many doses per day?

Q21 : How long have you been taking this medication?
- less than 3 months
- more than 3 months
- don't know

Fig. 55.2 The diagnostic questionnaire.

CDH. The algorithm will also enable us to determine whether CDH is accompanied by excessive drug intake. This algorithm has been implemented in a computer software program installed at all the centres taking part in the study. This software also permits follow-up of patients throughout the study (automatic print-out of personalized accompanying letters, entry of data recording documents) and provides the key indicators for conduct of the study (number of patients included per type of headache, descriptive dynamic reports of the population included).

The *estimated number of subjects* that need to be screened to meet our study objectives is 265 000 employees. This number has been calculated to guarantee a 95% confidence interval with a precision of 10 per 100 000 of the prevalence of the cluster headache (the lowest prevalence among idiopathic headaches), estimated to be 69 per 100 000.[5]

Data collection and analysis

The data gathered at the time of inclusion include sociodemographic features, case history, impact on work, quality of life, and the state of anxiety and/or depression of the patient. Follow-up data include a diary of attacks for migraine patients and headache diary for CDH patients, a description of the various health-care networks available, and an assessment of patients' quality of life and anxiety and/or depression state after 6 months. The tools used for this assessment are the 'Qualité de Vie et Migraine' (Quality of life and Migraine) questionnaire (QVM), which is a specific instrument for evaluating the quality of life of migraine sufferers[6] and the Hospital Anxiety and Depression scale (HADS), which is a self-administered questionnaire to assess the current level of anxious and depressive symptoms, disregarding somatic symptoms.[7]

Statistical analysis will include an estimation of prevalence rates, with the corresponding 95% confidence interval, of migraine, CDH, and CH.

The QVM and HADS will be analysed by comparing patients newly diagnosed during the study and those who had already been diagnosed within the three groups: migraine, CDH, and CH. The health-care networks used by patients—newly diagnosed or otherwise—will be described using the follow-up data.

References

1. Lipton RB, Stewart WF, Von Korff M. The burden of migraine: a review of cost to society. *PharmacoEconomics* 1994; **6**: 215–21.
2. Von Korff M, Stewart FW, Simon DJ, Lipton RB. Migraine and reduced work performance: a population-based diary study. *Neurology* 1998; **50**: 1741–5.
3. Warshaw LJ, Burton WN. Cutting the costs of migraine: role of the employee health unit. *J Occup Environ Med* 1998; **40** (11): 943–53.
4. Headache Classification Committee of the International Headache Society. Classification and diagnosis criteria for headache disorders, cranial neuralgias and facial pain. *Cephalalgia* 1988; **8**: 1–96.
5. Ekbom K, Ahlborg B, Schèle R. Prevalence of migraine and cluster headache in Swedish men of 18. *Headache* 1978; **18**: 9–19.

6. Richard A, Henry P, Chazot G, Massiou H, Tison S, Marconnet R, Chicoye A, D'Allens H. Qualité de vie et migraine. *Therapie* 1992; **48**: 89–96.

7. Razavi D, Delvaux N, Farvacques C, Robaye E. Validation de la version française du HADS dans une population de patients cancéreux hospitalisés. *Rev Psychologique* 1989; **39**: 295–308.

56
HIT-6™ scores discriminate among headache sufferers differing in headache-associated workplace productivity loss

M.S. Bayliss, M. Kosinski, M. Diamond, S. Tepper,
W.H. Garber, J.E. Ware Jr, and A.S. Batenhorst

Introduction

Diminished work productivity, which is common among patients with headache, has economic, social, and personal costs. Lost workplace productivity attributed to headache is due to both absenteeism and to reduced performance and output while on the job. The concept of reduced effectiveness while working is often denoted as *presenteeism*. Health-care providers recognize lost workplace productivity as a relevant marker of the functional consequences of headache syndromes.[1,2] While research suggests a hierarchy of functional activity loss with patients missing time in the following order: time lost from work < time lost from social and family responsibilities < time lost from household responsibilities,[3–5] doctors are responsive to patients' concerns about missing time from work due to their headaches.

The literature also questions the reliability of patients' recollections of time missed from work and their reports of reduced effectiveness. Valid tools that provide reliable, precise, and accurate scores that reflect lost productivity aspects may have value to clinicians when assessing the full impact of headache.

For use in clinical practice, tools for assessing headache impact should be evaluated in terms of their ability to differentiate among patients with respect to their functioning in the workplace. To that end, this study evaluated the ability of HIT-6, a short, self-administered paper-based questionnaire developed to quantify the impairment associated with headache, to discriminate among headache sufferers differing in productivity loss attributed to headache.

Background

HIT-6 measures the impact of headache on patients' lives with only six questions (Fig. 56.1). The HIT-6 items were selected from the Headache Impact Test (HIT) item pool, which was developed using modern psychometric methods to confer exceptional precision in measuring headache impact with either static, paper-based or dynamic, computer-adaptive assessments.[6]

HIT-6 is useful and effective in measuring headache impact because the questionnaire is precise, reliable, and valid. It measures the full range of headache impact and responds to change in headache impact over time. HIT and HIT-6 cover six aspects of headache impact including pain frequency and severity, role functioning, social functioning, energy/fatigue, cognition, and emotional distress. HIT-6 is easily interpreted by clinicians and patients because it quantifies headache impact on an easily understood, norm-based scale (mean score for headache sufferers, 50; SD, 10). HIT-6 scores can be interpreted as representing the following degrees of impact (Fig. 56.2): little to no impact (scores < 50); some impact (scores 50–55); substantial (scores 56–59); or very severe (scores ≥ 60).

Methods

A general population sample of recent headache sufferers completed, via either internet or telephone, a survey including HIT-6 and questions to assess workplace productivity loss in the 4 weeks prior to the survey. Headache-related lost workplace productivity, measured in hours, was calculated as

Absence from work + [time worked with symptoms × (100% − % effectiveness while working with symptoms)].

Mean hours of lost workplace productivity were calculated for participants whose HIT-6 scores reflected little to no, some, substantial, or very severe impact of headaches.

A one-way analysis of variance (ANOVA) was conducted to test the significance of differences in mean hours of lost workplace productivity estimated across the four categories of headache impact.

Results

Participants ($N=648$) were 18 to 65 years old and had a headache within the last 4 weeks that was not due to a cold, flu, head injury, or hangover. The mean number

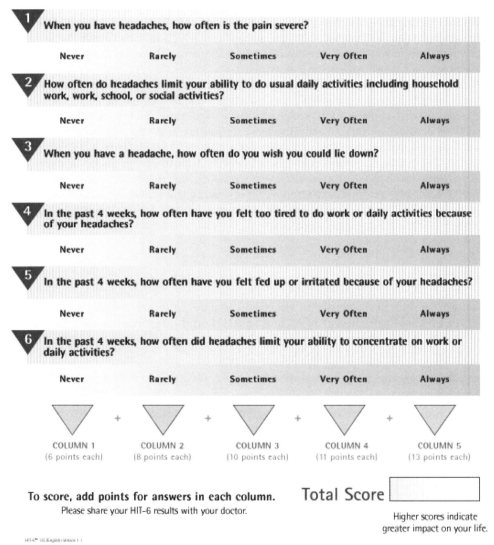

Fig. 56.1   HIT-6 questionnaire.

of hours of lost workplace productivity in the past 4 weeks was directly related to degree of headache impact measured by HIT-6 (Fig. 56.3). The difference in lost workplace productivity across the four headache impact groups was highly significant: $F = 30.43$, $p < 0.00001$.

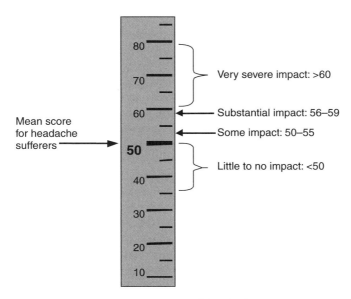

Fig. 56.2 HIT-6 scores in relation to the degree of headache impact.

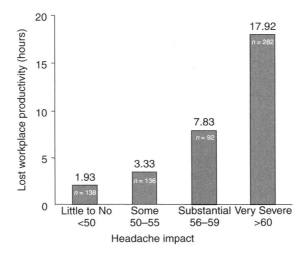

Fig. 56.3 Lost workplace productivity as a function of headache impact. $F = 30.54$; $p < 0.00001$ for difference in lost workplace productivity across the four headache impact groups.

Conclusions

HIT-6 scores are directly related to self-reported workplace productivity loss. These data demonstrate the practicality of HIT-6 for assessing a form of role disability that is personally, socially, economically, and clinically relevant. HIT-6 provides a comprehensive assessment of the effect of headaches on patients' functioning and well-being in an easily interpretable score. The ability to gauge efficiently the degree to which headaches impact patients' lives can help the health-care provider identify patients in need of intervention and tailor treatment strategies to patients' individual needs.

Acknowledgements

The authors gratefully acknowledge the contributions of B. Bowers and J. Carranza Rosenzweig from GlaxoSmithKline, Inc. to this manuscript.

References

1. Schulman EA, Cady RK, Henry D, *et al*. Effectiveness of sumatriptan in reducing productivity loss due to migraine: results of a randomized, double-blind, placebo-controlled clinical trial *Mayo Clin Proc.* 2000; **75**: 782–9.
2. Cady RK, Ryan R, Jhingran P, *et al*. Sumatriptan injection reduces productivity loss during a migraine attack: results of a double-blind, placebo-controlled trial. *Arch Intern Med.* 1998; **158**: 1013–18.
3. Stewart WF, Lipton RB, Whyte J, *et al*. An international study to assess reliability of the Migraine Disability Assessment (MIDAS) score. *Neurology* 1999; **53**: 988–94.
4. Adelman JR, Sharfman M, Johnson R, *et al*. Impact of oral sumatriptan on workplace productivity, health-related quality of life, health care use, and patient satisfaction with medication in nurses with migraine. *Am J Man Care* 1996; **2**: 1407–16.
5. Clarke CR, MacMillan L, Sondhu S, *et al*. Economic and social impact of migraine. *Quart J Med* 1996; **89**: 77–84.
6. Ware JE, Bjorner JB, Kosinski M. Practical implications of item response theory and computerized adaptive testing: a brief summary of ongoing studies of widely used headache impact scales. *Med Care* 2000; **38** (9 Suppl.): 1173–82.

57 Guidelines and interventions: discussion summary

Hans-Christoph Diener

....

In Chapter 48, the evidence-based treatment guidelines for headache of the American Academy of Neurology[1] were discussed by Silberstein. These guidelines are very sophisticated and targeted at headache specialists. What is needed more urgently is to translate these complicated guidelines, tables, and schemes into simple algorithms that can be used by primary care physicians in the 6–8 minutes per patient they have in their practice. Another unresolved issue is to measure the impact of guidelines on treatment patterns and outcome. Pfaffenrath and colleagues performed a study in which he investigated the impact of treatment guidelines on prescription patterns in Germany.[2] What he basically found was that treatment guidelines had no impact on prescriptions. The most depressing part of this study was the fact that drugs that were ineffective according to controlled trials were still prescribed. Methodological aspects of treatment recommendations include the way in which the literature is screened and evaluated. Meta-analysis as performed by the Cochrane collaboration is not informative in cases where all the studies that are included are of low quality or if the meta-analysis lacks the power to come to a conclusion. Unfortunately, many recommendations for the prophylaxis of headaches are based on small and poorly designed trials.[3]

In Chapter 49, Maizels showed that care for headache patients at the level of the general practitioner can be improved without referral to secondary or tertiary headache centres. In this way one could increase the number of patients who do not get ignored or temporized. Group settings like those in the USA offer a unique opportunity to test these integrated models including patient groups and specialized nurses.

In Chapter 50, Stewart and Lipton presented ways in which to implement programmes for the diagnosis and treatment of headache in the workplace and to show that treatment can be cost-effective and save lost work days. Important information will be gained by a prospective study that is now starting in France, the so called NOEMIE study (Chapter 55).

An important prerequisite for an optimal treatment is the correct diagnosis. Robert Smith (Cincinnati) analysed clinical records kept by general practitioners (GPs). Almost 75% of patients who fulfilled the International Headache Society (IHS) criteria for migraine or migrainous headache were not diagnosed. Chapter 51 reports a French prospective study on patients visiting pharmacies with headaches. One-third of the patients visited the pharmacy because of an acute attack of headache. In 25% no diagnosis had been made beforehand by a physician. These results show that pharmacists have to be trained to deal with headache and to select patients with frequent headaches, medication overuse, and those in whom medication has lost its efficacy for referral to a physician.

M.G. Bousser (Paris) set up an emergency service for patients with acute headaches. More than 10 000 patients were seen in 1 year. The percentage of patients with symptomatic headache including those with dissection or sinus-venous thrombosis who were undiagnosed before is frightening and justifies this set-up. Unfortunately, there is no follow-up system in place to monitor how the treatment recommendations given by the emergency service influence the outcome in the long run.

References

1. Silberstein SD, for the US Headache Consortium. Practice parameter: evidence-based guidelines for migraine headache (an evidence-based review). Report of the Quality Standards Subcommitee of the American Academy of Neurology. *Neurology* 2000; **55**: 754–63.
2. Krobot KJ, Steinberg HW, Pfaffenrath V. Migraine prescription density and recommendations. Results of the PCAOM study. *Cephalalgia* 1999; **19**: 511–19.
3. Tfelt-Hansen P. Prophylactic pharmacotherapy of migraine; some practical guidelines. In *Neurologic clinics* (*advances in headache*) (ed. Mathew NT). Philadelphia: Saunders, 1997: 153–67.

Section
VI

Improving health-care systems for headache

58
Integrating headache services across the primary/secondary-care interface

T.J. Steiner

Introduction

> Primary care has become a favourite of politicians, who regard it as a mechanism for containing technology-driven demand for medical care, for balancing the costs and consequences of care, and for fostering self-reliance in individuals.[1]

Van Weel's essay, which these words introduce, went on to question whether the public would be pleased with or, indeed, well served by the 'medicopolitical promotion of primary care'. He was not the first to do so. Coulter had already suggested that primary care might not be an acceptable substitute for secondary care in the popular imagination.[2] Van Weel cited evidence of better outcomes—in relation to costs—where there was greater orientation of care towards primary care,[3] and of economic benefits from the 'gate-keeper' role and personal lists of primary care.[4] He remained doubtful, nonetheless. 'Experience of modern life', he argued, 'tells us that the best buy is usually from the specialist, and we find it hard to imagine that what is true in general would not hold also for medicine.' General practitioners (GPs) and other health-care providers working in primary care might respond that they *are* specialists—in primary care. What *is* primary care is a crucial question.

I will give an answer to this first, then briefly consider the sometimes problematical interface between primary and secondary care in compartmentalized health-care systems. Health services are rarely highly successful in meeting the needs of people with headache disorders, who everywhere are low in the priority queue. Assuming that additional resources can be secured, the solution does not appear to lie in expanding specialist headache centres in secondary care to which most people with needs fail to gain access. Improved service provision in primary care, with facilitated referral to secondary-care specialists for the fewer people who then require it, is in line with the political climate (although not, as I shall argue, necessarily because it is cost-effective). An illustrative proposal is outlined in this chapter with specific details based on an inner-London borough.

Characterizing primary care

The UK in particular has a strong system of primary care.[5] The term dates back to 1920, but only in the 1960s came to denote GPs' settings and services, and was introduced to the world another decade later.[6] The World Health Organization's (WHO) definition of primary care, somewhat broader than 'what GPs provide', makes it the backbone of health care, delivering 'preventive, promotional, curative and rehabilitative health measures and community development activities...aimed at improving the living conditions of individuals, families and communities'. In the Alma-Ata declaration,[6] primary care is '...essential health care based on practical, scientifically sound and socially acceptable methods/technology, made universally accessible to individuals and families in the community through their full participation, and at a cost that the community and country can afford to maintain at every stage of their development, in the spirit of self-reliance and self determination'.[7] The declaration goes on to describe primary health care as 'the first level of contact of individuals, the family and community with the national health system bringing health care as close as possible to where people live and work', which perhaps conveys more of what primary care *is*.

Ambiguity arises because the term may refer to the nature or type of services provided, or to access to and the structure of them.[8] Starfield's[3] definition of primary care as 'first-contact, continuous, comprehensive and co-ordinated care, provided to populations undifferentiated by gender, disease or organ system' perhaps better encapsulates these main elements that primary-care systems aim to preserve. I believe primary care is distinguished by five features (Table 58.1). But there are variations. GPs in France and Germany, for example, do not have a gate-keeping role: patients may go directly to a consultant for a specialist opinion, who therefore becomes the first contact.

Returning to van Weel's conundrum,[1] assessment of needs, in his view, is the speciality of general practice. Decisions in primary care take account of patient-related factors such as family medical history and patients' individual expectations and values of which the continuity and long-term relationships of primary care generate awareness. Continuity of care engenders trust and satisfaction amongst patients,[9] although limited formal evidence establishes its importance otherwise.[10]

Table 58.1   The differentiating features of primary care

- First contact with the health system
- Offering continuity of care
- Comprehensive, therefore generalist
- Provided in or close to the community
- Triage and gate-keeping to specialist services

GPs 'treat a variety of illnesses in any one patient in contrast to secondary care, where many patients are treated for the same disease.'[1] Furthermore, patients value highly and wish to remain in 'their trusted home environment' and are enabled to do so through the social networks that primary care fosters.

Secondary care

In this conception, secondary care becomes whatever is behind the gate (although the gate is always open to emergency services), and where, as in France and Germany, the gate is optional, there is lack of clarity in distinction between primary and secondary care. Thus, often, secondary care is seen as synonymous with specialist care. By its nature, specialist care is usually provided in a hospital environment that has the complex technological facilities necessary to perform clinical investigations, surgery, and postoperative care. And it is technology, by and large, that has driven the expansion and ever-increasing specialization of secondary care, and with it a disempowerment of generalists in primary care.

The ambiguous purpose of gate-keeping

Undoubtedly this issue[11] underlay van Weel's doubts. Ferris *et al.* defined the gate-keeping system as 'one that requires the authorisation of referral to specialists by designated primary care providers'.[12] Embodied in the UK National Health Service (NHS) in a more paternalistic era, gate-keeping ostensibly guides patients efficiently and in their best interests through the system according to their needs rather than their demands. Even in America, patients have found the medical care system a 'nightmare to navigate'.[13] In addition, at least in systems built around personal lists, gate-keeping increases patients' contacts with their GPs who are thereby enabled to provide more comprehensive, coordinated, and continuous prevention and care, which patients value.[9]

Whatever the merits of this in terms of improved outcomes, gate-keeping developed in the USA in the 1980s as a means by which managed-care organizations controlled costs and the inappropriate utilization of resources.[14] And, whatever its original purpose, gate-keeping by GPs in the UK is believed to have contributed to maintaining low levels of expenditure on the NHS in comparison with health-care systems abroad. Today, the gate-keeping role of primary care is regarded as essential for cost containment, in part because of evidence that suggests that unrestricted access to specialists induces a demand for costly and sometimes unnecessary services. The effectiveness of this system,[15] and the equity of it, rely to a great extent on what happens at the *interface* between primary and secondary care, a seam in service continuity at which breakdowns generate a state described as 'limbo' in which patients feel that progress towards recovery ceases.[16] It has received attention recently partly because of concern about variations between GPs in their referral rates to specialist care.[17]

Why be concerned with cost-effectiveness?

The assumption underlying health-needs assessment, and the purchase by health authorities of the most appropriate services to meet those needs, is related to prioritization, given that needs always exceed supply. Cost-effectiveness in health care is now seen as crucial to the efficient use of limited resources. Cost-effectiveness analysis (CEA) ostensibly offers a framework by which the relative costs and consequences of different health-care interventions may be assessed as a rational basis for priority-setting and the allocation of resources to some needs rather than others when they are insufficient for all.

Many studies have therefore endeavoured to measure cost-effectiveness, for example in comparisons of drug or intervention A with B for a specific illness. They reveal great deficiencies in methodology, very often in measurement of outcome to establish the effectiveness side of the equation but also in deciding the context of cost and what to include within it. Guidelines are supported by three distinct groups—governments, pharmaceutical agencies, and peer-reviewed journals—and the conclusion is that the methodology, if not the meaning, of CEA differs according to the target audience.[18]

The shift to primary care

There is clear evidence that countries undertaking reform are shifting away from secondary care towards primary care.[2] The *key drivers* of this change can be incorporated into a 'PEST' analysis of environmental influences (Table 58.2).

If the main driver is cost-effectiveness, however, there is little formal evidence to support it. For example, availability of minor surgery in primary care only encouraged demand for it, and did nothing to reduce hospital-based minor surgery.[20] A study of shared care for diabetes found no advantage for patients receiving treatment at their local surgery rather than in hospital, but it included no outcome data for the cost-effectiveness of the new service.[21] The Grampian study of patients with asthma also found no difference in clinical outcomes between those receiving a new integrated care and those having conventional out-patient management, although costs were slightly lower for the shared-care group.[22] Outcomes of treating low back pain in North Carolina, USA, were similar whether patients received care from

Table 58.2   PEST analysis of drivers of the shift to primary care

---

◆ *Political*: government-imposed reforms (e.g., the NHS plan in the UK (ref. 19))
◆ *Economic*: cost minimization and cost-effectiveness as means of achieving more with less in a context of scarcity
◆ *Socio-cultural*: increasing consumerism and demand for accessibility, continuity, comprehensiveness, and equity in health care
◆ Technological: advancements in technology in the drive for efficiency, re-empowering primary care

---

a primary-care practitioner, chiropractor, or orthopaedic surgeon; the primary-care practitioners provided the least expensive care for acute low back pain, but not necessarily the most cost-effective.[23]

All that is clear from these examples is that the ongoing shifts in the balance of care are not easily justified on the basis that they will prove cost-effective.

Shifting the balance in the UK

Economic forces, cost-effectiveness, and political will

NHS hospitals once provided virtually all secondary-care services to patients in the UK. Although they were, presumably, profit-minimizing organizations, they could be seen acting as *price makers*,[24] not subject to competition over costs. The Conservative government reforms of 1990[25] diverted resources from the hospital sector,[15] creating fund-holding GPs whose contracts offered financial incentives for them to replace some hospital-based services with practice-based provisions. With new methods of commissioning and contracting, fund-holders were able to pay themselves or other health professionals to provide a specified list of traditionally secondary-care services, whilst being held accountable for their allocation of funds. *Competition*, it was believed, had the potential to bring patients a better service—a higher quality of care delivered cost-effectively.[24]

These changes had some impact, in parts of Britain at least, on the pattern of service provision to patients[20] and, amongst other developments, brought hospital specialists into outreach clinics in the community.[26] Unfortunately, the changes had little discernible effect on the demand for specialist care in hospitals,[2] nor did they have any objectively measurable impact on efficiency, equity, effectiveness, and choice for patients.[5] GPs, on the other hand, complained bitterly of increased workload,[27] although evidence of cause and effect was noted to be lacking.[26]

The drive towards primary care was more explicit in the most recent strategic review of the NHS, the *NHS plan* published in the summer of 2000.[19] Fund-holding was swept away. The Labour government this time intended that this document set out a radical and ambitious vision for the NHS redesigned around the patient and making full value of promised additional financial investment. Crucially, the NHS plan laid out bigger roles for GPs, both clinically and managerially.

Empowering and broadening primary care

Thus, firstly, the NHS plan envisaged significant expansion in numbers—an extra 2000 GPs would help achieve, by 2004, the 48-hour target wait-time to see a GP. The plan also foresaw that GP-specialists would be developed[28]—primary-care physicians who would have special expertise in areas, such as dermatology, orthopaedics, and ear, nose, and throat (ENT), that often had long waiting times to be seen by hospital specialists.

Secondly, the NHS plan envisaged a power-shift away from health authorities to primary care trusts (PCTs), 'led by clinicians' and not only responsible for primary care but also managing many community health services and commissioning services from secondary-care providers such as acute hospitals. By 2004, 75% of NHS funds will flow directly to PCTs. As paymasters, PCTs should have a powerful influence over the shape of secondary services and will doubtless use it to continue the shift of some of them into primary care. In fact, the NHS plan set a target of 4 million out-patient consultations moved into primary- and community-care settings by 2004, which may be a desirable development in terms of patients' convenience but there was no reference to any evidence that this is an effective or efficient alternative to secondary care. Indeed, there is no published evidence to support it on any other grounds.[26] Anecdotally, when specialist consultations in primary care were encouraged under GP fund-holding, the result was that specialists who participated in the scheme saw fewer, less ill patients than they would have done in their hospitals.

Finally, an important theme of the NHS plan was the need not just for 'more of the same': there would be a fundamental review of working practices to ensure that different steps in the process of treatment added value instead of being simply 'hand-offs' from one care-giver to another. The plan envisaged whole-service reviews of care pathways from GP to hospital, which, if they crossed the interface between primary and secondary care, would inevitably need to address what might or should be done in primary care and what needed to be done in secondary care.

So, in summary, the new 'primary-care-led NHS' takes emphasis, and potentially money, away from the acute hospital sector and moves them to a more broadly defined primary care.[24] Although one commentary described the changes as 'the "redisorganisation" of the NHS'[29] involving unhappy managers and able only to worsen the service, the expected result is the appearance of different models of integrated care, shared care schemes, specialist outreach services, intermediate hospital care, and other forms of substitution for hospital care together with community services focused on prevention and education of the public on health-related issues. An opportunistic proposal is presented below.

Headache services in Southwark

The WHO recognizes headache disorders as a high-priority public health concern[30] in a worldwide context of significant need arising from headache disorders but low priority given to them in the queue for health care.[31] Headache disorders are common and in many cases lifelong conditions.[32–35] Up to 5% of some populations have daily or near-daily headache.[36,37] Headache disorders are associated with recognizable burdens that include personal suffering, disability, and impaired quality of life.[38–42] Their impact extends beyond those immediately affected.[43] Estimates of the financial cost of headache disorders relate principally to lost work-time and reduced productivity due to impaired working effectiveness. On any working day in the UK, 90 000 people are absent from work or school because of migraine alone.[32]

Consequently, large numbers of people with headache are seen by GPs and by neurologists.[44,45] Of a sample of patients aged 16–65 years registered in a large general practice, 17% consulted because of headache at least once in 5 years and 9% of these were referred to secondary care.[46] Far more patients are referred to secondary care than need be: up to a third of all patients consulting neurologists in the UK do so because of headache, more than for any other neurological condition, and numbers are increasing.[47] In fact, only a small minority of cases of primary headache are *not* best managed in primary care with skills expected to be generally available.[48]

Whilst the large numbers of headache referrals to neurologists are difficult to justify, at the same time most migraine sufferers are not seeing any doctor for headache, many remain undiagnosed, and most do not receive prescription drugs.[49] The same goes for other headache disorders. Barriers to access to headache care—at appropriate levels and overall—exist within the NHS, which are reflected globally.[30, 31] Unmet needs are enormous as many headache sufferers have high disability, whilst effective therapies exist that relieve pain and restore ability to function.

Southwark

Health-care needs in Southwark, an inner-London borough, must be considered in the context of social deprivations and other inequalities that exist locally. These increase rather than reduce the requirement for effective headache services.[50] There are 280 000 people registered with 140 GPs in Southwark.[51] Within this number, according to national data,[32] about 31 000 adults have migraine, of whom some 25 000 have significant disability attributable to it.[49] Over 100 000 working days per year are lost to migraine, and up to twice that number to other headache disorders. About 168 000 adults have occasional other headaches, mostly episodic tension-type headache, which is rarely disabling. An estimated 9000 have headache every or nearly every day; most of these are disabled and, in at least half of these cases, medication misuse is a major (and remediable) factor in causation.[52]

If a distinction is made between *need* and *demand*,[53] the former determined by capacity to benefit from effective intervention and the latter being expressed as wants (not necessarily with underlying need), at least 34 000 adults in Southwark (15% of the total adult population) and over 4000 children are likely to benefit directly from headache care. More will benefit indirectly since larger numbers of people are adversely affected by headache disorders than actually have them.[43]

Proposals for change

Opportunity for change—doing things differently and better, establishing the right structure for headache services with the optimum involvement of primary care—arises because of the government's commitment, described above, to a more efficient, primary-care-led NHS.[19] As noted, the development of GP-specialists, able to provide more complete care for patients outside hospital,[28] is an expected consequence of this reorganization.[54] In this context the British Association for the Study of Headache (BASH), following a national consultation process, has made draft recommendations for change.[48] The essential elements are that the role of primary care in the management of headache disorders should be expanded, incorporating a multidisciplinary approach, with headache services reorganized on three levels. Each general practice, with better education, should provide front-line headache services for their patients (*level one*). Within each PCT, one or more primary-care headache centres (PCHCs) should be established (*level two*) to which local GPs at level one may refer their patients requiring more skilled care. Hospital-based specialists (*level three*) should provide necessary support to level two, and facilitated access for the relatively few patients from levels one or two needing secondary-care management.

The proposals for Southwark build eclectically on these recommendations, seeking to patch the seam in headache services at the primary/secondary-care interface. Headache service development in Southwark is planned around a PCHC that will be established, staffed, operated, and evaluated during a pilot phase of 3 years. Specific proposals are made on siting the PCHC centrally within the community, the range of services to be provided and by whom (a multidisciplinary mix of GP- and nurse-specialists, physiotherapists, psychologists, and community pharmacists), aspects of governance including leadership, integration with level-one primary-care headache services and with level three in secondary care, and use of protocols and care pathways. The *aims* of the project are:

(1)   to reduce waste and improve efficiency of service delivery by pulling inappropriate headache referrals to secondary care back into primary care, thereby freeing resources;
(2)   to use these to improve quality of service, *and* to discover and meet unrecognized headache-related health-care needs, in the community.

Will they work? The problem of evaluation

This project is not readily amenable to controlled evaluation: for example, comparing north Southwark with a PCHC and south Southwark without, or randomizing at practice/GP/patient level within all Southwark so that one group of the population is offered the service and another group is not. Concerns exist about the equity of this approach. There are ethical difficulties in seeking to make comparisons between, for example, Southwark and adjacent Lambeth, where patients in Lambeth become a control group without the opportunity to consent to being observed. Ultimately, persuasive arguments are that the existence of the service, and observation, will change practice even where the service is not directly available (Hawthorne effect) and that there are no objective outcome measures on which power calculations may be based.

Evaluation, in part qualitative, is necessary in several domains but in no case easy.

Clinical effectiveness (has the service improved?)

Standard outcome measures exist for some headache disorders for use in clinical trials, but they have recognized limitations. In the case of service development it is not sufficient to assess outcomes only in those with known headache: this will not measure success or failure in identifying and diagnosing those not complaining of or not already receiving treatment for headache (unrecognized need), who are likely to be numerous and in whom burden may nevertheless be significant.[49] Evaluation must measure *population* headache burden over time, before and during intervention. The management recommendations of the British Association for the Study of Headache[55] suggest an adaptation of Migraine Disability Assessment (MIDAS)[56] for this purpose.

There are problems with this. All methods of longitudinal evaluation assume a certain stability of the local population whereas, in Southwark, annual turn-over of the population is up to 30%.[57] Such a highly fluid population has a limited opportunity to benefit from interventions over time, and then is not available for measuring outcome. It may be that these measures can be applied only to the stable segment. Local issues of language (120 are spoken in the area[58]) and illiteracy are also a factor.

Patient satisfaction (do patients agree?)

An increasingly consumerist approach to the NHS accompanies expanding demand. Patients are rightly arbiters of whether change to service delivery constitutes improvement, and headache patients have clearly expressed views on what aspects of a headache service are highly important (Table 58.3).[59]

Interestingly, these aspects are all related to *process* rather than *outcome*. Patients believe that, if the process is good, so will be the result.

Cost-effectiveness (is the service affordable?)

Service development requires either the investment of further resources or improved cost-effectiveness in applying those currently allocated. This project will be cost-effective if it improves the service without added cost or maintains standards whilst reducing costs. Whereas neurologists are a scarce and relatively costly resource to be used no more than is necessary (and there is opportunity gain in removing workload from them), GPs are in no position to add to their own workloads.

Table 58.3 Features of a headache service that patients rate as important (ref. 59)

- Timely access to services nearby, in primary care rather than hospital-based
- Interested staff who take them seriously
- Sufficient information and explanation
- Follow-up when needed

The PCHC is expected, eventually, to consume 1.8 whole-time equivalents of GP-time, requiring an increase in this resource allocation of approximately 1.3%.

Cost evaluation will measure direct treatment costs—the overall and *per capita* costs of providing care (that is, the costs to the health-care system): primary-care consultations at levels one and two; use of investigations including computerized tomography (CT); referrals to secondary care; and prescriptions. Some of the added costs of enhancing headache services in primary care will be offset by savings both within this setting and elsewhere, for example, costs should be recovered to primary-care budgets by cut-backs on wastage through mismanagement including prescriptions of inappropriate medication, and to commissioning budgets through avoided referrals to secondary care. Where neurologists' work loads are reduced, analysis must include how they utilize released time (opportunity gain). An important issue is that assessable costs are not limited to direct health-care costs but widened to include the much larger non-health-care costs (for example, 100 000 lost working days per year attributable to migraine in Southwark), where savings are more likely to accrue.

Tackling inequality (is the service equitable?)

There is evidence that the more socially deprived experience greater difficulty in accessing health-care services and obtain less good care with poorer outcomes.[60] This is relevant to Southwark. Improving access does not guarantee benefit to the subgroups of the population who most need to be reached.[61] Factors likely to affect access (for example, patient characteristics such as socio-economic status and ethnicity) need to be monitored in order to be aware of, and endeavour to remedy, special problems that may apply to certain groups.

Who will benefit?

Primary care has generally lower overheads. GPs may be less resource-consuming than consultant neurologists, but more GPs are needed if headache services are relocated to primary care. Nurses can take over some aspects of headache care, but again more will be needed. Almost inevitably, if services are improved or merely moved to where patients are, more patients will seek care. Demand will rise, as will costs if any of this new demand is met.

Neurologists may be freed of work, but will not stand idle; they will see other patients. Paradoxically, as a result of this opportunity gain, benefits accruing from shifting headache services to primary care may be seen in better secondary-care management of epilepsy, multiple sclerosis, and parkinsonism!

Conclusions

The complications of evaluation are described because they illustrate how difficult it is. Evidence-based policy-making is in its infancy. Cost-effectiveness is a topical subject, and health-care decision-makers are beginning to use tools such as CEA in resource allocation. But there is very little evidence to support cost-effectiveness as a principal driver for the widely observed shifts of secondary-care services to primary care, whilst efficiency measurement needs to be balanced by considerations of equity.

In this context, it is uncertain whether cost-effectiveness will justify the proposed changes to headache services but there are other influential arguments to support them. There are many problems with the compartmentalized *status quo* in headache services, and in the UK there is opportunity for change. These problems, and the priority that should be accorded to headache services, must be acknowledged if change is to be made to happen and resistance to it resolved. *Education* is necessary at a number of levels. A GP-specialist service bridging the seam between primary and secondary care may provide solutions to (some) current failures, but measuring the benefits of change is a challenge. Whilst major improvement to services requires significant investment, there are opportunities for substantial savings to offset it.

Acknowledgements

I am grateful to the following for assistance in researching or preparing parts of this manuscript: Ms Tracy Davies, Mr Mark Easton, Dr Dmitry Feoktistov, Ms Julie Harris, and Mrs Niamh Lennox-Chhugani.

References

1. Van Weel C. Primary care: political favourite or scientific discipline? *Lancet* 1996; **348**: 1431–2.
2. Coulter A. Shifting the balance from secondary to primary care. *Br Med J* 1995; **311**: 1447–8.
3. Starfield B. Is primary care essential? *Lancet* 1994; **344**: 1129–33.
4. Badia JG. General practice/family medicine in the new Europe—changes and challenges. *Allmanmedicin* 1996; **17** (Suppl. 18): 22–5.
5. Dixon J, Holland P, Mays N. Developing primary care: gatekeeping, commissioning, and managed care. *Br Med J* 1998; **317**: 125–8.
6. World Health Organization International Conference on Primary Health Care. *Declaration of Alma-Ata*. Geneva: WHO, 1978.
7. Hertzel BS. *Basic health care in developing countries. An epidemiological perspective*. Oxford: Oxford University Press, 1978.
8. Ritsatakis A, Barnes R, Dekker E, Harrington P, Kokko S, Makara P (eds). *Exploring health policy development in Europe*. Copenhagen: WHO Regional Publications, 2000.
9. Mainous AG, Baker R, Love MM, Gray DP, Gill JM. Continuity of care and trust in one's physician: evidence from primary care in the United States and the United Kingdom. *Family Med* 2001; **33**: 22–7.
10. Freeman G, Shepperd S, Robinson I, Ehrich K, Richards S. *Continuity of care. Report of a scoping exercise Summer 2000* (draft). London: NCCSDO, 2001 at http://www.sdo.lshtm.ac.uk.
11. Tarino E, Webster EG. *Primary health care concepts and challenges in a changing world. Alma-Ata revisited*. Geneva: WHO, 1995.

12. Ferris TG, Chang Y, Blumenthal D, Pearson SD. Leaving gatekeeping behind—effects of opening access to specialists for adults in a health maintenance organization. *New Engl J Med* 2001; **345**: 1312–17.

13. Picker Institute. *Eye on patients: a report of the American public.* Chicago: American Hospital Association, 1996.

14. Lawrence D. Gatekeeping reconsidered [editorial]. *New Engl J Med* 2001; **345**: 1342–3.

15. Jones R, Lamont T, Haines A. Setting priorities for research and development in the NHS: a case study on the interface between primary and secondary care. *Br Med J* 1995; **311**: 1076–80.

16. Preston C, Cheater F, Baker R, Hearnshaw H. Left in limbo: patients views on care across the primary/secondary interface. *Qual Hlth Care* 1999; **8**: 16–21.

17. Pringle M, Heath I. Primary care: opportunities and threats: distributing primary care fairly. *Br Med J* 1997; **314**: 595.

18. Walker D. Cost and cost-effectiveness guidelines. *Hlth Policy Planning* 2001; **16**: 113–21.

19. Department of Health. *The NHS plan. A plan for investment. A plan for reform.* Norwich: HMSO, 2000.

20. Lowy A, Brazier J, Fall M, Thomas K, Jones N, Williams B. Minor surgery by general practitioners under the 1990 contract: effects on hospital workload. *Br Med J* 1993; **307**: 413–17.

21. Naji S. Integrated care for diabetes: clinical, psychosocial and economic evaluation. *Br Med J* 1994; **308**: 1208–12.

22. Grampian Asthma Study of Integrated Care. Integrated care for asthma: a clinical, social and economic evaluation. *Br Med J* 1994; **305**: 599–604.

23. Carey TS, Garrett J, Jackman A, *et al.* The outcomes and costs of care for acute low back pain among patients seen by primary care practitioners, chiropractors, and orthopedic surgeons. *New Engl J Med* 1995; **333**: 913–17.

24. Hossain M. *The provision of secondary care services in primary care.* Diploma dissertation: Imperial College London, 1998.

25. *NHS and Community Care Act 1990.* London: HMSO, 1990.

26. Pederson LL, Leese B. What will a primary care led NHS mean for GP workload? The problem of the lack of an evidence base. *Br Med J* 1997; **314**: 1337–41.

27. Helliwell CD, Carney TA. General practitioners' workload in primary care led NHS [letter]. *Br Med J* 1997; **315**: 546.

28. Department of Health. *Shifting the balance of power within the NHS: securing delivery.* London: Department of Health, 2001.

29. Smith J, Walshe K, Hunter DJ. The 'redisorganisation' of the NHS [editorial]. *Br Med J* 2001; **323**: 1262–3.

30. World Health Organization. *Headache disorders and public health. Education and management implications.* Geneva: WHO, 2000.

31. American Association for the Study of Headache, International Headache Society. Consensus statement on improving migraine management. *Headache* 1998; **38**: 736.

32. Steiner TJ, Scher AI, Stewart WF, Kolodner K, Liberman J, Lipton RB. The prevalence of adult migraine in England and its relationships to major sociodemographic characteristics. *Cephalalgia*, in press.

33. Rasmussen BK, Jensen R, Schroll M, Olesen J. Interrelations between migraine and tension-type headache in the general population. *Arch Neurol* 1992; **49**: 914–18.

34. Rasmussen BK, Jensen R, Schroll M, Olesen J. Epidemiology of headache in a general population—a prevalence study. *J Clin Epidemiol* 1991; **44**: 1147–57.

35. Jensen R. Pathophysiological mechanisms of tension-type headache: a review of epidemiological and experimental studies. *Cephalalgia* 1999; **19**: 602–21.

36. Scher AI, Stewart WF, Liberman J, Lipton RB. Prevalence of frequent headache in a population sample. *Headache* 1998; **38**: 497–506.
37. Castillo J, Munoz P, Guitera V, Pascual J. Epidemiology of chronic daily headache in the general population. *Headache* 1999; **39**: 190–6.
38. Osterhaus JT, Gutterman DL, Plachetka JR. Healthcare resource and lost labour costs of migraine headache in the US. *PharmacoEconomics* 1992; **2**: 67–76.
39. Kryst S, Scherl E. A population-based survey of the social and personal impact of headache. *Headache* 1994; **34**: 344–50.
40. Rasmussen BK. Epidemiology of headache in Europe. In *Headache classification and epidemiology* (ed. Olesen J). New York: Raven Press, 1994; 231–7.
41. Stewart WF, Lipton RB, Simon D. Work-related disability: results from the American migraine study. *Cephalalgia* 1996; **16**: 231–8.
42. Schwartz BS, Stewart WF, Lipton RB. Lost workdays and decreased work effectiveness associated with headache in the workplace. *J Occup Environ Med* 1997; **39**: 320–7.
43. Steiner TJ. Headache burdens and bearers. *Funct Neurol* 2000; **15** (Suppl. 3): 219–23.
44. Hopkins A, Menken M, De Friese GA. A record of patient encounters in neurological practice in the United Kingdom. *J Neurol Neurosurg Psychiatry* 1989; **52**: 436–8.
45. Wiles CM, Lindsay M. General practice referrals to a department of neurology. *J Roy Coll Physicians* 1996; **30**: 426–31.
46. Laughey WF, Holmes WF, MacGregor AE, Sawyer JPC. Headache consultation and referral patterns in one UK general practice. *Cephalalgia* 1999; **19**: 328–9.
47. Hopkins A. Neurological services and the neurological health of the population in the United Kingdom. *J Neurol Neurosurg Psychiatry* 1997; **63**: 553–9.
48. British Association for the Study of Headache. *Review of the organisation of headache services in primary care and recommendations for change*, 1st edn (consultation draft). London: BASH, 2000.
49. Lipton RB, Scher AI, Steiner TJ, Kolodner K, Liberman J, Stewart WF. Patterns of health care utilization for migraine in England and in the United States: a comparative study. In preparation.
50. Lipton RB, Stewart WF, Diamond S, Diamond ML, Reed M. Prevalence and burden of migraine in the United States: data from the American Migraine Study II. *Headache* 2001; **41**: 646–57.
51. Lambeth, Southwark and Lewisham Health Authority. *Proposal to create a primary care trust in Southwark*. London: LSLHA, 2001.
52. Steiner T. Daily grind. *Chemist & Druggist* 2000; **253**, no. 6225 (5 February), Continuing Education Programme supplement: v–viii.
53. Wright J, Williams R, Wilkinson J. The development and importance of health needs assessment. In *Health needs assessment in practice* (ed. Wright J). London: BMJ Books, 1998; 1–11.
54. UK Department of Health. *Making a difference. Integrated working in primary care*. London: Department of Health, 2000 at http://www.doh.gov/nurstrat/primarycare.htm.
55. British Association for the Study of Headache. *Guidelines for all doctors in the diagnosis and management of migraine and tension-type headache*. London: BASH, 2001 at http://www.bash.org.uk.
56. Sawyer J, Edmeads J, Lipton RB, *et al.* Clinical utility of a new instrument assessing migraine disability: the Migraine Disability Instrument (MIDAS) questionnaire. *Neurology* 1998; **50**: A433–4.
57. Information provided by Lambeth, Southwark and Lewisham Health Authority.
58. Lambeth, Southwark and Lewisham Health Authority, 2001 at http://www.lslha.nhs.uk/ha.
59. Information provided by Migraine Action Association.

60. Acheson D. *Independent inquiry into inequalities in health* [the Acheson Report]. London: The Stationery Office, 1998.
61. Shaw R, Smith P. Allocating health care resources to reduce health inequalities. In *Health care UK Spring 2001* (ed. Appelby J, Harrison A). London: King's Fund, 2001: 7–13.

59 Comprehensive academic headache centres

Hartmut Göbel

Need for and availability of specialized headache therapy

Figures for the year 2000 in Germany show that headache is a widespread problem and that the patients affected make very heavy use of health-care services. For example, 8.7% of women and 5.1% of men in Germany take headache medication several times a week, and 51.4% of women and 43.8% of men use headache medication 1 to 4 times a month. Only 39.5% of women and 50.9% of men never use headache medication. Migraine alone is responsible for 900 of 100 000 insured persons a year having to take time off work. On average this incapacity to work lasts 6 days. About 1% of insured persons have to take early retirement because of headaches. Their average age is around 51 years. According to the German hospital statistics for 1998, 0.02% of women and 0.01% of men require acute in-patient treatment for conditions diagnosed as migraine. In 1998 a total of 88 588 days in hospital were due to migraine. It was primarily patients aged between 15 and 55 years who had to be hospitalized because of migraine. The figures show clearly that a considerable number of patients with headache require intensive and specialized therapy to avoid individual suffering and economic consequences.[1,2]

No systematic studies existed of the need for specialized pain therapy. In order to clarify this question an exact analysis of hospitalization cases in the German state of Schleswig-Holstein was undertaken in 1995. It was found that, in the course of a year, 2.8% of the population had to be given in-patient treatment in a hospital because of chronic pain. The average length of stay was around 14.3 days. For the diagnosis of headache alone, 1% of the population had to be admitted to hospital in the course of a year. The average length of stay for headache therapy was 12 days. The average cost per case totalled 3061 euros. Treatment of medication-induced continuous headache made hospitalization necessary for 0.14% of the population during the year. Here the average length of stay was 16 days, and the average cost per case 3079 euros. An analysis of these figures showed that chronic pain syndromes were the third most frequent reason for full in-patient treatment. An analysis extending over several years also showed an annual increase of around 11% in the number of cases treated for chronic pain syndromes. Most of these patients were treated in non-specialized general hospitals without any specialized therapeutic concepts, especially for complex headache problems. An examination of the data to identify the most expensive headache syndromes revealed that tension-type headache is the most expensive pain syndrome in view of the lengthy treatment in a non-specialized setting. Here the average treatment costs work out at 7785 euros. Other particularly expensive syndromes are basilar migraine, thalamic neuralgia, atypical facial neuralgia, trigeminal neuralgia, cervicogenic headache, and migraine. An analysis of existing health-care structures shows that, at present, diagnosis and therapy are largely non-specialized, and that the great fund of existing knowledge in the field of headache therapy is generally not available for the patients. As a rule, the patients are treated on a monodisciplinary basis. Comprehensive and multidisciplinary therapeutic strategies are not generally available to the patients. On the basis of these analyses it can be calculated that there is, roughly speaking, a need for one specialized headache therapy centre for every million of the population.

Health-care levels

It is essentially possible to distinguish a number of stages in the care of headache patients. A large proportion of patients take care of themselves, without any professional diagnosis or therapy. Self-medication is the rule here. The next stage is the general practitioner. If therapy at this level is not effective, the patients are usually referred to a neurological practice. If specialized in-patient treatment is required, the patients are then admitted to a general neurological clinic. The patient may also be referred to a regional multidisciplinary headache out-patient clinic, if one exists. The highest level in the health-care scale is an academic multidisciplinary headache centre. The following description gives an idea of how such an establishment works.

Academic multidisciplinary headache centres

Out-patient and in-patient setting

In principle, such a headache centre can treat patients on an out- or an in-patient basis. Admission may be preceded by a preliminary out-patient examination to clarify the indication for admission, or possibly to initiate an effective out-patient therapy plan and thereby avoid unnecessary hospitalization. The out-patient facility is also necessary for postclinical follow-up and progress monitoring and, if necessary, for subsequent therapy adjustment in the course of time.[3–5]

Admission criteria

Typical admission criteria[6] for a headache centre are: unclear diagnosis; ineffective treatment at lower levels in the health-care structure; excessive medication intake;

complex physical or psychological comorbidity; and, in individual cases, emergency pain therapy cases such as therapy-resistant exacerbation of an active cluster period or the onset of therapy-resistant trigeminal neuralgia.

Experience at the Kiel Pain Clinic

The following description outlines the working methods and the functions of a specialized multidisciplinary pain clinic, taking the Kiel Neurological and Behavioural Pain Clinic as an example. As a result of the analyses described, a specialized neurological and behavioural pain clinic was established in Kiel pursuant to Section 63 ff. of the German Social Code, as adopted by the German Bundestag, in order to implement specialized therapeutic measures and investigate the clinical and economic effects of treatment. The clinic works in cooperation with the University of Kiel and the Allgemeine Ortskrankenkasse (AOK) Schleswig-Holstein, the largest statutory health insurance fund in the state of Schleswig-Holstein. The facility emerged from the long-standing headache and pain working group at the university's neurological clinic. Criteria for the establishment of the model projects were an innovative medical strategy and cost-effective provision of services.

Admissions

Admission to the clinic is only possible by medical referral, which presupposes prior treatment at lower health-care levels. The example of the Kiel Pain Clinic shows that general practitioners, at 45%, account for the most referrals. The next largest groups referring patients are neurologists (21%), anaesthesiological pain therapists (10%), orthopaedic specialists (8%), internal specialists (7%), and neurosurgeons (also 7%). The rest come from a wide range of medical specialisms. The distribution of the diagnoses shows that the largest group of patients admitted have primary headaches. Some 30% of patients have migraine or tension-type headache. They are followed by 13% with medication-induced headache. Further diagnoses in declining order of frequency are: backache (12%); failed back surgery syndrome (8%); painful neuropathia (7%); somatoform disorders (6%); posttraumatic headache (7%); central pain (6%); cluster headache (4%); postherpetic neuralgia (4%); cervical distonia (3%); and others. Ninety-five per cent of patients display at least two diagnoses; as a rule these involve psychological comorbidity,[7,8] and with over 50% there is a depressive reaction. Fifty-eight per cent of the patients have more than five different diagnoses. The patients are referred from all over Germany. More than 60% of the patients admitted come from other German states or from neighbouring countries. The patients are most commonly aged between 30 and 60 years.

Organizational structure

A multidisciplinary organizational structure was created in the Kiel Pain Clinic for the treatment of such complex pain syndromes. The Kiel Pain Clinic is an independent clinic that can concentrate exclusively on the needs of chronic pain patients. For preclinical admission examination and postclinical follow-up, the clinic cooperates closely with the out-patient pain department of the Neurological Clinic of the University of Kiel. Staff of the pain clinic work both in the out-patient department and in the clinic, to permit continuous treatment in the out- and in-patient sectors. The clinic operates as a totally hospitalization-based acute clinic. It has an inter-disciplinary staff structure made up of neurologists, psychiatrists, specialist pain therapists, psychologists, behavioural therapists, orthopaedic specialists, and inter-nal specialists. The team also includes nursing staff with special training in pain therapy, physiotherapists, and experts in rehabilitation and welfare counselling. If invasive diagnostic or therapeutic measures are necessary, these are undertaken in the multidisciplinary setting of the various specialized clinics of the University of Kiel. These in turn belong to an alliance of specialist doctors in the form of the interdisciplinary pain centre, which is a regular conference of representatives of the individual specialisms who discuss and deal with problem situations on a multidis-ciplinary basis. Thus the entire field of maximum medical care is available to the patients.

The core staff of the Kiel Pain Clinic consists of academically qualified specialists whose aim is to place the entire fund of pain therapy knowledge at the patient's disposal. As an independent clinic, the establishment is devoted entirely to pain therapy. To this end specialized accommodation is also guaranteed, ensuring that the needs of pain therapy are not subordinated to other aspects. The clinic maintains a highly structured and specialized diagnosis and therapy programme for the care of neurological pain syndromes. It also maintains an active research programme and an active teaching programme for students. Moreover, it holds ongoing further training events for doctors and public relations events for sufferers.

This organizational basis allows the extensive present-day knowledge in the fields of headache diagnosis and treatment to be made available to the headache patient. It also makes it possible in particular to provide specific treatment for pain syndromes where therapeutic results to date have been unsatisfactory. This also applies espe-cially to rare headache syndromes that frequently cannot be treated effectively in non-specialized establishments. Complex pain syndromes and multiple additional health problems can also be given comprehensive specialized treatment. Other possibilities are a particularly specialized diagnosis that gives greater precision to the neurological and psychological findings and updates and supplements them, and a complete analysis of the biological, psychosocial, and economic conditions of the pain syndrome. Diagnostic differentiation down to the fourth level of the Interna-tional Headache Society (IHS) classification can be guaranteed as standard. Items registered for tension-type headache, for example, are muscular pain sensitivity, using a variety of diagnostic therapy methods such as pressure algometer, electro-myography, or palpation, and aggravating factors. Simultaneous registration of these parameters, especially oromandibular dysfunction, psychosocial stress, anxiety, depression, muscular stress, and excessive use of medication, and their simultaneous and multidisciplinary treatment are an important key to achieving therapeutic successes in hitherto frustrating cases.

A multidisciplinary headache centre is in a position to offer particularly sophisticated medication therapy for complex syndromes. This applies both to acute treatment and to headache prevention. Cases of rare diseases, complex comorbidity, contraindications, and medication interactions call for specialized knowledge and experience that can usually only be offered at a specialized centre.

All occupational groups at a specialized pain centre must be trained for the needs of chronic pain patients. This also applies to the nursing staff. Many rules that apply to other groups of patients are not appropriate to headache patients. Migraine and headache patients should not have to beg for the necessary medication, but must be provided with them just as normally as diabetes mellitus patients are given their insulin. Patients should not have to fetch triptans and other acute medication from the nursing staff when an attack starts, but should always have this medication with them. Medication for treating secondary headache or preventing primary headache must not be given on demand, but on a fixed time basis. The nurses must also ensure that active behaviour is reinforced and that pain behaviour is not rewarded with attention.

Special organizational requirements are also important. For example, peace and a dark room must be possible during the acute phase of migraine attacks or the acute phase of rebound headaches. Patients with cluster attacks at night cannot be accommodated in a room with others until the therapy has started to take effect. Non-specialized centres are usually unable to cater for these and other special requirements of migraine or headache patients, since the usual daily routine with acute admissions takes priority in everyday practice. A headache centre must also have facilities for taking in and caring for small children in cases of mothers with headaches.

Behavioural therapy

One very important element in a multidisciplinary headache team is specialized psychologists and behavioural therapists. They are essential for informing and educating headache patients. The therapeutic measures can be performed in group therapy or in individual treatments. Important diagnostic and therapeutic tasks are: information about pain conditions (education); patient workshops; discussion groups; introduction to patient-oriented literature; headache advice books, etc. (bibliotherapy); familiarization with and avoidance of trigger mechanisms; nutritional counselling and adjustment; daily planning; progressive muscle relaxation; biofeedback methods; psychiatric therapy measures; operant therapeutic measures (identification and elimination of positive amplifiers for pain behaviour, increasing physical activity, medication withdrawal); cognitive methods (management of pain-maintaining contingencies); stress-management training (relaxation training, counselling for effective stress management, self-regulating medication programme, information on stress and pain, individual and group therapy, family therapy, therapeutic setting that attaches value to maximum relaxation and self-involvement); self-assurance training (reducing anxieties and increasing social competence with the aim of controlling situations that trigger pain attacks); pain inoculation training (situational analysis through daily recording of pain episodes, their triggers, and intensity); analysis of pain behaviour with regard to the connection between cognition, coping strategies, and pain episodes; presentation of pain stimulation and discussion of thoughts and feelings; comparison of experimental and clinical pain; discussion of patients' individual pain strategies; learning new coping strategies, for example, focusing attention, relaxation, imagination, self-instruction; transfring training content to everyday life (video feedback, etc.).

Physiotherapy

Another indispensable core element is physiotherapists with special training in specialized headache therapy. This includes activation and mobilization of patients with aggravating factors such as muscular stress or oromandibular dysfunction, informing and educating patients, and treating elevated pericranial pain sensitivity. Specific treatment of muscular factors such as trigger and tender points in particular is also the province of the physiotherapist.

Other medical disciplines

In many cases it is necessary to integrate diagnosis and treatment methods of other disciplines in the concept in an academic multidisciplinary setting. These include neuroradiology, cardiology, orthopaedics, ophthalmology, anaesthesiology, neurosurgery, and dentistry.

Research and teaching

An active research programme and an active training programme for medical students, psychologists, physiotherapists, and nursing staff permit the further development and dissemination of high-quality diagnosis and treatment programmes. Regular further training programmes for neurologists, general practitioners, psychologists, physiotherapists and other groups transfer the knowledge into the general health-care sector and permit direct communication between referring doctors and the multidisciplinary pain centre.

International exchange in the development of therapy programmes through reciprocal visits by a wide variety of specialist groups from headache centres in other countries provides an important stimulus for further improvements in the individual programmes.

Effectiveness: relieving pain and reducing costs

Both the clinical effectiveness and the economic effectiveness of multidisciplinary headache centres have been examined in studies. There was found to be a significant reduction in individual suffering, a marked reduction in social and occupational incapacity with an increase in social and occupational performance,[9–19] and a significant reduction in costs for the persons affected, for the public, and for the insurance funds.[20–26] This can be seen in a marked reduction in time off work, a reduction in the need for early retirement, a reduction in use of medication, and a reduction in the use of medical services. The scientific analysis of the therapeutic effectiveness of the Kiel Pain Clinic was performed by an independent external institute; its cost-effectiveness was determined directly by analysing the costs incurred by the health insurance fund in the out- and in-patient sectors. It transpires that some 80% of patients achieve a marked clinical improvement despite many years' history of therapy resistance. The improvement is maintained for an observation period of 12 months and increases steadily during the posthospitalization period. After treatment, more than 75% of the patients were able to engage in normal social and occupational activities, whereas before treatment 88% of the patients suffered from marked impairment (Fig. 59.1). The highly specialized diagnostic and therapeutic measures make it possible to achieve much higher treatment quality than in a non-specialized treatment setting. Moreover, the treatment can be performed considerably more cost-effectively, resulting in substantial cost-saving potential for the health insurance funds.

Thanks to intensive international research results in recent years, a large fund of knowledge about pain therapy is currently available. The application of this knowledge calls for specialization in specially equipped multidisciplinary centres. If this requirement is met, the treatment programmes can be implemented extremely effectively and result in a distinct reduction in pain-induced incapacity, often even in cases that have proved resistant to therapy for many years. Comprehensive

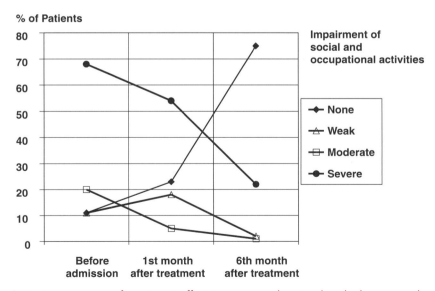

Fig. 59.1 Improvement of treatment effect in a comprehensive headache centre during the posthospitalization period. After treatment, more than 75% of the patients were able to engage in normal social and occupational activities, whereas before treatment 88% of the patients suffered impairment.

multidisciplinary headache centres are essential for innovative and intensive research, teaching, and further training.

References

1. Crook J, Tunks E, Rideout E, Bowne G. Epidemiologic consideration of persistent pain sufferers in specialty pain clinics and the community. *Arch Phys Med Rehabil* 1986; **67**: 451–5.
2. Göbel H, Buschmann P, Heinze A, Heinze-Kuhn K. Epidemiology and socioeconomic consequences of migraine and headache diseases. *Versicherungsmedizin* 2000; **52** (1): 19–23.
3. Csordas TJ, Clark JA. Ends of the line: diversity among chronic pain centers. *Soc Sci Med* 1992; **34**: 383–93.
4. Deardorff WW, Rubin HS, Scott DW. Comprehensive multidisciplinary treatment of chronic pain: a follow-up study of treated and non-treated groups. *Pain* 1991; **45**: 35–43.
5. Göbel H, Buschmann P. Schmerzen lindern—Kosten senken. *Schmerz* 2001; **15** (2): 79–80.
6. Turk DC, Rudy TE. Neglected factors in chronic pain treatment outcome studies—referral patterns, failure to enter treatment, and attrition. *Pain* 1990; **43**: 7–25.
7. Roberts AH, Reinhardt L. The behavioral management of chronic pain: long-term follow-up with comparison groups. *Pain* 1980; **8**: 151–62.
8. Romano J, Turner JA. Chronic pain and depression: does the evidence support a relationship? *Psychol Bull* 1985; **97**: 18–34.
9. Aronoff GM, McAlary PW, Witkower A, Berdell MS. Pain treatment programs: Do they return workers to the workplace? *Spine* 1987; **2**: 123–36.
10. Becker N, Sjögren P, Olsen AK, Eriksen J. Therapeutic results in chronic, non-malignant pain in patients treated at a Danish multidisciplinary pain center compared with general practice. A randomized controlled clinical trial. *Ugeskr Laeger* 2001; **163** (22): 3078–82.
11. Catchlove R, Cohen K. Effects of directive return to work approach in the treatment of workman's compensation patients with chronic pain. *Pain* 1982; **14**: 181–91.
12. Caudill M, Schnabble R, Zuttermeister P, *et al.* Decreased clinic use by chronic pain patients: responsiveness to behavioral medical intervention. *Clin J Pain* 1991; **7**: 305–10.
13. Chapman SL, Brena SF, Bradford LA. The treatment outcome in a chronic pain rehabilitation program. *Pain* 1981; **11**: 255–68.
14. Dieudonne I, Richardson PH, Williams AC deC, Featherstone J, Harding V. Can pain management enable severely impaired chronic pain patients to return to work? In *Abstracts: 7th World Congress on Pain*. Seattle: IASP Publications, 1993: 138.
15. Malec J, Cayner JJ, Harvey RF, Timming RC. Pain management: long-term follow-up of an inpatient program. *Arch Phys Med Rehabil* 1981; **62**: 369–72.
16. Newman RI, Seres JL, Yospe LP, Garlington B. Multidisciplinary treatment of chronic pain: longterm follow-up of low back pain patients. *Pain* 1978; **4**: 283–92.
17. Parris WCV, Jamison RN, Vasterling JJ. Follow-up study of a multidisciplinary pain center. *J Pain Symptom Managment* 1987; **2**: 145–51.
18. Peters J, Large RG, Elkind G. Follow-up results from a randomized controlled trial evaluating in and outpatient pain management programmes. *Pain* 1992; **50**: 41–50.
19. Sturgis ET, Schaefer CA, Sikora TL. Pain center follow-up study of treated and untreated patients. *Arch Phys Med Rehabil* 1984; **65**: 301–3.
20. Cicala RS, Wright J. Outpatient treatment of patients with chronic pain: an analysis of cost savings. *Clin J Pain* 1989; **5**: 223–6.
21. Cohen MJM, Campbell JN (ed.). *Pain treatment centers at a crossroads: a practical and conceptual reappraisal. Progress in pain research and management*, Vol. 7. Seattle: IASP Press, 1996.

22. Göbel H, Buschmann P, Heinze A, Heinze-Kuhn K. Value of specialized pain treatment. *Versicherungsmedizin* 2000; **52** (2): 57–65.

23. Göbel H. Specialised pain therapy: does it pay for patients and health authorities? *Schmerz* 2001; **15** (2): 103–9.

24. Göbel H. Value of organized headache care. *Eur J Neurol* 1999; **6** (Suppl. 2): 43–55.

25. Stieg RL, Turk DC. Chronic pain sydrome: the necessity of demonstrating the cost-benefit of treatment. *Pain Management* 1988; **1**: 58–63.

26. Turk DC. Efficacy of multidisciplinary pain centers in the treatment of chronic pain. In *Pain treatment centers at a crossroads: ca practical and conceptual reappraisal. Progress in pain research and management*, Vol. 7 (ed. Cohen MJM, Campbell JN). Seattle: IASP Press, 1996.

60 Headache clinic or pain centre: together or separate

Hans-Christoph Diener

There are basically two ways to organize patient care for patients with headache. Patients can be seen at a specialized headache out-patient clinic or at a general pain clinic. The author is not aware of prospective studies investigating the quality of patient care and outcome in terms of improvement of headache in these two structures. The author, however, has personal experience in running a dedicated headache clinic and a general pain centre.

Arguments in favour of treating headache patients in a pain centre

Pain centres by their very nature are based on the interdisciplinary cooperation of many specialities such as anaesthesiology, neurology, psychiatry, psychosomatic medicine, psychology, orthopaedic surgery, internal medicine (rheumatology, oncology), radiology, dentistry, paediatrics, and pharmacology. *De novo* patients are usually seen first by the specialist who has the adequate expertise for the particular pain. Other specialists, depending on whether the diagnosis is easy or complex and whether comorbidity exists, will then see the patient. Difficult patients are presented in discussion rounds, and an integrated treatment plan will be worked out.

Patients who should be diagnosed and treated in a pain centre are those with non-primary headache, neck pain, or facial pain. This includes patients with chronic pain and psychiatric comorbidity (anxiety, depression, bipolar disease).[1-5] Pain centres have more sophisticated diagnostic tests and procedures. These include special imaging procedures to rule out symptomatic headache and special psychological testing. An anaesthetic block of the root C2, a procedure that should be performed by an anaesthetist or an interventional neuroradiologist, can diagnose patients with cervicogenic headache.[6] Dentists are needed in cases of temporomanibular disorders.

Due to their very nature, pain centres can provide complex treatment strategies combining drug therapy and behavioural therapy. Chronic pain patients will not improve with drug treatment alone. Pain centres have experience with the long-term use of opioids, drugs that sometimes are needed in hemicrania continua, refractory trigeminal neuralgia, and postherpetic neuralgia. Patients in whom the head or facial pain is caused by malignant tumours or metastases sometimes require destructive surgery in addition to radiation, chemotherapy, and slow-release opioids.

Arguments in favour of treating headache patients in headache clinics

For most headache patients headache clinics are appropriate. Headache clinics are usually run by neurologists in collaboration with psychologists. In some countries, anaesthetists with a special training primarily in pain therapy see headache patients. An integral part of any headache clinic should be physical therapy. The ideal patient for headache clinics is a patient with a primary headache or facial pain, for example, patients with migraine, tension-type headache, cluster headache, and other trigemino-autonomic headaches. Most headache centres are able to diagnose and treat medi-cation overuse headache.[7] The treatment approach for patients with posttraumatic headache is similar to the one used in chronic tension-type headache. Therefore, these patients can be treated in a headache clinic. Physicians from other disciplines (dentistry, psychiatry) can be consulted if necessary. For most patients with migraine and episodic tension-type headache as well as cluster headache this is not necessary. Diagnostic procedures include imaging, in rare cases electroencephalo-graphy (EEG) and ultrasound, psychological testing, and blood tests. Headache clinics have a longstanding experience with the drug treatment of episodic headache as well as headache prophylaxis in migraine or chronic headaches.[8–9] Patients with chronic headache should be treated, whenever possible, with a combination of drug therapy and behavioural therapy.[10] Physical therapy or exercise are useful, but not yet proven to be effective in randomized trials.

The organization of a headache clinic is much easier than that of a pain centre. The small team involved facilitates communication and avoids long delays in treatment decisions. Patients in pain centres sometimes have to wait for 1 or 2 weeks until the whole team has joined and discussed the case.

Conclusion

As usual, there is no easy solution to the question. Different patients with different histories and different chronologies as well as different comorbidities require different structures for diagnosis and long-term treatment. Table 60.1 summarizes patient characteristics that would predict whether treatment should be performed in a headache clinic or a pain centre.

Table 60.1 Patient stratification and organizational features of headache clinics versus pain centres for the treatment of headache and facial pain

Headache clinic	Pain centre
Patients with primary headache	Secondary headache
Patients with minimal comorbidity	Major comorbidity
Short or medium duration of condition	Long duration
Need for opioids	
Need for surgery	
Small team	Interdisciplinary team
Easy to organize	Complex infrastructure

References

1. Bahra A, Goadsby PJ. The comorbidity of migraine and depression: a review. *Neurol Psychiatry* 1998; **2**: 23–7.
2. Juang K-D, Wang S-J, Fuh J-L, Lu S-R, Su T-P. Comorbidity of depressive and anxiety disorders in chronic daily headache and its subtypes. *Headache* 2000; **40**: 818–23.
3. Lipton RB, Silberstein SD. Neurologic and psychiatric comorbidity with migraine. *Neurology* 1994; **44**: S1–S47.
4. Merikangas KR, Stevens DE. Comorbidity of migraine and psychiatric disorders. *Neurol Clin N Am* 1997; **15**: 115–23.
5. Wang S-J, Liu H-C, Fuh J-L, Liu C-Y, Wang P-N, Lu S-R. Comorbidity of headaches and depression in the elderly. *Pain* 1999; **82**: 239–43.
6. Sjaastad O, Bovim G. Cervicogenic headache. The differentiation from common migraine. An overview. *Funct Neurol* 1991; **6**: 93–100.
7. Katsarava Z, Fritsche G, Muessig M, Diener HC, Limmroth V. Clinical features of withdrawal headache following overuse of triptans in comparison to other antimigraine drugs. *Neurology* 2001; **56** (Suppl. 3): A220.
8. Goadsby PJ, Mathew NT. Clinical approach to the headache patient. In *The headaches*, 2nd edn (ed. Olesen J, Tfelt-Hansen P, Welch KMA). Philadelphia: Lippincott Williams & Wilkins, 2000: 41–2.
9. Goadsby PJ, Lipton RB, Ferrari MD. Drug therapy: migraine—current understanding and treatment. *New Engl J Med* 2002; **346**: 257–70..
10. Holroyd KA, O'Donnell FJ, Stensland M, Lipchik GL, Cordingley GE, Carlson BW. Management of chronic tension-type headache with tricyclic antidepressant medication, stress management therapy and their combination. *J Am Med Assoc* 2001; **285**: 2208–15.

61
The first year of the Lariboisière emergency headache centre: a series of 10510 patients

D. Valade, A. Ducros, M. El Amrani, L. Ben Slamia, C. Roos,
R. Djomby, V. Domigo, L. Morin, V. Besançon, and M.G. Bousser

Introduction

An emergency headache centre (EHC) was opened on 9 December 2000 in the emergency department of Lariboisière hospital, Paris, France. The population was informed by various media that the EHC would be open 24 h/24 h all year long for adults suffering an acute recent heachache. It was established in answer to a real public health need and was intended for patients with specific headaches that needed an urgent diagnosis and rapid treatment rather than for patients suffering from chronic headaches for whom specific structures already existed.

We will describe the main characteristics of all patients seen in the EHC during its first year. The files of all those patients who were seen during the year were reviewed for the following data: sex; age; origin; final diagnosis at discharge; and diagnosis requiring hospitalization. A total of 10 510 patients were seen during the year, of whom the majority were females (68.2%). The mean age was 36.9 years, and only 17.8% patients were aged above 50 years. As regards origin, 39.9% came from Paris, 52.9% from the Paris suburbs, 6.4% from other French regions, and 0.8% from the French islands and abroad. Two hundred and fifty patients were hospitalized.

Types of headache diagnosed

Primary headaches were diagnosed in 8253 cases (79.3%), secondary headaches in 1157 (10.3%), cranial neuralgias in 153 (1.3%), and no precise diagnosis could be made on an emergency basis in 947 (9.1%). There was a trend over the year towards a decrease in primary and an increase in secondary headaches.

Primary headaches (Table 61.1)

Attacks of migraine accounted for 50.2% of cases, mostly in females (77.5%). Migraine with aura accounted for 7.1% of migraine attacks. All varieties of aura symptoms were found, including transient unilateral motor deficit (three patients). Episodic or chronic tension-type headache accounted for 23% of cases.

A total of 644 patients (6.1%) came for cluster headache, mostly not previously diagnosed.

Secondary headaches (Table 61.2)

Sinusitis (149 patients; 1.4%) and head trauma (154 patients; 1.5%) were the most frequent causes of secondary headache followed by cerebrospinal fluid (CSF) hypotension (117 patients; 1.1%). Vascular disorders were detected in 118 patients (1.1%), 60 males and 58 females having a mean age of 45.9 years (range 21–87 years). Various vascular causes were identified including subarachnoid haemorrhage (75), dissection of cervical arteries (12), cerebral venous thrombosis (12), transient

Table 61.1   Causes of primary headaches (8277 patients)

Headache	Number of patients
Migraine without aura	4484
Migraine with aura	736
Tension-type headache	2389
Cluster headache	644
Miscellaneous	24

Table 61.2   Causes of secondary headaches (1203 patients)

Causes	Number of patients (%)
Sinusitis	149 (12.4)
Other disorders of neck, eyes, ear, nose	35 (2.8)
Head trauma	154 (12.8)
CSF hypotension	117 (9.5)
Trigeminal neuralgia	153 (12.8)
Vascular disorders	118 (9.5)
Meningitis	34 (2.8)
Tumour	16 (1.3)
Noncephalic infection	47 (3.9)
Miscellaneous	380 (31.6)

ischaemic attack (9), arteriovenous malformation (6), and bilateral carotido-cavernous fistula (1).

For the remaining 361 patients (3.5%) with secondary headaches, as many as 20 different causes were identified as various as severe anaemia, optic neuritis, or cerebral toxoplasmosis revealing HIV infection.

727 patients (6.9%) have come back from two to six times of whom 49 came for detoxification.

Discussion

Some interesting features may be discussed. Firstly, the majority of patients are females aged 21 to 50 years old, reflecting the female preponderance in migraine. Secondly, the high frequency of cluster headache was totally unexpected, suggesting that cluster headache may be more frequent than usually thought. Finally, serious vascular conditions such as cervical artery dissection or cerebral venous thrombosis were rare but often misleading, presenting only with headache and without the other classical signs of these conditions. Recent and new headaches should always prompt neuroimaging, CSF studies, and/or cervical duplex scanning and transcranial Doppler before considering a primary headache.

62
Headache symptoms and other headache features in non-specified headaches in primary care

R. Smith, L.A. Hasse, P.N. Richey, A.E. Cassedy, and D.J. Rudawsky

Introduction

The purpose of the study reported in this chapter was to measure the extent of migraine symptoms and other migraine features recorded at headache visits by family physicians and diagnosed as 'headache NOS' (headache, not otherwise specified, International Classification of Diseases (ICD)-9:784). For this purpose, headache visit clinical data, recorded by a group of family physicians ($N=30$) over the period 1 July 1995 to 31 December 1999, were gathered retrospectively and analysed. A headache patient was defined as a patient who made at least one headache visit during the study period.

The practice population consisted of 23 470 patients of whom 1623 (7%) were headache patients who made 3434 visits for headache during the study period. A diagnosis of headache NOS was made at 69% of these visits (1112/1623). A random sample of headache NOS patients ($n=201$) who made 289 headache visits in all was studied.

Data from the patient clinical records were collected by trained reviewers. Accuracy and consistency in data collection were maintained by cross-checking between reviewers and adherence to a set of decision rules concerning the words, phrases, abbreviations, and clinical acronyms used by the recording physicians. A template consisting of 20 headache items based on the International Headache Society (IHS) diagnostic criteria and other headache features was used for data collection and analysis.

Results

Migraine symptoms and other headache features were recorded in over 80% of headache NOS visits. The number of headache symptoms and headache features ranged from 1 (20.3% of NOS visits) to 9 (0.4% of NOS visits).

As the number of migraine symptoms and other headache features per NOS visit increased, the number of NOS visits tended to decrease (Table 62.1). This indicated, with one exception, that the greater the number of migraine symptoms and other headache features recorded, the less likely it was that a headache NOS diagnosis would be made. At nearly 30% of NOS visits, four or more migraine symptoms or other headache features (listed in Table 62.2) were recorded, suggesting that a significant amount of migraine may have been missed. The percentage of headache NOS visits at which various symptoms and other headache features are recorded was measured (Table 62.2). Many migraine symptoms and other headache features are recorded at headache NOS visits (Table 62.2). More generalized headache features are more frequently recorded than more specific migraine symptoms.

No headache pain data were recorded at 70.6% of NOS visits. Mild pain was recorded at 4.5% of NOS visits, moderate at 9.3%, and severe at 15.6%.

Secondary headaches were recorded at 6.9% of NOS visits, and disability data were recorded at 4.2% of NOS visits. Evidence from a physical examination, including some neurological screening data, was recorded at 70.2% of NOS visits.

Conclusions

This study shows that 69% of patients who visited family physicians ($N=30$) for headache were not given a specific headache diagnosis. During these visits many symptoms and other headache features, suggestive of migraine or migrainous

Table 62.1 Number of migraine symptoms and other headache features recorded per visit versus the number of visits resulting in a diagnosis of headache NOS

Number of migraine symptoms/ other headache features per visit	Percentage of visits resulting in diagnosis 'headache NOS'
0	17.6
1	20.3
2	18.0
3	15.3
4	9.6
5	11.1
6	4.2
7	2.3
8	1.1
9	0.4

Table 62.2 Percentage of visits resulting in a diagnosis of 'headache NOS' on which a particular migraine symptom or other headache feature was recorded

Migraine symptom/ other headache feature	Percentage of headache NOS visits on which symptom recorded
Chronicity	64.4
Frequency	57.4
Duration	31.1
Previous headache history	29.1
Unilateral location	26.6
Nausea	18.3
Migraine mentioned	17.0
Pulsating/throbbing	10.7
'Vision problems'	9.7
Photophobia	9.3
Family history of headache	6.6
Vomiting	6.2
Phonophobia	4.2
Movement worsens headache	4.2
Aura	2.8

headaches, were recorded. This finding supports results of the American Migraine Study II, which concluded that, though the diagnosis of migraine has increased over the past decade, approximately half of migraine patients continue to remain undiagnosed.[1] We found little data recorded on the level of headache pain, or disability, at NOS visits.

At 70% of NOS visits we found data on physical examination, including neurological screening. This suggests that priority is given in family practice to eliminating possible secondary headaches. Secondary headaches were recorded in 6.9% of NOS visits.

Given the increased availability of improved methods of migraine treatment, raising standards of physician headache diagnosis is urgently needed.

Acknowledgements

Funding was provided by GlaxoSmithKline.

Reference

1. Lipton RB, Diamond S, Reed M, Diamond ML, Stewart WF. Migraine diagnosis and treatment: results from the American Migraine Study II. *Headache* 2001; **41**: 638–45.

63
Headache treatment outcome: a proposed paradigm for quantitative analysis

M.C. Borrell-Wilson, and C. Cahill-Wright

Introduction

Numerous specialized centres have established protocols for the treatment of chronic, disabling headache. This specialized treatment involves diverse combinations of known therapeutic interventions, which may include abortive and preventive medications, diet changes, biofeedback, sleep hygiene, identification and elimination of headache triggers, lifestyle changes, and cognitive–behavioural modification. This use of a multimodal approach has proven successful in gaining control of headaches.[1] Although a plethora of functional disability measures exist, a Medline search demonstrates that there is currently no paradigm by which to quantitatively measure the outcomes of these assorted combination therapies as a whole. Outcome measurement to document the efficacy of interventions is especially important in the current environment of enhanced accountability for the utilization of costly health-care resources. Outcome data in the management of headaches serves a dual purpose; it provides third-party payers with validation for expended resources and supports improvements in programme processes.[2] Therefore, we have developed a composite paradigm, which we call the Quantitative Evaluation of Headache Intervention paradigm or QEHI, for the quantitative analysis of treatment programme outcomes.

The QEHI paradigm

Table 63.1 outlines the QEHI paradigm. The first column denotes six areas of measurable programme objectives that we utilize in the treatment of refractory headaches. We propose, in the second column, that the percentage of patients meeting each programme objective be calculated and compared to a predetermined

Table 63.1 The quantitative evaluation for headache interventions (QEHI) paradigm

Prioritized objectives	Measures*	Application to	Documentation†	Goal (%)
1. Reduce number of migraine headaches	Patients (%) with ≤6 migraine headaches/week	All patients who complete the in-/out-patient programme with refractory migraines/ rebound headaches	≤6 migraines/month from baseline to discharge and at all follow-up intervals	80
2. Reduce dependence on abortive analgesics	Patients (%) not using OTC and/or prescribed analgesics more than once/week for headaches	All patients who complete the in-/out-patient programme with rebound headaches using daily abortive analgesics	Analgesic use no more than 1 day/ week from baseline to discharge at all follow-up visits at 3, 9, 24, 52 weeks	80
3. Increase overall sense of physical well-being and physical functioning	Patients (%) with increased activity levels as evidenced by daily exercise; patients (%) working at their desired capacity	All patients who complete the in-/out-patient headache programme	Daily exercise from baseline to discharge and maintenance of increase at follow-up at 3, 9, 24, 52 weeks; Employed with negligible time missed due to migraine and/or returned to desired functional tasks	80
4. Enhanced psychological functioning	Patients (%) with decreased scores on HIT-6; patients (%) with decreased BDI scores; improvement on global scale	All patients who complete the in-/out-patient headache programme	Decreased HIT-6 scores from baseline to 3-week follow-up and maintenance of increase at 9, 24, 52 weeks; decreased BDI from baseline to discharge; improvement in global response to treatment scale	80
5. Decreased utilization of the health-care system	Patients (%) who used emergency care system for headaches	All patients who complete the in-/out-patient headache programme	Patient does not use emergency rooms/walk-in clinics for headache from discharge to end of follow-up	80
6. Customer satisfaction with services provided	Patients (%) who report satisfaction with programme and its elements on a questionnaire	All patients who complete the in-/out-patient headache programme	Patient documents satisfaction with programme at discharge on patient satisfaction questionnaire; patient afforded anonymity	80

*OTC, Over-the-counter.
†Baseline discharge to postdischarge.

threshold as indicated in the last column. While most of the programme objectives are applicable to all patients, some objectives (for example, to reduce dependence on abortive analgesics) may only be applicable to a subset of patients, as indicated in the third column. The proposed documentation methods for treatment outcomes are indicated in the fourth column. Outcomes are determined through patient interview and report, the use of several standardized instruments, including the Headache Impact Test (HIT-6),[3] the Beck Depression Inventory (BDI),[4] a global response to treatment scale, and the use of a non-standardized patient satisfaction questionnaire.

The QEHI was developed after identifying desired outcomes, which were converted into measurable programme objectives. These objectives were prioritized, as opposed to weighted, in degree of importance. This prioritization was arrived at with the entire treating team's input. The return to work threshold is set at 50%, consistent with the return to work average in chronic pain patients. The threshold of no less than 80% for the other objectives is set in keeping with the treatment facility's quality improvement standards. The threshold, however, could be adjusted if the outcomes consistently exceeded this value. If less than 80% of patients achieved the outcomes, and a trend was noted, this would indicate the possible need to examine the relevant clinical protocol. The paradigm is dynamic as it allows for the redefining of objectives, adjustment of thresholds, and updating of instruments in data collection.

The first primary objective identified in the paradigm calls for a reduction in the number of headaches. Each patient is initially interviewed and the headache frequency recorded. A reduction in headache frequency to no more than six headaches per month meeting International Headache Society (IHS) criteria for migraine per month is considered attainment of the objective.

The second objective requires a reduced dependence on specific and non-specific abortive agents. As with objective 1, patients are initially interviewed and the number of days per week on which abortive analgesics are utilized is documented. A reduction in abortive analgesic use to no more than 2 days per week would indicate a successful treatment outcome.

The third objective is to increase the level of physical functioning. Assessment procedures include simply asking the patient 'Are you functioning at full capacity in your job or as a full-time homemaker?' If the patient has returned to a functional capacity in either their job, or their role as student or homemaker the objective is attained. Employment status can be further explored if the patient is receiving worker's compensation, as a case manager can validate employment. Another aspect of increased physical functioning involves leisure activities. If the patient reports that he or she is now engaged in leisure pursuits identified as disrupted at the outset of treatment then the objective is obtained. Report of daily exercise is also an indicator of physical functioning. Each patient is provided with an individualized daily exercise programme for use at home and compliance with the programme can be assessed by patient report. It is important to note that, in the self-report areas, it is useful to obtain feedback from a spouse or significant other regarding the patient's level of functioning.

Objective 4 requires an increase in psychological functioning. Standardized instruments are utilized to measure outcomes of this objective. The indicator of attainment is threefold. Psychological functioning is measured with the HIT-6, the BDI, and the global response to treatment scale. The HIT-6 is a headache-specific quality of life measure that assesses an individual patient's progress over time. Not a diagnostic tool, it provides feedback on the impact headaches have on the patient's ability to function at home, at work, and in social settings. The BDI is a 21-item screening instrument found to be effective in identifying depression symptoms across treatment. It has been widely accepted as an assessment for depression in chronic pain patients and has been used as an outcome measurement in this diagnostic group. The global response to treatment scale encompasses a percentage of improvement or worsening derived from the treatment plan. The team psychologist administers the BDI scale. Improvement in psychological functioning is attained by a decrease in the BDI and HIT-6 scores and an improvement in the global response to treatment scale.

Objective 5 assesses whether patients utilize emergency care systems following discharge. A system is established by which the personnel of the emergency room report any of our patients requesting treatment for headaches. Additional feedback is gleaned from insurance adjusters, and external case managers. This, along with patient report, is how this objective is measured.

Finally, objective 6 involves satisfaction with the treatment programme. The objective is measured using qualitative as well as quantitative data. A non-standardized instrument is used to measure the outcome of this objective. The Patient Satisfaction Questionnaire is specific to the elements of the programme and the programme in general. Each discipline and the programme are represented in the questionnaire with a total of 31 items and a Likert scale of 1–5 utilized. Anonymity and confidentiality are assured and the patient is afforded the opportunity to suggest improvements to the programme.

We applied these objectives prospectively to 42 patients who completed our in- or out-patient headache programme. The programme consisted of 1 week of hospitalization for evaluation and interventions utilizing a multimodal, interdisciplinary approach designed to consistently reduce headache frequency. A repetitive use of intravenous (IV) protocols was utilized, including but not limited to dihydroergotamine (DHE), chlorpromazine, prochlorperazine, corticosteroids, droperidol, or magnesium sulfate. Intensive training in non-pharmacological interventions is provided along with the use of standard headache abortive and preventive medication. Upon completion of the interdisciplinary programme patients are scheduled to return for nine additional sessions of biofeedback and/or physical therapy.

Programme follow-up assessment is performed at our clinic 3, 9, 24, and 52 weeks postdischarge, at which time each patient is evaluated and the assessment scales provided. Once the patient has completed the questionnaires, they are interviewed by the advanced registered nurse practitioner (ARNP). Questions related to compliance with their prescribed daily exercise regimen, use of relaxation techniques, employment/leisure functioning, number of headaches, analgesic use, and use of the emergency care system are posed at the interview. The responses are documented on a database tool that is implemented at the time of admission and follows each patient through the programme to the prescribed follow-up visits. The patient response is checked against their ongoing prescription record and validated with insurance case managers when appropriate. The data collected at baseline and postdischarge visits is then examined using the QEHI paradigm to assess overall programme outcome.

Testing the paradigm

Sample

The sample for the pilot of the proposed paradigm consisted of 42 patients with chronic daily headache with or without analgesic overuse who completed the in- or out-patient programme. The same programme was applied for both the in- and out-patient settings and so the patient data were analysed together.

Interventions

Interventions were provided in a daily consistent manner to all patients in the sample. The 1-week programme consisted of:

- physical therapy for postural re-mediation, cervical modalities, and tailored exercise programme;
- occupational therapy for energy conservation, pacing, functional task simulation, and leisure exploration;
- psychological therapy provided in individual and group settings;
- IV protocols and other pharmacological strategies directed at breaking the chronic cycle;
- biofeedback and relaxation therapy.

Data collection

Baseline data once captured are recorded on each patient's cumulative database. At the time of discharge each patient is scheduled for the initial follow-up visit for comparative data collection. At the end of each visit, subsequent visits are scheduled for ongoing data collection to evaluate outcome durability.

Outcomes

Forty-two patients who have completed the standardized interdisciplinary, multimodal headache programme are prospectively evaluated utilizing the proposed outcome paradigm. The data reflect outcomes at baseline and at 3 and 9 weeks follow-up from programme completion (Table 63.2).

Table 63.2 Outcomes of the interdisciplinary headache programme

Outcome	Number of patients/N (%)
≤6 migraines/month	36/42 (86)
Analgesics used on ≤2 days/week	28/30* (93)
Increased physical functioning	40/42 (95)
Desired functional status/return to work	31/42 (74)
Decreased BDI scores	36/38† (95)
Decreased HIT-6 scores	36/42 (86)
Improvement reported by patient	31/42 (74)
Emergency care system not used for headache	42/42 (100)
Satisfaction with care reported by patient	40/42 (95)

*Number of patients using medication for acute attacks >2 days/week at baseline.
†Number of patients with elevated baseline BDI.

Conclusion

The proposed QEHI paradigm is a composite of objective, valid measurements of headache quality of life and depression. The paradigm determines the overall efficacy of combination protocols, irrespective of the exact components comprising the treatment plan. The paradigm can be used to assess both initial outcomes and the durability of said outcomes. We have found the paradigm to be efficient in approaching the analysis of treatment outcomes provided in an interdisciplinary setting. In addition, the paradigm is dynamic, affording flexibility in the establishment of programme-related objectives, which may be adapted for alternative diagnostic groups.

Disability from headache is difficult to measure when dealing with quality of life as an outcome domain. While the practitioner can clearly document disability within this domain, payers ignore such findings as there is no mechanism by which to rate disability as a result of migraine. The American Medical Association's *Guides to the evaluation of permanent impairment* (p. 570) does not assign a permanent impairment rating for headache, which is noted as a 'well-established pain syndromes without significant, identifiable organ dysfunction to explain the pain'.[5] The World Health Organization has developed an International Classification of Impairments, Activities, and Participation (ICIDH-2) that provides yet another conceptual framework for outcome assessments.[6] The ICIDH-2 defines impairment, activity limitation, and participation restriction in terms that are relevant to the headache population. The QEHI paradigm can be further adapted within the ICIDH-2 framework for further studies focusing on migraine-specific quality of life as a measure of outcome.

Acknowledgements

We appreciate the skilful assistance of Theresa Chisholm, PhD, in the review of this manuscript.

References

1. Lake AE III, Saper JR. Prospective outcome evaluation of an accredited inpatient headache program. *Headache*, 1998; **28**: 315–16.
2. Abrams HB, Hnath-Chisholm T. Outcome measures: the audiologic difference. In *Audiology practice management* (ed. Hosford-Dunn H, Roeser RJ, Valente M). New York: Thieme Medical Publishers Inc., 2000: 69–83.
3. Kosinski M, Bjorner JB, Bayliss MS, Ware J. Measuring the impact of migraine and severe headache with the Headache Impact Test (HIT): using item response theory (IRT) models to score widely-used measures of headache impact. Presented at the 52nd Annual Meeting, American Academy of Neurology, San Diego, California, 4 May 2000.
4. Beck AT, Ward CH, Mendelson M, Mock N, Erbaugh I. An inventory for measuring depression. *Arch Gen Psychiatry* 1961; **4**: 561–71.
5. Cocchiarella L, Anderson GBJ (ed.). *Guides to the evaluation of permanent impairment*, 5th edn. Chicago: AMA Press, 2000.
6. World Health Organization. *Towards a common language for functioning and disablement: ICIDH-2 beta-draft for field trials*. Geneva: World Health Organization, 1997.

64
Development of HIT-6™, a paper-based short form for measuring headache impact

M.S. Bayliss, J.B. Bjorner, M. Kosinski, C.G.H. Dahlöf,
A. Dowson, R.K. Cady, J.E. Ware Jr, and A.S. Batenhorst

Introduction

It is well documented that migraine and other severe headaches cause suffering, reduce productivity, and lead to high health-care costs and it is recognized that patients are the best source of information about how their headaches affect their functioning and overall well-being.[1–3] At issue is whether headache impact surveys used successfully in research can be made more practical while maintaining accepted standards of reliability and validity. To be most useful in clinical practice and research, health assessment questionnaires should meet psychometric and clinical criteria for reliable, valid measurement. The internet-based Headache Impact Test (HIT), a dynamic computerized adaptive questionnaire, has demonstrated evidence of precision, reliability, validity, and clinical relevance in the measurement of the impact of headache on sufferers' lives. A paper-based, standardized version of the HIT questionnaire was desirable for clinicians and patients without access to the internet. Our objective was to develop a new short form for assessing the impact of headaches that is brief as well as reliable and valid for use in screening and monitoring patients in clinical research and practice.

Methods

This study was conducted in independent developmental and validation phases. First, we analysed 54 items in the Headache Impact Test (HIT) item pool administered by telephone interview to a representative sample of recent headache sufferers participating in the US National Survey of Headache Impact (NSHI) ($N=1016$). Item response theory (IRT) estimates of item parameters (difficulty, slope) and content validity were considered in selecting a subset of items for a fixed-length survey of headache impact (HIT-6). Using NSHI data, the 'best' candidate items were evaluated on the basis of psychometric standards of content validity (in relation to widely used surveys, clinician's judgements), item internal consistency, and distributions of scores (skewness and 'ceiling' and 'floor' effects) and IRT-based information functions. Second, psychometric tests were carried out and test–retest (2-week) reliability and construct validity were evaluated in an internet-based survey of headache sufferers ($N=1103$) who were members of America Online, an internet service provider with more than 33 million members worldwide. Construct validity was evaluated in terms of HIT-6 correlations with a generic health-related quality of life (HRQoL) measure, the SF-8™ Health Survey[4], and in clinical tests of discriminant validity (diagnosis, headache severity). For purposes of group-level tests of discriminant validity, relative validity (RV) estimates for HIT-6 were based on comparisons of F-ratios for the score based on all 54 items in the pool (total score). The responsiveness of HIT-6 scores in detecting clinically mean-ingful change was evaluated for randomly selected mild, moderate, and severe headache sufferers in the NSHI ($N=245$) who were classified as better, same, or worse in terms of change scores and compared across groups who reported being the same or with more or less limited change at the time of a 6-month follow-up survey.

Results

HIT-6 includes one item from each of the six content categories represented in widely used surveys of headache impact. In the developmental sample, items correlated highly (0.64 to 0.76) with the HIT-6 score and reliability coefficients ranged from 0.78 to 0.90 (median=0.81) across samples and estimation methods (see Tables 64.1 and 64.2). HIT-6 IRT thresholds covered most (53%) of the total HIT (HIT-TOT) range measured by all 54 items and HIT-6 scored less than 1% at either the ceiling or floor (see Table 64.2). This pattern of favourable psychometric results was replicated in the validation sample.

Further, all correlations with HRQoL measures were negative, as hypothesized, and all were below 0.40 (Table 64.2). HIT-6 correlated 0.908 with the total score in an analysis that was only possible in the developmental sample. In tests of validity in discriminating across diagnostic groups, RV coefficients of 0.83 and 0.87 were observed for HIT-6, in comparison with the total score. In the test of validity in discriminating across mild to severe groups, HIT-6 was equivalent to the total score (RV=1.00, see Table 64.3). For all three criteria of group-level changes in headache impairment, HIT-6 was, as hypothesized, significantly responsive in the follow-up study (see Fig. 64.1).

Table 64.1 Item descriptive statistics, item-to-scale and scale-to-scale correlations

	HIT1	HIT2	HIT3	HIT4	HIT5	HIT6	HIT-6 score
Descriptive statistics							
Mean	3.11	2.77	3.79	2.85	3.26	3.12	59.53
SD	0.88	0.91	0.95	0.99	1.09	0.97	7.58
% Ceiling	4.9%	3.1%	24.6%	3.6%	12.2%	7.0%	0.9%
% Floor	3.4%	7.6%	1.6%	10.5%	7.5%	5.7%	0.5%
Correlations with HIT-6 and SF-8 scales							
HIT-6 score	0.67*	0.73*	0.64*	0.75*	0.68*	0.76*	—
Physical functioning	−0.32	−0.24	−0.28	−0.25	−0.32	−0.22	−0.27
Role physical	−0.36	−0.26	−0.33	−0.24	−0.35	−0.29	−0.32
Bodily pain	−0.25	−0.19	−0.20	−0.19	−0.26	−0.20	−0.22
General health	−0.32	−0.24	−0.27	−0.22	−0.30	−0.23	−0.27
Vitality	−0.29	−0.21	−0.24	−0.18	−0.31	−0.24	−0.25
Social functioning	−0.38	−0.27	−0.31	−0.26	−0.37	−0.32	−0.31
Role emotional	−0.35	−0.24	−0.29	−0.23	−0.35	−0.30	−0.29
Mental health	−0.27	−0.17	−0.21	−0.20	−0.27	−0.25	−0.21
Physical component score	−0.33	−0.25	−0.29	−0.23	−0.32	−0.24	−0.29
Mental component score	−0.30	−0.20	−0.24	−0.21	−0.31	−0.28	−0.24

*Item-scale correlation corrected for overlap (relevant item removed from its scale for correlation). Starred correlations also hypothesized to be highest in same row.

Table 64.2 Reliability of the HIT-6

Reliability test	Result
Internal consistency reliability (Cronbach's α)	
Time 1	0.89
Time 2	0.90
Alternate-forms reliability: HIT-6 versus HIT-TOTAL)	
Time 1	0.78
*Test–retest scale reliability (total sample)**	
Pearson correlation coefficient	0.81
Intraclass correlation coefficient	0.78
Test–retest scale reliability (stable sample)†	
Pearson correlation coefficient	0.83
Intra-class correlation coefficient	0.80
Test–retest item-level reliability (ranges)	
Pearson correlation coefficient	0.60–0.71
Intra-class correlation coefficient	0.57–0.70

*Entire sample who completed both time 1 and time 2 questionnaires.
†Stable sample—completed both time 1 and time 2 questionnaires and reported no change on self-report transition items.

Table 64.3 Validity of three headache impact scales in relation to headache diagnosis and severity (N=1016)

	Score (SD) for diagnosis			Relative validity
	No migraine	Migraine	F-statistic	
Migraine diagnosis based only on presence of nausea and light and sound sensitivity (migraine, n=621; no migraine, n=395)				
HIT-TOT	54.11 (7.1)	62.37 (6.0)	449.22*	1.00
HIT-6	54.60 (7.1)	62.81 (6.0)	392.36*	0.87
Migraine diagnosis based on all International Headache Society symptom criteria (migraine, n=421; no migraine, n=595)				
HIT-TOT	54.22 (6.0)	62.64 (5.9)	487.69*	1.00
HIT-6	54.80 (7.0)	63.03 (5.9)	405.72*	0.83

	Score (SD) for headache severity				Relative validity
	Mild (n=77)	Moderate (n=677)	Severe (n=262)	F-statistic	
HIT-TOT	50.47 (6.3)	57.76 (5.9)	65.25 (6.2)	231.95*	1.00
HIT-6	50.30 (7.1)	58.24 (6.4)	65.92 (95.7)	232.89*	1.00

*$p < 0.001$.

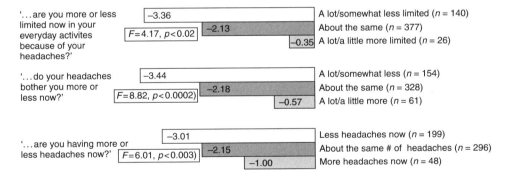

Fig. 64.1 Responsiveness of HIT-6 in relation to change in headache severity.

Conclusions

The IRT model estimated for a 'pool' of items from widely used measures of headache impact was useful in constructing an efficient 'static' short form for use in screening and monitoring patient outcomes. Although HIT-6 is much shorter than most widely used measures of headache impact, it demonstrated satisfactory reliability and validity for use in group-level studies throughout the entire range of headache impact studied. HIT-6 was also very accurate in detecting individual patients for severe headache impact and in detecting important changes in headache impact. Further research is necessary to determine whether smaller changes in HIT-6 are important to headache sufferers and the interpretation of differences that can be detected. Further, the HIT-6 was has been translated into more than 28 languages using a method developed for the International Quality of Life Assessment (IQOLA) project.[5] Psychometrically sound, clinically useful, and cross-nationally adaptable, HIT-6 provides clinicians with a practical, precise measure of headache impact that can be used to tailor treatment to disease severity and facilitate patient and physician communication.

References

1. Clouse JC, Osterhaus JT. Healthcare resource use and costs associated with migraine in a managed care setting. *Ann Pharmacother* 1994; **28**: 659–64.
2. Pryse-Phillips W, Findlay H. Tugwell P, *et al*. A Canadian population survey on the clinical, epidemiological and societal impact of migraine and tension-type headache. *Can J Neurol Sci* 1992; **19** (3): 333–9.
3. Hu XH, Markson LE, Lipton RB, Stewart WF, Berger ML. Burden of migraine in the United States: disability and economic costs. *Arch Intern Med* 1999; **159** (8): 813–18.
4. Ware JE, Kosinski M, Dewey JE, Gandek B. *How to score and interpret single item health status measures: a manual for users of the SF-8™ health survey*. Lincoln, Rhode Island: Quality Metric Incorporated, 2001.
5. Bullinger M, Alonso J, Apolone G, Leplege A, *et al*. Translating health status questionnaires and evaluating their quality: the International Quality of Life Assessment project approach. *J Clin Epidemiol* 1998; **51** (11): 913–23.

65
Low socio-economic status is associated with increased risk of frequent headache: a prospective study of 22718 adults in Norway

Lars Jacob Stovner, Knut Hagen, Lars Vatten, John-Anker Zwart, Steinar Krokstad, and Gunnar Bovim

Introduction

Conflicting results exist regarding the relationship between headache and socio-economic status (SES). In the USA, headache and migraine were more frequent among groups with low income and low education (for example, refs 1–3), but such an inverse relationship between headache and SES has not been reported in studies outside the USA.

In Nord-Trøndelag County in Norway, two population-based cross-sectional surveys (the HUNT study) have been performed. The first survey (HUNT-1) took place in 1984–86, and the second (HUNT-2) in 1995–97. SES at baseline in HUNT-1 was defined by education level, occupation, and income, and the subsequent risk of migraine, non-migrainous headache, and frequent headache (>6 headache days/month) was estimated at follow-up 11 years later (HUNT-2).

Material and methods

In HUNT-1 and HUNT-2, all residents aged ≥20 years were invited. In HUNT-1, of 85 100 eligible individuals, 77 310 (91%) answered the questionnaire that was sent with the invitation. The participants were divided into three categories of SES according to: (1) duration of education (≤9 years, 10 to 12 years, and ≥13 years); (2) occupation (*high*: white-collar workers; *medium*: routine non-manual workers, farmers, and other self-employed workers in primary production; *low*: blue-collar workers); and (3) income (three categories based on the 33 and the 66 percentiles).

We wanted to establish a relatively headache-free population at baseline. The HUNT-1 questionnaire did not include headache items, but 59 471 persons responded to a question on use of analgesics ('How often have you taken pain-relieving medication during the last month?'). A total of 41 581 responded that they 'never' used analgesics. For the purpose of the present study, we have assumed that, among those who had never used analgesics, the proportion of headache sufferers would be relatively small. Among the 41 581 individuals, 33 694 were available for HUNT-2, and, of these, 22 718 (67%) responded to a headache questionnaire. Among the latter group, income data were available in 22 005 individuals, education level in 20 627, and current or last held occupation in 19 246.

The HUNT-2 questionnaires included 13 questions on headache. Those who answered 'yes' to the question 'Have you suffered from headache during the last 12 months?' were classified as 'headache sufferers'. Participants were also categorized according to headache frequency, and 'frequent headache' was defined as having headache on more than 6 days per month. Migraine was diagnosed in those who reported themselves as suffering from migraine *or* who fulfilled a modified version of the International Headache Society (IHS) migraine criteria.[4] Non-migrainous headache was diagnosed in those who did not satisfy the criteria for migraine. The headache diagnoses were mutually exclusive. In a validation study, the diagnoses based on questionnaire information were compared to diagnoses made in a clinical interview in a sample of participants.[4] The positive and negative predictive values were respectively 84% and 78% for migraine, 68% and 76% for non-migrainous headache, and 68% and 86% for frequent headache.[4]

In multivariate analyses, using multiple logistic regression, we used information about SES in HUNT-1 to estimate the relative risk of different headache categories, as registered at follow-up in HUNT-2. We evaluated potential confounding by age, current smoking, alcohol consumption, body mass index, and physical activity.

Results

Whereas non-frequent headache showed no relation to SES, low SES defined by education level and occupation at baseline was associated with increased risk of frequent headache. This was evident for both sexes and for both migraine and non-migrainous headache. Since there was no difference between the diagnostic categories (migraine and non-migrainous headache) as to the association with SES, these groups were combined, as shown in Table 65.1. Among individuals with less than 10 years of education, the relative risk of frequent headache was 1.8 (95% confidence interval (CI), 1.5–2.4) as compared to that in individuals with ≥13 years of education. This relation was most evident in those aged between 30 and

Table 65.1   Age-adjusted risk ratio (with 95% confidence interval) of frequent headache (≥7 headache days per month) by education, occupation, and income

	Risk ratio (95% confidence interval)	
	Women	Men
Years of education		
≤13	1.0	1.0
10 to 12	1.3 (0.9–1.9)	1.4 (1.0–2.0)
≤9	2.0 (1.4–2.9)	1.6 (1.1–2.2)
Social class by occupation		
High	1.0	1.0
Medium	1.4 (1.0–1.8)	1.5 (1.1–2.0)
Low	2.0 (1.5–2.8)	1.8 (1.4–2.5)
Income		
High	1.0	1.0
Medium	1.0 (0.8–1.2)	1.3 (1.0–1.7)
Low	1.0 (0.8–1.3)	1.4 (1.1–1.9)

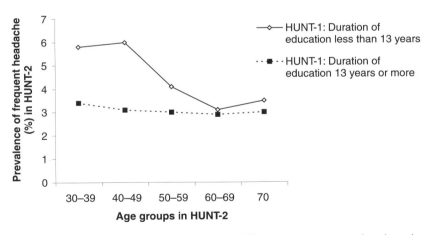

Fig. 65.1   Headache prevalence in HUNT-2 in different age groups related to duration of education in HUNT-1.

50 years (Fig. 65.1). Low social class defined by occupation was also associated with higher risk of frequent headache in both sexes (Table 65.1). Low SES defined by income was also related to higher risk of frequent headache, but only among men (Table 65.1). Adjustment for body mass index, smoking, alcohol consumption, or physical activity did not change the results.

Discussion

In this prospective study, low SES defined by education and occupation at baseline was associated with increased risk of frequent headache 11 years later. This was evident for both sexes and for migraine as well as for non-migrainous headache. The risk of frequent headache decreased with increasing individual income, but only among men.

No previous studies concerning SES and headache have had a prospective design, but our main finding is in agreement with cross-sectional studies from the USA.[1-3] With the latter study design, the temporal (and possible causal) relation between factors cannot be determined, since information about SES is obtained at the same time as the information on headache. Accordingly, an inverse relation between headache prevalence and SES may be explained by headache interfering with scholarly achievements and job career, as suggested in the social selection model.[5] In our prospective study the information about SES was obtained in a presumably headache-free population. Therefore, it was less likely that headache had interfered with education or job career as registered at baseline. Our results indicate that other factors associated with low SES, such as stress, poor diet, or poor medical care, may influence headache risk (the social causation model).[5] Because SES seems to be a relatively strong predictor of frequent headache, it is important to consider and adjust for this factor in epidemiological studies on headache.

Conclusion

Low socio-economic status at baseline was associated with higher risk of frequent headache 11 years later. It would seem important to identify more closely which factors related to low SES are responsible for the increased risk of frequent headache.

References

1. Stewart WF, Lipton RB, Celentano DD, Reed ML. Prevalence of migraine headache in the United States. Relation to age, race, and other sociodemographic factors. *J Am Med Assoc* 1992; **267**: 64–9.
2. Schwartz BS, Stewart WF, Simon D, Lipton RB. Epidemiology of tension-type headache. *J Am Med Assoc* 1998; **279**: 381–3.
3. Scher AI, Stewart WF, Liberman J, Lipton RB. Prevalence of frequent headache in a population sample. *Headache* 1998; **38**: 497–506.
4. Hagen K, Zwart JA, Vatten L, Stovner LJ, Bovim G. Head-HUNT: validity and reliability of a headache questionnaire in a large population-based study in Norway. *Cephalalgia* 2000; **20**: 244–51.
5. Dohrenwend BP, Levav I, Shrout PE, *et al*. Socioeconomic status and psychiatric disorders: the causation–selection issue. *Science* 1992; **255**: 946–52.

66

Reducing the burden of headache by communicating treatment strategies for employees

Hartmut Göbel, Peter Buschmann, Axel Heinze, Elke Püffel,
Joachim Krüger, Frank Meyer, Bertold Nicola, and Frederico Polano

Introduction

In addition to the individual suffering, headache syndromes give rise to extremely high costs for the health-care system and for society as a whole. These costs are made up in particular of the direct costs of medical care and the indirect costs resulting from loss of working time and premature pensioning. It has been calculated that the costs due to headache problems in the European Community come to 20 billion euros a year.[1] Headaches are one of the most common reasons for unfitness for work. Through direct and indirect costs, headaches also result in a considerable burden on the financial resources of employers and health insurance funds. To date, there are very few figures available on quantitative analyses of the socio-economic significance of headache syndromes in Germany. In recent studies in France,[2,3] a survey of some 20 000 employees of the French national gas and electricity supply companies showed that similar numbers of days were lost as a result of headache and backache. If employees have both headache and backache, an average of 58.1 days work a year taken over a 4-year period are lost through unfitness for work due to these disorders. If they have either backache or headache, the number of days off work comes to 38.4 or 31.8, respectively. Headache and migraine at work have a particularly strong impact on quality of life.[3] An extensive representative German study on the epidemiology of headache found that employees with migraine have an average of 34 days a year off work and those with tension-type headache have 32 days off work.[4] A recent survey[5] found that, in cases of chronic tension-type headache, an average of 27.4 days a year were lost through unfitness for work and labour productivity was reduced on a further 27.4 days.[5,6]

Some 270 working days a year per 1000 employees are lost through migraine alone, and 920 working days per 1000 employees are lost as a result of tension-type headaches.[1,7,8] An analysis of patients of an out-patient pain clinic in 1995 showed that 22% of the patients treated there had submitted or intended to submit an application for a pension on the grounds of their headache problems. Since the average age of this sample was 46 years, this figure means that in a large subgroup of patients nearly half their working life is lost as a result of headaches. Before the progression with time of headache disorders ultimately leads to a pension application or occupational disability, there are many years of reduced productivity, disability, suffering, and pain.[9]

Against the background of the considerable burden on the financial resources of employers and health insurance funds caused by headache disorders, the regional health insurance fund Allgemeine Ortskrankenkasse (AOK) Schleswig-Holstein and the shipbuilders Howaldtswerke Deutsche Werft AG (HDW), the biggest industrial employer in the Kiel region, ran a concerted campaign in cooperation with the Kiel Pain Clinic. The main objective of HDW was to make an active contribution to improving the quality of life of its employees and their families. The idea was to give employees and their families the chance of providing anonymous information about their personal headache problems and obtaining up-to-date information. The aim of the regional health insurance fund AOK Schleswig-Holstein was to provide information to its insured persons about modern ways and means of headache prevention and treatment. The background to this motive was that headache therapy is almost exclusively a field of self-medication and that most people affected by headaches do not have any up-to-date knowledge for effective headache treatment with a minimum of side-effects. Communicating information about up-to-date headache therapy was of special importance because headache is a large-scale widespread disease that frequently persists for years or even decades. Another objective from an epidemiological point of view was to analyse the affected persons' knowledge of how to treat headaches and to analyse and describe the impact of chronic headache problems on everyday life and on health habits. To date there are no figures of this kind in Germany for the employees and their families of a large industrial company like HDW and the structure of the insured community of the AOK health insurance fund. The campaign gained special significance from the fact that it was not merely an employer and a health insurance fund that were making efforts to organize improvements in the health care of their employees or insured persons, but the doctors, pharmacists, and the media of the region were also actively integrated in the project.

Methods

The project consisted of three phases. In the first phase, a survey of how employees and their families deal with headache was initiated using a questionnaire. In the second phase, specific information offers, treatment, and training programmes relating to up-to-date headache intervention strategies were implemented for headache sufferers, doctors, and pharmacists. In the final phase the changes induced in the burden of headache were analysed.

Measurement at the commencement of the project

Standardized questionnaires about health habits relating to headache were sent to 1946 shipyard employees who were insured with the AOK. The employees and their families were asked to complete and return the questionnaires if they had headache problems.

Intervention phase

In the intervention phase the participants were offered specific information on preventing and managing headache. Accompanying media reports in the regional press also provided information on headaches, and especially about the dangers of unconsidered self-medication. In addition, the respondents were sent material in the form of information brochures in German and Turkish, thereby creating a basis of knowledge of up-to-date headache therapy. Furthermore, active courses on pain management, relaxation training, and various forms of compensatory exercise were offered by the company medical service and the AOK. In addition, in order to promote effective and up-to-date treatment of headache by doctors or pharmacists, upgrading training for these occupational groups was to be offered in the course of the campaign. The pharmacists and doctors in Kiel and the surrounding region were invited to headache workshops at which up-to-date therapy standards were communicated and generous time was devoted to discussion about their practical implementation.

Measurement of the effects of the project

A standardized questionnaire about health habits relating to headache was used as a follow-up 6 months later to document any change in the health and health habits of the participants. Table 66.1 gives an overview of all project events.

Results

Three hundred and forty-one questionnaires were returned, which means that 17% or roughly one in five of the questionnaires distributed reached individuals with headaches. The headache problem most commonly encountered was migraine. The reason for this is probably that migraine results in very acute suffering and sufferers are therefore particularly motivated to take an active part in such a measure. The headaches had been going on for an average of 10 years or more. The average frequency of headache days was 5–8 days per month. In spite of this considerable incidence of headaches, most of the respondents did not possess any specific information on adequate measures for preventing and managing headaches. Regardless

Table 66.1 Overview of the project events offered by AOK, HDW, and the Kiel Pain Clinic

---

For patients
Evaluation of headache questionnaires
Information brochures in German and Turkish
Courses in pain-coping strategies
Courses in relaxation training
Examination and treatment in the out-patient department of Kiel Pain Clinic
Information via the media

For doctors
Training courses in headache therapy
Information via medical articles

For pharmacists
Seminars on headache therapy
Information via medical articles

---

of the nature of the headache, most sufferers merely took self-medication in the form of painkillers. The respondents had hardly any knowledge of specific precautionary measures or non-medication-based behavioural measures for preventing headache. A total of 183 respondents stated their address when returning the initial questionnaire and were prepared to take part in the final survey.

On request, the respondents received an individual reply that discussed the characteristics of their headaches on the basis of the Kiel headache questionnaire and suggested behavioural rules and preventive measures. In parallel with this, workshops were held to inform the doctors and pharmacists in the region about modern treatment methods. Thus, participants who consulted a doctor because of the severity of their suffering were able to find doctors and pharmacists with up-to-date information. The headache questionnaire also made it possible for the respondents to describe their headache type precisely when consulting the doctor. A large proportion of the respondents displayed considerable difficulty in stating the symptoms of their headaches. This is probably one of the reasons why most of the respondents had difficulty in finding a specific therapy differentiated by headache type.

The final analysis (Fig. 66.1) reveals that the health condition of about 30% of the respondents was improved at the end of the project. Of those who returned the final questionnaire, 43.1% said that they had had fewer headaches, 38.9% reported that the headache attacks were shorter, and 50% said that they had not had to visit the doctor so often as a result of the information from the project. A health-conscious lifestyle was also achieved by reducing alcohol and nicotine consumption. Of the participants in the final survey, 70% took monopreparations to treat their headaches and used various information sources to achieve effective headache therapy. Health-conscious behaviour became a topic of conversation at work, among friends, and in the family.

Figure 66.2 shows what individual initiatives were taken by the employees of HDW suffering from headache during the project. Almost without exception the

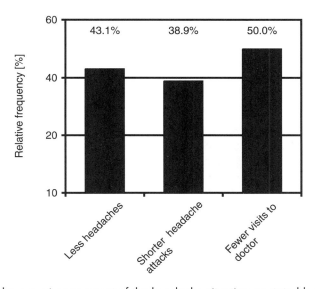

Fig. 66.1 Final survey: improvement of the headache situation as stated by the 183 employees of HDW suffering from headache who completed the questionnaires at the beginning and at the end of the project.

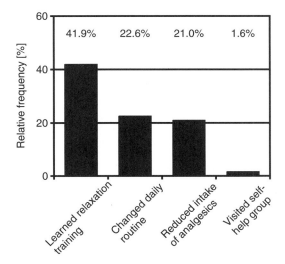

Fig. 66.2 Final survey: individual initiatives taken by the 183 employees of HDW suffering from headache who completed the questionnaires at the beginning and at the end of the project.

project received a very positive reception from the respondents. The campaign supplemented a number of other extensive health-care measures by the company medical service of HDW. While these projects were running, time off work due to illness was down by about 20%.

Discussion

Because of the high prevalence of migraine and headache disorders, prevention and treatment is particularly important at the working environment. The results of this study show that a high headache frequency can be prevented to a large extent, resulting in positive effects on both the quality of life and productivity. It is estimated that over 25% of the population suffer from moderate to severe attacks of headache characterized by pain and other debilitating symptoms. These result in impaired functional capacity and diminished quality of life. Since the prevalence peaks during the age range 25–55 years, the prime working years, migraine and other headaches place a tremendous burden on employers, primarily in the form of lost productivity as well as increased health benefits costs.[10] This clearly favours therapeutic and preventive programmes against chronic headaches in the workplace. These interventions may include identifying migraineurs and other headache patients in the workforce, educating them about their problem and ensuring that they are receiving optimal care, controlling exposures to factors in the workplace that may trigger headache attacks, and managing disability to minimize loss of productivity. Which individual factors can be identified as responsible for this improvement remains an open question. In this study it was, however, evident that specific organized intervention by the company medical service, health insurance fund, and a specialized headache clinic can achieve an significant improvement in health.

In conclusion, the availability of a systematic comprehensive programme for headache treatments resulted in fewer headache attacks, improved quality of life, and increased work productivity. Also it had a net benefit for the employer and the health insurance fund.

References

1. Olesen J (ed.). *Headache classification and epidemiology*. New York: Raven Press, 1994.
2. Dartigues JF, Michel P, Lindoulsi A, Dubroca B, Henry P. Comparative view of the socioeconomic impact of migraine versus low back pain. *Cephalalgia* 1998; **18** (Suppl. 21): 26–9.
3. Michel P, Dartigues JF, Lindoulsi A, Henry P, Loss of productivity and quality of life in migraine sufferers among French workers: results from the GAZEL cohort. *Headache* 1997; **37** (2): 71–8.
4. Göbel H, Why patients with primary headache illnesses do not consult a doctor. In *Headache classification and epidemiology* (ed. Olesen J). New York: Raven Press, 1994: 267–72.
5. Schwartz BS, Stewart WF, Lipton RB. Lost workdays and decreased work effectiveness associated with headache in the workplace. *J Occup Environ Med* 1997; **39** (4): 320–7.

6. Schwartz BS, Stewart WF, Simon D, Lipton RB. Epidemiology of tension-type headache. *J Am Med Assoc* 1998; **279** (5): 381–3.
7. Lipton RB, Stewart WF. Prevalence and impact of migraine. *Neurol Clin* 1997; **15** (1): 1–13.
8. Göbel H. *Die Kopfschmerzen. Ursachen, Mechanismen, Diagnostik und Therapie in der Praxis.* Berlin: Springer-Verlag, 1997.
9. Lipton RB, Stewart WF, von Korff M. Burden of migraine: societal costs and therapeutic opportunities. *Neurology* 1997; **48** (3, Suppl. 3): S4–S9.
10. Warshaw LJ, Burton WN. Cutting the costs of migraine: role of the employee health unit [review]. *J Occup Environ Med* 1998; **40** (11): 943–53.

67 The usefulness of the publication, *Patient-centered strategies for effective management of migraine*, in primary care

Roger K. Cady, Kathleen Farmer, Curtis P. Schreiber, and Robert Kaniecki

Background

Headache is one of the most common complaints encountered in general practice. There are an estimated 28 million migraine sufferers in the United States, approximately 10% of the population worldwide, but fewer than half are appropriately diagnosed and even fewer are adequately treated.[1] Family physicians are consulted more frequently than any other medical speciality for headache care. Yet these physicians treat patients with diverse complaints under short time constraints, making the diagnosis and management of the headache patient a challenge.

Primary Care Network is a non-profit organization that links nearly 10 000 primary care practitioners via the internet and is dedicated to continuing medical education that is patient-oriented and clinically relevant. During the annual training programme in 2000, the 82 faculty members unanimously requested a document that summarized the principles of recognition and management of migraine that have been central to the educational programmes presented nationwide in the USA over the past 4 years.

Overview of *Patient-centered strategies for effective management of migraine*

An advisory committee consisting of 17 physicians and psychologists with training and experience in managing migraineurs was formed to write *Patient-centered strategies for effective management of migraine*. The subject matter was divided into the following categories: (1) impact-based recognition of migraine; (2) acute treatment strategy; (3) preventive treatment strategy; (4) behavioural and physical treatments; (5) special considerations; and (6) system management. These individuals reviewed the National Headache Foundation's standards of care for headache diagnosis and treatment,[2] the evidence-based guidelines for migraine headache in the primary care setting of the US Headache Consortium,[3] and the Canadian guidelines for headache management of the Canadian Headache Society.[4] Besides extracting from these guidelines an abbreviated but useful way to manage patients in primary care, the authors included consensus clinical experience, judgement, and research findings that had not yet been published when the above guidelines were written. *Patient-centered strategies for effective management of migraine* was published with the intention of providing an effective framework to approach the patient with disabling headaches.

Impact-based recognition of migraine[5]

The recognition of migraine can be achieved by asking four questions.

(1)   How do headaches interfere with your life?
(2)   How frequently do you experience headaches of any type?
(3)   Has there been any change in your headache pattern over the last 6 months?
(4)   How often and how effectively do you use medication to treat headaches?

Recurrent headaches that produce significant disability should be considered migraine until proven otherwise. The frequency of headaches alerts the clinician to chronic headache disorders, migraine transformation, and the need for preventive medication. A patient who uses acute treatment medications more than 2 days a week may require a preventive medication. If the headache pattern has changed, a more in-depth evaluation is necessary. The goals of acute treatment are to be pain-free and fully functional within 2 to 4 hours. If these goals are not being reached, medication needs to be changed.

Comfort signs are the presence of characteristics commonly associated with migraine that support the impression that the headache is primary, not a secondary symptom of a serious underlying disorder. These include the existence of prodrome, aura, and postdrome; family history; and menstrual association. Also, if the headaches fulfil International Headache Society (IHS) criteria or respond to a treatment plan over time, the headaches are likely to be primary. In addition, patients should have normal vital signs, physical examination, and screening neurological examination.

Acute treatment strategy

The strategy for acute treatment consists of five components: (1) identify phases of migraine symptomatology that allow for intervention as early as possible in the migraine process; (2) select the best pharmacological options for each patient; (3) instruct patients on the proper use of medications; (4) encourage use of a headache diary to monitor treatment and medication usage; (5) provide information resources for patient education.

The goals of acute therapy are the following: (1) safely abort the symptoms of migraine; (2) prevent or stop disability and maintain function; and (3) use medication that accomplishes these goals within 2 to 4 hours.

Preventive treatment strategy

Preventive treatment should be initiated when: (1) headache frequency is more than twice a week; (2) despite acute treatment, recurring migraines are significantly interfering with the patient's daily routines; (3) contraindication to, failure or overuse of, or adverse events with acute therapies; (4) presence of complex auras (basilar or hemiplegic), prolonged aura, or migrainous infarction; (5) use of rescue medication for more than one migraine a month; (6) consistent use of acute treatment medication more than 2 days per week; (7) patient preference.

The goals of preventive therapy include: (1) reduce attack frequency, severity, or duration; (2) improve responsiveness to treatment of acute attacks; (3) improve function and reduce disability; (4) deter the evolution of episodic headaches into chronic daily headache; (5) treat comorbid disorders.

Behavioural and physical treatments

Behavioural therapy should be a proactive part of managing all headache patients, whether it is as simple as words of encouragement or as formal as psychological consultation. When behavioural therapy is combined with drug therapy, patients often achieve additional clinical improvement for headache relief. Behavioural therapy includes biofeedback, relaxation training, and stress management as well as cognitive interventions.

Physical treatments too have proven effective for prevention of disabling headaches. These range from acupuncture/acupressure to manipulative procedures, massage, and exercise.

Special considerations

Special considerations address the management of headaches that may be more complicated than migraine, such as chronic headache disorders. Also, headaches that are hormonally associated or that occur during pregnancy, childhood and adolescence, and mature adulthood may require a different management style.

System management

System management explores situations and resources available for management of patients with needs beyond the scope of office-based primary care. These include neuroimaging, consultation and referral, in-patient management, and working with third-party payers.

Study of the usefulness of *Patient-centered strategies* in primary care

The objective of the study was to measure the usefulness of the publication, *Patient-centered strategies for effective management of migraine*, in the primary care setting. Over 200 000 copies of the publication were sent to primary care physicians in the USA. The first 1000 physicians who returned the post-test, which qualified them for 1.5 hours of continuing medical education, were sent a survey that measured the usefulness of the publication in their practices.

The survey was returned by 315 physicians. The results indicated that 95% found that the publication helped them become better prepared to treat patients with migraine (Fig. 67.1); 65% had begun to screen for migraine (Fig. 67.2); 98% were

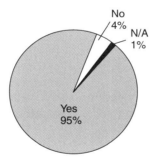

Fig. 67.1 Results of a survey asking physicians (N=315) whether reading *Patient-centered strategies for effective management of migraine* made them better prepared to treat patients with migraine. N/A, Not answered.

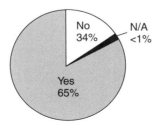

Fig. 67.2 Results of a survey asking physicians (N=315) whether reading *Patient-centered strategies for effective management of migraine* had led them to begin to screen patients for migraine. N/A, Not answered.

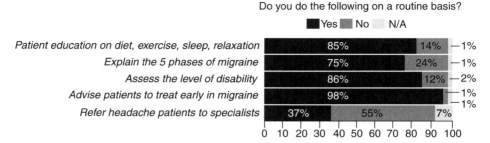

Fig. 67.3 Results of a survey asking physicians (N=315) who had read *Patient-centered strategies for effective management of migraine* whether they took certain actions on a routine basis. N/A, Not answered.

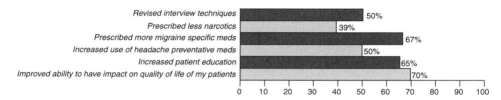

Fig. 67.4 Results of a survey asking physicians (N=315) who had read *Patient-centered strategies for effective management of migraine* what changes they had made in their daily practice.

advising their patients to treat migraine early, before the pain intensity reached moderate to severe (Fig. 67.3); and 67% now prescribed migraine-specific medication rather than analgesics (Fig. 67.4).

Conclusion

On the basis of these findings, primary care physicians find *Patient-centered strategies for effective management of migraine* helpful in recognizing and managing individuals with disabling headaches.

References

1. Lipton RB, Diamond S, Reed M, Diamond M, Stewart WF. Migraine diagnosis and treatment: results from the American Migraine Study II. *Headache* 2001; **41**: 638–45.
2. Standards of Care Committee. *Headache diagnosis and treatment*. Chicago: National Headache Foundation, 1999.
3. US Headache Consortium (2000). Evidence-based guidelines for migraine headache: overview; pharmacological management of acute attacks; pharmacological management for

prevention of migraine; neuroimaging in patients with nonacute headache; behavioral and physical treatments. *Neurology* 2000; **54**: 1553; also available at www.aan.com.
4. Canadian Headache Society (1998). Canadian guidelines for headache management. *Can Med Assoc J* 1998; **159**: 47–54.
5. Cady R, Farmer-Cady K (2000). Migraine: changing perspectives on diagnosis and management. *Consultant* 2000; **40**: S13–S19.

68
Improving health-care systems for headache: discussion summary

Stephen D. Silberstein

We have read in many chapters about migraine underdiagnosis and undertreatment. How can this be corrected?

Timothy Steiner told us about the tremendous shortage of neurologists in the UK. There are fewer than 400 in the whole country and the waiting list to see a neurologist is months long. After a patient goes to a general practitioner (GP) and the GP decides that there is nothing more he or she can do, the patient is in limbo. A recommendation has been made to train GPs to deliver disease-specific headache care. Thus the GP would deliver primary care, the new breed GP specialist would deliver secondary care, and the neurologist would deliver tertiary care. This system creates potential problems, as there are few headache speciality or tertiary headache centres in the UK, unlike the situation that exists in many other countries. Thus, true tertiary care does not exist. In addition, once someone has specialized in the treatment of a disorder, that individual becomes an expert in that disorder and is no longer, by definition, a GP. To diagnose and treat headache patients in a secondary care setting requires neurological expertise. This requires a knowledge of the neurological history, the physical examination, and the diagnosis and treatment of secondary headache disorders. Who is best able to do this?

Hartmut Göbel described the comprehensive academic pain and headache centre in Kiel, Germany. In the German system, patients are treated at different levels in the health-care system. Most headache patients can be, and are, treated by their GPs, just as in the UK. The next level of care is a neurological practice or a neurological clinic. In Germany there are enough neurologists to meet this need. Multidisciplinary tertiary headache and pain care, while limited, is available. Kiel is one of the few academic headache centres in the world.

Both Drs Göbel and Diener pointed out the difference between headache and pain centres. A headache centre requires neurologists, psychiatrists and/or psychologists, and trained nurses. A comprehensive pain centre requires, in addition, internists, rheumatologists, anaesthetists, social workers, physiotherapists, pain therapists, and often orthopaedic surgeons and neurosurgeons. The goal of pain centres is to decrease pain and improve function. The goal of headache centres is to eliminate head pain.

In addition to patient care, a multidisciplinary academic headache centre is involved in research, student education, and advanced training for doctors and other health-care providers. Evidence suggests that the German centres are cost-effective. Dr Gobel's epidemiological data suggest that there is a great worldwide need for further centres (possibly one for every 2 million people).

A major debate emerged over who should care for headache patients. Some felt that the primary care physician was best suited. All agreed that the GP is adequate at the primary level of care, but primary care physicians need additional training and more support.

The debate moved on to secondary level of care. In most countries, this would be, and is, performed by neurologists. Some stated that neurologists in the USA do not care about headache patients and do not screen for psychological morbidity and that specialized GPs would do a better job. Others argued that GPs have less training and little interest in headache. The issue is interest and training.

The fundamental problem is the level of headache expertise in academic medical centres and residency training programmes. There is hardly anyone who can train neurologists about headache and pain. The situation is even worse in most primary care residencies, where the trainees have little neurological training. Many primary care physicians do not even do a complete neurological examination or examine the ocular fundi.

What is needed is a network or alliance where jurisdictional barriers can be broken down. This occurs in comprehensive headache and pain centres. Another model is the City of London Migraine Clinic, where neurologists work side by side with their primary care colleagues. A network would provide support to neurologists to upgrade their education and allow them to act as a resource to the primary care provider.

One solution is the use of nurse practitioners trained in headache to help educate and treat patients in a primary care situation under the supervision of a headache expert. A pilot programme of education followed by evaluation has been established at the Kaiser-Permanente group in California. Duke University, Kaiser-Permanente, and the Jefferson Headache Center are beginning a controlled trial of this concept. Patients who attend a primary care physician's office at each of these sites will be randomized to standard care or to specialized care by a nurse practitioner under the guidance of a headache expert using the principals of the US Headache Consortium Guidelines. Outcome measures are being developed.

An animated discussion took place about the use and misuse of opioids in pain and headache management. The observation that slow-release (and long-duration) opioids are not associated with medication overuse headache was made by several participants. In contrast, immediate-release opioids, particularly when combined with other agents, are often associated with medication overuse headache.

The use of opioids for acute as opposed to maintenance therapy was energetically debated. Some never use them. Others argue that they are needed as rescue therapy and when first-line treatments fail or are contraindicated.

Index

Note: Headache and migraine have not been indexed as they appear throughout but specific entries eg tension-type headache; migraine with aura are entered.